CT SCANNING – TECHNIQUES AND APPLICATIONS

Edited by **K. Subburaj**

CT Scanning – Techniques and Applications
Edited by K. Subburaj

Published by InTech
Janeza Trdine 9, 51000 Rijeka, Croatia

Publishing Process Manager Davor Vidic

Technical Editor Teodora Smiljanic

Cover Designer InTech Design Team

Additional hard copies can be obtained from orders@intechopen.com

CT Scanning – Techniques and Applications, Edited by K. Subburaj
p. cm.
ISBN 978-953-307-943-1

For EU product safety concerns:
IN TECH d.o.o., Prolaz Marije Krucifikse Kozulić 3, 51000 Rijeka, Croatia,
info@intechopen.com or visit our website at intechopen.com.

Meet the editor

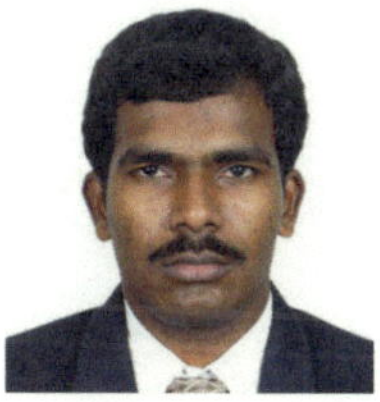

Dr. K. Subburaj is a postdoctorial fellow at the Department of Radiology and Biomedical Imaging, University of California San Francisco (UCSF). He completed his engineering degree from Manonmaniam Sundaranar University, India in 2003, followed by PhD from the Indian Institute of Technology Bombay in 2009. He worked as a Research Specialist-Surgical outcomes research at OrthoCAD laboratory, IIT Bombay before joining UCSF. His areas of research include CT/MR Imaging, medical image analysis, 3D geometric data processing and visualization, and lower-limb biomechanics. His current research focused on developing voxel-based statistical methods for measuring knee osteoarthritis progression and studying effect of physical exercise on knee health.

Contents

Preface

Since its introduction in 1972, X-ray computed tomography (CT) has evolved into an essential diagnostic imaging tool for a continually increasing variety of clinical applications. The original systems were dedicated to head imaging only, but "whole body" systems with larger patient openings became available in the late 1970's. Technical advancements in developing high-power x-ray tubes and computing technologies led to two major evolutionary leaps in CT imaging during the past decade. The first of these occurred in the early 1990's with the introduction of CT scanners with simultaneous patient translation and data acquisition ("spiral" or "helical"). The second leap occurred mid-decade, with the introduction of multiple row detectors capable of multiple slices per x-ray tube rotation. These advances improved volume coverage and/or longitudinal spatial resolution, and creating new applications that could not have been attempted before, such as CT angiography, virtual endoscopy, CT-guided surgery/radiation therapy, and computer integrated surgery.

The goal of this book was not simply to summarize currently available CT imaging techniques but also to provide clinical perspectives, advances in hybrid technologies, new applications other than medicine and an outlook on future developments. Major experts in this growing field contributed to this book, which is geared to radiologists, orthopedic surgeons, engineers, and clinical and basic researchers. Each of us has written different part of this book, obviously depending on our areas of expertise. We believe that CT scanning is an effective and essential tools in treatment planning, basic understanding of physiology, and and tackling the ever-increasing challenge of diagnosis in our society.

I would finally like to acknowledge our publishing process manager Davor Vidic's hard work and support during the preparation of this book.

K. Subburaj, PhD
Department of Radiology and Biomedical Imaging
University of California, San Francisco
USA

Part 1

Imaging

1

State-of-the-Art Multi-Detector CT Angiography in Acute Pulmonary Embolism: Technique, Interpretation and Future Perspectives

IJC Hartmann, PJ Abrahams-van Doorn
and C Schaefer-Prokop
Erasmus MC University Medical Center Rotterdam,
Meander Medisch Centrum Amersfoort
The Netherlands

1. Introduction

Since the first application of CT angiography (CTA) for the diagnosis of acute pulmonary embolism (PE) in the early nineties (1), CTA has become the first imaging technique of choice in the workup of patients with suspected PE.

Though the considerable inherent limitations of CTA with single-detector CT (SDCT) systems, its diagnostic potential for direct visualization of arterial clots was instantaneously appreciated by the radiological community. Limited by a maximum breath hold of 30 s and a single detector row data acquisition, image quality and thus diagnostic efficiency was limited by the trade off between the need to cover a certain scan length and the spatial resolution determined by the slice collimation: e .g., with a slice collimation of 5 mm only a scan range of 15 cm could be covered within 30 s. Even with use of 3 mm collimation and a pitch of 1.7, a confident detection of acute PE was only possible down to the segmental level. With the newest generation CT scanners the full chest can be scanned in less than 4 s with sub-millimeter collimation which has become the standard nowadays (see table 1). Small thrombi can be identified in subsegmental arterial branches and elaborate post-processing techniques can be executed, resulting in a significant increase of both sensitivity and specificity in PE detection. This substantial gain in image acquisition speed and spatial resolution also lead to novel image interpretation concepts including the assessment of perfusion defects of the lung parenchyma and the evaluation of cardiac dysfunction, both of which are important determinants for the clinical outcome of the patient.

Besides the significant increase of detectors in the most recent generations of CT scanners a complete novel concept has been developed: dual-source CT. Although the main gain of the use of two radiation sources is the steep increase in temporal resolution, which is especially of benefit for cardiac scanning, this new technique can also be used for PE detection by performing either a dual-source CT protocol resulting in CTA and CT perfusion datasets obtained during one image acquisition, or as a fast track protocol resulting in a dataset obtained within 1 s and without disturbing breathing artifacts, even in very dyspnoeic patients.

The development of faster CT scanning techniques has resulted in a substantial decrease of the percentage of non-interpretable scans (overall from 10% using SDCT techniques to up to 6% for multi-detector CT (MDCT)) (2, 3). However, the very fast data acquisition in a few seconds carries also new risks and new down-sides such as scans with suboptimal image quality due to a sub-optimal contrast medium injection protocol or a sudden Valsalva maneuver by the patient almost inevitably resulting in inadequate vessel enhancement. An examination with suboptimal quality and, as a result, ambiguous or completely impossible interpretation, is still the most important drawback of CT in the workup of patients with suspected PE. Many of these qualitatively suboptimal CT scan results can be avoided when acquisition and contrast medium injection protocols are optimized and proper patient instruction is executed, with special attention to specific subgroups such as ICU and pregnant patients. Furthermore, interpreters of the CT datasets should be familiar with a good interpretation protocol taking benefit of the appropriate post-processing techniques and should keep in mind the potential pitfalls.

In the following, we will focus on the optimization of CTA protocols using most modern MDCT systems, with special attention to the acquisition and contrast medium injection techniques and with potential adaptation of these protocols for specific patient subgroups. On the other hand, we will discuss options for display optimization of the datasets using post-processing techniques and recently developed computer aided detection (CAD) systems. Finally potential pitfalls, related to the technique, the patient and the interpreter will be explained.

2. Image acquisition protocols

2.1 Scanning parameters

Due to the continuous and rapidly advancing MDCT technology, scanning protocols need to be continuously adapted, too (table 1). The optimal scan protocol depends on the generation of scanner (e.g., the number of detector rows being used) and the vendor of the CT machine. Using MDCT scanners with ≥ 16 detector rows, the scan time is reduced to < 10 s, resulting in a significant decrease of movement artefacts and an increase in spatial resolution, obviating an adaptation of the scan protocol even in very dyspnoeic patients. Therefore, the use of CT scanners with less than 16 detector rows cannot be advocated anymore for obtaining CT pulmonary angiography (CTPA).

Scanner type (number of detector rows)	**Collimation** (mm)	**Rotation time** (s)	**Scan duration** (s, 24 cm)
4	1-1.25	0.5	≤ 20
4 (dyspnea)	2-2.5	0.8	≤ 10
16	0.625-1	0.37-0.42	≤ 8
64	0.5-0.625	0.35-0.42	≤ 4
128	0.6	0.30	< 3
128 DS	0.6	0.28	< 1
256	0.625	0.33	< 2
320 (160)	0.5	0.35	< 4

DS = dual source, 320 detector snap shot imaging, 160 detector row spiral data acquisition

Table 1. Scan parameters for the different types of scanners.

2.2 kV and mAs

Lowering the kV from 120-130 kV to 100 kV or even 80 kV substantially decreases radiation dose roughly up to 60% (4-7). The resulting increase in image noise is compensated by the improved absorption of iodine with lower kV resulting in higher HU of the enhanced vessels. Several studies could show that visualization especially of small vessels was improved with lower kVp (8).

This 80 kV scanning technique, however, can only be applied in patients weighting less than 75 kg (7). In large patients (body weight > 90 kg) and in patients of whom the arms cannot be brought above the head (e.g., in ICU patients), lowering the kV usually results in such an increase in image noise that image quality is substantially decreased and diagnostic quality not guaranteed anymore.

The use of dose modulation software should be routinely used. Dose modulation techniques as offered by all manufacturers modulate the mAs as function of the body dimension along the xy-axis and along the z-axis of the patient. That way data are acquired with lowered dose during the mid part of the chest as compared to the upper thoracic inlet at the level of the shoulders and the lower thoracic outlet, where the liver is already included into the scan. Similarly radiation is lowered for ventro-dorsal transmission direction as compared to the right-to-left direction. These techniques are quite effective with a dose reduction of up to 50% in the chest (9, 10), however, depending on the dose level originally determined by the 120 kVp and the region of the chest, e.g., shoulders central part, thorax outlet/upper abdomen. Further dose reduction is possible by lowering the kV as function of body weight and body dimensions. In table 2, a guideline is provided for the adaptation of kV and reference mAs to the body weight of the patient.

Weight	kV	mAsref
<50 kg	80	1.5 mAs/kg
50-70 kg	100	120
70-90 kg	100(120)	150
>90 kg **	120	150

** kVp may not be lowered in patients which are scanned with arms along the body.

Table 2. Dose protocols adapted to the patient's body weight.

A low signal-to-noise ratio may deteriorate the image quality significantly, impeding a reliable interpretation of especially the subsegmental and more peripherally located pulmonary arteries. This may cause diagnostic problems in obese patients. Therefore, in patients > 120 kg image quality may be further improved by using slower rotation times to increase the amount of delivered dose. Also reconstruction of thicker slices (e.g., 2 mm instead of 1 mm) may be helpful to allow a more meaningful interpretation of too noisy images.

2.3 Dose aspects

The radiation dose of a CTPA is described in DLP (in mGy x cm) which takes into account the individual scan length. It is calculated using the equation: dose-length product (DLP) = scan length x $CTDI_{vol}$. The resulting effective dose *E* (in mSv) is calculated using the specific conversion factor of 0.014 (11) or 0.017 (12) mSv per mGy x cm for a CTPA covering the whole chest. For simplification, the conversion factor is the same for men and women, although the individually received dose is higher for women because of radiation to the breasts. The $CTDI_{vol}$ is given on the scanner console after each examination. As a rule of

thumb it can be said that for a total CTPA with a scan length of 30 cm the effective dose amounts to about 40% of the $CTDI_{vol}$ for men and to about 50% of the $CTDI_{vol}$ for women.
If the scan range is reduced, the effective dose decreases proportionally. As a consequence, effective dose may vary substantially despite the fact that the same mAs and kVp settings have been chosen. The European Guidelines for Quality in Computed Tomography EUR 16262 suggest a maximum effective dose level for the chest of 9 mSv. In our experience, the required dose levels are lower and the $CTDI_{vol}$ does not exceed 5-7 mGy in a standard size patient (70 kg, 170 cm).
Lowering the kV has the important advantage of considerably decrease radiation dose for the patient. The absorption of iodine increases with lower kVp resulting in higher intravascular enhancement (figure 1). This effect can be used to compensate for the higher image noise resulting from lowering the kV. This increased noise is the reason that lowering the kVp is only recommended for children and low to normal weight persons but not in patients > 75 kg (7), unless the tube current is increased to keep the image noise constant. In slim patients and children, use of an 80 kVp protocol (without adaptation of the tube current) decreases the radiation dose to as low as 1.5-2 mSv.

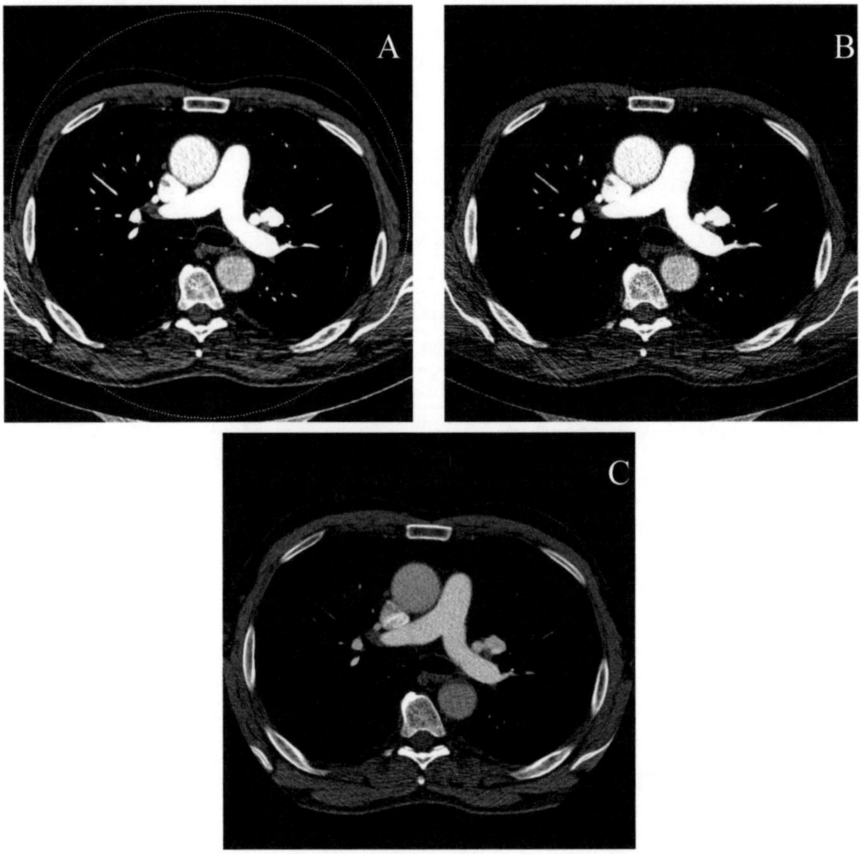

Fig. 1. Dual-energy CT of a 46-year-old male patient with acute PE, performed with 75 mL contrast medium with 400 mg/mL iodine concentration injected at 5 mL/s.
Axial 1-mm virtual 120 kV slice (A), 2-mm 80 kV slice (B) and 2-mm 140 kV slice (C), with mean contrast enhancement at the main PA of 541 HU, 709 HU and 284 HU, respectively.

In a recent study, comparing simulated low-dose CT scans, generated by the superimposition of computer-calculated noise, to a reference standard of 90 mAs in non-obese patients found no statistically significantly differences in the visualization of peripheral PE and inter- and intraobserver agreement (13).

2.4 Scan length and direction

The first CTPA protocols proposed a scan range between 2 cm above the aortic arch to 2 cm below the pulmonary veins. This protocol allowed for coverage of the central part of the lung with an appropriate spatial resolution at the time of slower data acquisition within a single breathhold. Today the whole chest can be easily covered within less than 5 s. Therefore, it becomes more important to pay attention to determine just the scan range needed without including too much of the neck or the upper abdomen to avoid unnecessary radiation. This seems to be especially important in young patients and in women. Though retrospective data analysis did not find a diagnostic disadvantage for determining or excluding PE if the lung tops and the lower costophrenic angles are spared (14) , this approach is not generally advocated but should be reserved to certain indications such as repeat examinations in young patients. It may lead to loss of information with respect to alternative diagnosis (e.g., extent of pleural effusion or pneumonia) and is therefore not considered useful in elderly patients or in patients with known or suspected comorbidity. This approach also seems to be less well definable within a standardized protocol that ideally should be the same independent of institutional, personal or time related effects.

With SDCT, a caudo-cranial scanning direction was in general preferred as breathing artefacts are less disturbing in the upper lung zones and to avoid beam hardening artefacts due to inflow of high density contrast medium. With shorter scanning times and use of a saline chaser bolus these issues have been overcome. Today, both caudo-cranial and cranio-caudal scanning directions are in use, depending on local preference.

2.5 ECG-gating

There are three potential indications why to obtain a CTA data set with ECG-gating, though all three of them have not yet found their way into clinical routine or have not been found to provide substantial advantages. Limiting factors for ECG-gated CTPA protocols are the increase of radiation dose and the prolongation of scan time.

a. Prospective ECG-gating diminishes motion artefacts due to cardiac pulsation, especially in the lingula and left lower lobe vessels. As a result, it may improve image quality as compared to non-ECG-gated CTPA. Whether ECG-gated CTPA indeed results in a clinically relevant increase of diagnostic accuracy remains questionable and studies on this topic are so far not available. Up to now, ECG-gating has not found its way into clinical routine in the workup of patients with potential PE (15).
b. The role of ECG-gated data acquisition may be more important in the context of the assessment of cardiac function rather than image quality. ECG-gated CTPA allows for functional assessment of the right ventricle (RV). Dysfunction of the RV has been proven to be an independent predictor of survival in patients with PE. Yet, assessment of the RV/LV (right ventricle / left ventricle) ratio on non-ECG-gated scans were found to equally well assess RV dysfunction as functional parameters based on ECG-gated CTPA, and
c. a triple or dual rule-out protocol to assess the presence of PE, coronary disease or aortic dissection in patients with acute chest pain, requires ECG-gating to obtain the necessary quality for the evaluation of coronary arteries (16).

2.6 Injection protocol

The injection protocol should be optimized to ensure a constant and high degree of pulmonary arterial enhancement during the complete data acquisition. A minimal attenuation of 300 to 350 HU (i.e., 250 to 300 HU net contrast enhancement) is considered optimal for the assessment of PE at CTPA (17, 18). Suboptimal vascular opacification is a major reason for non-diagnostic scans and further aggravates other artefacts such as partial volume effects or movement artefacts potentially causing false positive interpretations.

Optimizing the injection protocol becomes more challenging the shorter the scan time is, as Valsalva maneuvers or inadequate scan delay time can completely destroy the whole scan.

The most important causes of general insufficient enhancement are: low injection rate, wrong bolus timing and decreased heart function. All these causes are in a way predictable and measurable and therefore can be overcome by appropriate steps.

1. A sufficiently high delivery of mg iodine per s should be obtained by choosing a high flow injection rate (4 - 6 mL/s) and/or a high concentration of the contrast medium (370-400 mg of iodine/mL). This will result in good visualization of small, peripherally located pulmonary arteries, eventually improving the overall sensitivity (19). Similarly as with radiation, more iodine is needed in large patients to achieve a comparable opacification of the pulmonary arteries as in a small patient. This can be achieved by either increasing the iodine flow rate (20) or by increasing the total volume of administered contrast medium (21) to overcome the inversely proportional relationship between opacification of the pulmonary arteries and body weight (17).
2. The duration of contrast medium injection should approximately be equal to the sum of the scan duration and the delay time. For very short scan durations, the delay time has to be increased. After reaching the trigger threshold 5-8 s of delay have to be added depending on the type of scanner (the faster the scanner and the shorter the acquisition time, the more delay time should be added). Importantly, if for some reason the injection time is increased, e.g., due to limited venous access, the scan delay has to be prolonged accordingly to avoid scanning and data acquisition when pulmonary arteries are not yet sufficiently opacified (22). The trigger level and the region of interest chosen for bolus triggering have to be chosen to allow for adequate contrast build-up down to the peripheral arteries during the complete scan acquisition (table 3). If scanning is started too early, especially in very fast high-end MDCT scanners, inhomogeneity in opacification can result in pseudo-filling defects. Narrowing the window settings is helpful to differentiate between pseudo-defects and true PE.

   As a consequence, contrast volume can be substantially reduced for CTPA with fast high-end scanners.

Scan duration (s)	**Scanner type**	**With saline** (ml) / (ml/s) / (s)	**Without saline** (ml)
≤ 5	16, ≥ 64	70 + 40 / 5 / 8-10P*	80
10	4 (dysp.), 16	80 + 40 / 5 / 5-8P*	100
20	4	100 + 40 /4 /5P*	120

* P is the time that should be added after a threshold of 150 HU is reached using bolus triggering. The region of interest (ROI) is placed in the pulmonary trunk.

Table 3. Injection protocols for the different types of scanners.

3. Frequently, a saline chaser of 30-60 mL is used. It is immediately injected with the same injection rate after the contrast medium bolus.
   The advantages of such a saline flush are threefold:
   a. it flushes the contrast medium out of the subclavian vein and superior vena cava (SVC), decreasing the risk of beam hardening artefacts. These artefacts are more frequently seen with use of high concentration and/or high flow rates and hamper the visualization of the right pulmonary artery and its branches in the right upper lobe.
   b. it prolongs the length of the contrast plateau resulting in a more homogeneous intravascular contrast, and
   c. finally, it decreases the total volume of contrast medium needed (23).
4. With the short and very short scanning times that result from the use of modern MDCT scanners, an individualized injection timing using bolus triggering has become essential. It compensates for unexpected changes in circulation time, which can be slowed down due to right-sided heart failure, pulmonary hypertension (PH) or low cardiac output, or on the other hand can be increased in case of a hypercirculatory status e.g., in adolescents or pregnant women.

The ROI for bolus triggering is usually localized in the pulmonary trunk or pulmonary artery (PA) but may as well be set in the RV or the ascending aorta. The preset trigger level is usually between 150 and 200 HU.

The right cubital vein is the preferred site for contrast medium injection in CTPA to avoid streak artefacts caused by the nearly horizontal course of the left brachiocephalic vein. In general, both arms are placed above the head. Some authors prefer positioning the left arm above the head and the right arm parallel to the body with right-sided contrast medium injection as this technique reduces the risk for hampered inflow of contrast medium due to compression of the brachiocephalic vein at the level of the thoracic inlet. As a consequence of placing the arm aside the body, however, the image noise in the scanned volume may increase especially when low-dose protocols are used.

In a subgroup of patients with suspicion of PE but contraindications for iodinated contrast medium injection, gadolinium may be used as an alternative to iodine containing contrast medium (24, 25). Diagnostic CTPA with adequate opacification of the complete pulmonary arterial tree up to the subsegmental level using gadolinium can only be obtained with fast data acquisition (MDCT with ≥ 16 detector rows) as the amount of gadolinium than can be injected for CTPA is limited to 0.3-0.4 mmol/kg. A high injection rate protocol has to be chosen also with gadolinium. As it is well known, gadolinium is contraindicated in patients with severe renal insufficiency and up-to-date guidelines for its use have to be followed (ESUR guidelines on contrast media; www.esur.org).

2.7 Filtered back projection and iterative reconstruction

Filtered back projection is currently the standard technique to reconstruct the image dataset from the raw scan data. Iterative reconstruction techniques are an alternative method to work with the raw data whereby image data are corrected using several different models. Iterative reconstruction is routinely used in PET and SPECT imaging. These techniques reduce image noise while preserving sharpness, which is especially useful in using low-dose CT protocols. In addition, the use of iterative reconstruction further improves image quality by reducing artefacts, i.e., spiral artefacts and beam hardening artefacts, the latter might be especially advantageous in the assessment of use of dual-energy CT (DECT) perfusion images (see below under 'Dual-source CT'). So far, these techniques were not used in CT as the algorithm requires significant computational time. Due to modification of the technique and the increased speed of processing, this technique has now become available in routine clinical practice for CT. A potential disadvantage of this technique may be a different image appearance, of which the potential effect on the detection of PE has so far not been studied. Whether the decrease of image noise by iterative reconstruction resulting in image quality improvement in low-dose CTPA protocols will balance the potential disadvantage of the different aspect of the structures at CT needs to be subject of further study.

2.8 Dual-source CT

Dual-source CT (DSCT) scanners can be used in two different ways for the detection of acute PE. Using the "Flash" technique, the chest can be scanned from the apex to the diaphragm with the thinnest collimation in less than 1 s. This will further reduce the risk for movement artefacts and increases the temporal resolution.

Alternatively, DSCT scanners offer the option to reconstruct "material specific images", e.g., images in which the distribution of iodine in the lung parenchyma is used to produce lung perfusion images (27-30). In DECT, lung perfusion does not correspond to blood flow analysis in its strict definition, but refers to the iodine enhancement at one point in a time (blood volume), which is related to the pulmonary blood flow or microcirculation of the lung. The distribution of the iodine within the pulmonary capillaries is influenced by various parameters such as the amount of contrast medium administered and the anatomic structures the contrast medium passes through, both, before and after the pulmonary capillary bed (31).

There had been attempts earlier to produce lung perfusion images using single-source CT scanners: They used dynamic scan protocols or assessed parenchymal density by means of color coded maps. Since these techniques have serious limitations, they never found their way into broad clinical application. Using the dynamic technique, additional serial scanning has to be performed with a rather limited coverage. Subtracting an enhanced from an unenhanced scan will further increase display of lung perfusion but requires a very long breathhold (to obtain both scans within one breathhold) and still suffers from subtraction artifacts.

These limitations could be overcome by dual-source / dual-energy CT technique. Using DSCT with dual-energy technique, two datasets obtained at two different kilovoltages are reconstructed. Fusion of the two image sets with an 80:140 kVp linear weighting of 0.3- 0.4 produces a "standard" CTA of 120 kVp (figure 2). Subtracting the lower kV from the higher kV images using dedicated processing software produces CT-perfusion colour-coded maps, resembling the distribution of iodine in the lung. The 80 kVp data set, although it suffers from an increased image noise, the contrast to noise ratio is optimised (see above under 'kV and mAs ') and therefore may be helpful for the assessment of PE in peripheral pulmonary arteries. To allow the contrast material to perfuse the complete lung, the delay time should not be too short (see below) and a saline flush is needed to limit streak artefacts from the SVC. The latter may be further reduced by using a split-bolus injection technique (32).

There are a number of new pitfalls in these perfusion images such as gravity dependent perfusion, pseudo/high perfusion due to dense contrast material in the thoracic veins, cardiac motion, or artefacts caused by underlying pulmonary disease especially emphysema and the reader has to become familiar with them when assessing CT perfusion images (33). Recent studies in small patient groups have found a good correlation between pulmonary perfusion defects seen by DECT perfusion imaging and the gold standard, pulmonary perfusion (SPECT) scintigraphy (34, 35).

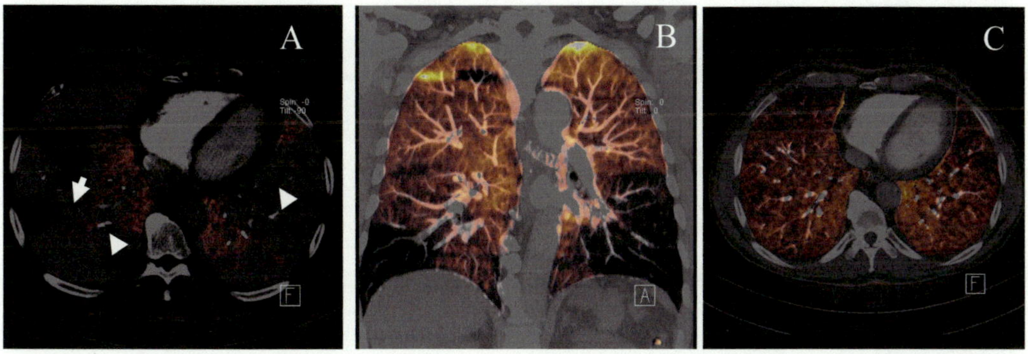

Fig. 2. Dual-energy CT of a 46-year-old male patient with acute PE. Fused color-coded and virtual 120 kV axial images (A) and coronal MPR (B) showing bilateral multiple segmental and sub-segmental thrombi (white arrows) obstructing the pulmonary arteries. As a result, multiple (sub) segmental perfusion defects are observed (black areas). A follow-up scan after 6 months of anticoagulant treatment revealed neither residual thrombi nor perfusion defects (C).

The disadvantage of the first generation DSCT scanners caused by a too small diameter of the field of view of the second tube (26 cm), resulting in incomplete truncated iodine maps in large patients, is now overcome in the second generation of DSCT scanners that provide a sufficient coverage also of the second tube (33 cm).

Besides the analysis of the distribution of iodine in the lung parenchyma, dedicated software algorithm visualizing the iodine content in the pulmonary vessels has been developed. This software was designed especially to differentiate true PE from other causes of low HU values such as low contrast enhancement and partial volume effects, especially in small pulmonary vessels. A first evaluation of this technique demonstrated that this algorithm may especially be helpful in the exclusion of PE (36).

Summarizing it can be said that although the perfusion technique seems promising for combining direct visualization of the thrombus with the functional consequences, namely perfusion defects (figure 1). The radiation dose of DECT technique is equivalent to or slightly higher than for the single tube CT technique, but the potential benefits of DECT are thought to balance the possible minor dose increase. However, the actual additional value of this technique for diagnosis, prognosis and therapy monitoring still needs to be determined in future studies.

2.9 Patient instruction

It is generally recommended to perform image acquisition for a CTPA during breathhold and in inspiration.

Breathing artefacts and a Valsalva maneuver by the patient hampering contrast-inflow are still major causes for sub-optimal scan quality. A careful patient instruction by the technologist is therefore very important: it should include an appropriate explanation of the effects of fast contrast-inflow (transient feeling of warmth and unusual oral taste), a performance of a trial breathhold for the required scan duration and a careful explanation not to increase intrathoracic pressure by a Valsalva maneuver. By watching the movement of the abdominal surface adequate suspension of respiration can be assessed. Patients usually require about 4 s between the breathhold command and the actual scan to obtain a full inspiration. Substantial movement artefacts may occur if scan delay is too short or patients are improperly instructed. In the elderly even more than 4 s may be needed. Individual instruction by the technologist instead of using the automatic command and start of scanning further reduces the chance of significant breathing artefacts. With slower CT scanners and scanning times of more than 15 s (below 16-row CT scanners) a short hyperventilation of 3-4 times before starting the data acquisition may be helpful to ensure breathhold capability.

Deep inspiration immediately prior to the image acquisition may lead to transient interruption of the contrast column in the pulmonary arteries. This is the result of variable inflow of non-opacified blood from the inferior vena cava as a normal response to the negative intrathoracic pressure (26). Valsalva maneuvers on the other hand, lead to diminished inflow of contrast medium as a result of increased intrathoracic pressure. Both may lead to inhomogeneous or inadequate contrast enhancement of the pulmonary arteries that becomes even more critical with faster scanners that require less than 5 s for full data acquisition. Some authors have therefore recommended obtaining CTPA in expiration (to avoid inflow of uncontrasted blood via the inferior vena cava). The disadvantage of crowded and compressed vascular structures in expiration and the substantially lowered display quality of the lung parenchyma, however, make this a technique that cannot be generally recommended. Some patients tend to 'gasp for air' internally against a closed glottis at the end of scan acquisition. This may result in motion artefacts due to the involuntary diaphragmatic movements and can also be avoided by careful patient instruction.

In severely dyspnoeic patients, shallow breathing is preferred over forced breathholding to avoid severe and uncontrollable movement artefacts. This will slightly reduce the quality of both the axial slices and multiplanar reformats (MPR's), but in the majority of cases a diagnostic scan can be obtained, at least of the central pulmonary arteries.

2.10 CTPA during pregnancy

Venous thrombo-embolic disease has a two- to fourfold increased incidence during pregnancy and is a leading cause of maternal mortality. Ultrasound of the leg veins has been advocated as the first clinical test for suspected non-life threatening thrombo-embolism (Statement of the Fleischer Society) because further radiographic imaging is only required if leg ultrasound is normal (37).

The question which technique to use next for pregnant patients with suspected thrombo-embolism has been hotly debated (38-41). There is no general consensus to which diagnostic technique is the most appropriate to diagnose acute PE in pregnant women. It is important to know that at no time point of the pregnancy (including the first three months) a CTPA delivers a radiation dose that poses a risk to the unborn child, and risks of an undiagnosed PE are much greater than any theoretical risk to the fetus from diagnostic imaging (42, 43).

Since diagnosis of a deep venous thrombosis represents a sufficient indication for treatment, the first diagnostic step should be an ultrasound examination of the deep leg veins. For evaluating the pulmonary arteries, a CTPA or a perfusion scintigraphy can be obtained. The latter is only useful if the chest radiograph excludes overlying parenchymal disease. The absorbed dose to the uterus (and fetus) is approximately 0.2-0.3 mGy for ventilation / perfusion imaging but varies dependant on the agents used (44). Recent estimations of the radiation dose absorbed by the fetus during CTPA have been reported to be as low as 0.026 mSv using SDCT and 0.014 mSv for MDCT (45).

More concern has been devoted to an increased risk of cancer induction after radiation exposure during CTPA to radiosensitive organs in pregnant patients, particular breast tissue. The calculated breast dose using organ-specific conversion factors have been calculated to range between 5.5-13.1 mGy (average 7.4 mGy) per breast. An exposure of 10 mGy to the breasts of a woman aged 35 years increases the risk of breast cancer by approximately 14% over the background rate for the general population (46). A perfusion scintigraphy provides less dose for the breasts at the expense of a slightly increased dose for the foetus especially since the radiopharmacon is eliminated through kidneys and bladder.

If a CTPA examination is planned to be carried out, it is important to adapt the protocol to reduce dose and to optimize contrast application.

As previously described the kV should be reduced to 100 kV, in very small patients to 80 kV to substantially reduce radiation dose. The scan range should be sharply limited to the lung parenchyma. Further on, the pitch and slice collimation can be increased to further reduce dose (pitch of 1.7-2 and slice thickness of 1-1.5 mm). Since pregnant women have a hypercirculatory state with increased cardiac output and increased plasma volume already at an early state of their pregnancy, the injection rate should be increased to 6 ml/s to ensure adequate vascular enhancement (47).

To avoid a valsalva maneuver in these usually very nervous patients, patients should be instructed to breath shallowly instead of holding their breath.

Last but not least, it seems to be the most important to obtain an examination of interpretable image quality that justifies the radiation given to patient and child. Thus per institution, that technique should be chosen for which interpretation experience and technical standard are highest.

2.11 ICU patients

In patients under respiratory ventilation the quality of a CTPA is highly dependant on the capacity of cooperation of the patient. If the scan quality is likely to be substantially improved when image acquisition is performed with full sedation of the patient and in full inspiration, it should be discussed with the clinicians before obtaining the scan. Such a procedure and dependant on the scanner type, it might require an interruption of the respiratory ventilation for a period of 15-20 s which poses no problem in most patients. When apnea during image acquisition is not an option, the frequency of ventilation can be reduced in order to minimize breathing artefacts.

In addition, as patients are frequently scanned with their arms parallel the body, the scan has to be obtained with a sufficiently high dose to ensure low noise and adequate signal (lowering kV and mAs is not an option in this patient group).

2.12 Repeating CTPA

Despite the use of an optimized protocol and careful patient instruction, the CTPA may still result in a non-diagnostic scan. One should only consider repeating the examination if a better result can be expected after adequate adaptation of the protocol or patient preparation, e.g., having a better venous access available, adapting contrast medium injection rate or dose, choosing a longer scan delay, or changing patient instruction (figure 3).

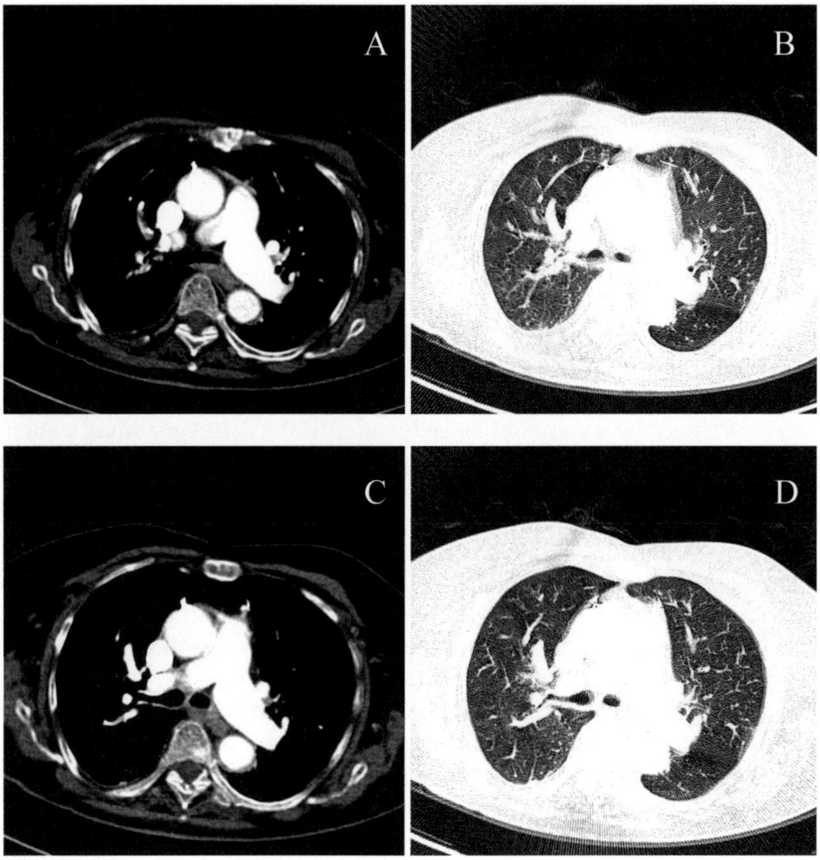

Fig. 3. CTPA of a 61-year-old female patient with severe dyspnea. The 1-mm axial slices in mediastinal (A) and lung parenchyma (B) window setting demonstrate severe breathing artefacts resulting in a non-interpretable scan result. The CTPA was repeated immediately after the first acquisition with a second contrast medium bolus injection, which resulted in a CTPA of diagnostic quality (C and D).

2.13 Thrombus load and right ventricular function: predictors of adverse outcome?

Besides diagnosing PE by direct visualization of the thrombus, a CTPA can also be helpful in predicting the outcome of patients with PE, which is assumed to be related to clot burden and RV function (48).

Several parameters in predicting right ventricular dysfunction (RVD) have been mentioned, like the RV/LV ratio, dilatation of the PA, SVC and azygos vein, bowing of the interventricular septum and the pressure in the right atrium. Of these, only a RV/LV ratio ≥ 0.9-1.5 obtained on the axial views has been shown to be directly correlated with RVD and adverse outcome (49).

For the quantification of thrombus load in the pulmonary vascular tree, several scoring systems have been proposed. The modified Walsh and Miller scores, which were primarily angiographic scores, but adapted to the needs of CT, both quantify the severity of PA obstruction (50). The CT derived scores proposed by the groups of Qanadli and Mastora not only give information about thrombus load, but also about the degree of obstruction (51, 52). However, despite the excellent clot imaging, the literature still shows contradicting results in the usefulness of the PA obstruction index as a predictor of RVD or short-term survival. Furthermore, since obtaining these scores is very time-consuming they have never found their entrance in clinical routine so far. The use of CAD software might overcome this limitation in the future (37).

3. Interpretation of CT: How it should be done

3.1 Slice reconstruction

Dependant on the slice collimation used during acquisition, slice reconstruction width varies from 0.9 to 1.5 mm, preferably 0.9-1.0 mm. Usually an overlapping reconstruction algorithm is applied with a reconstruction index of 0.7-1.0. Thinner slice thicknesses do not further contribute to the diagnosis and will unnecessarily decrease signal-to-noise ratio. In obese patients, a smoothing reconstruction algorithm and thicker slices of 1.5 or 2.0 mm might be advantageous to increase the signal to noise ratio. It is not recommended to use a slice thickness thicker than 2.0 mm to ensure optimal evaluation of peripheral pulmonary arteries (figure 4).

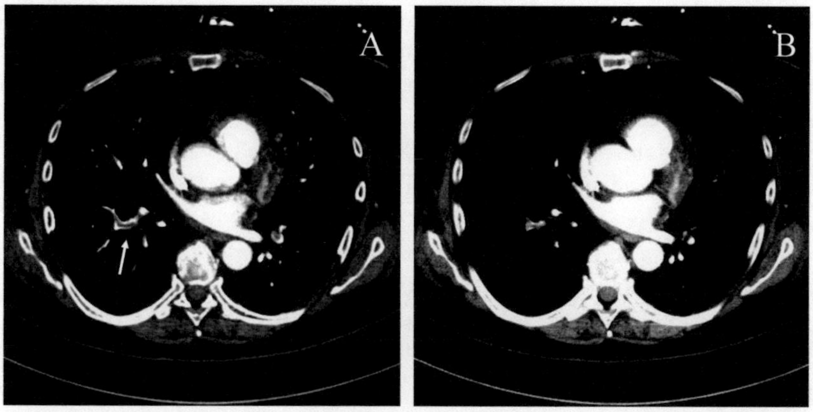

Fig. 4. CTPA in a 56-year-old female patient with progressive dyspnea. Axial 1-mm reconstruction revealing a PE in a subsegmental vessel surrounded by contrast medium (white arrow), a so-called 'railway track sign' (A), which is less well depicted on the 5-mm reconstruction (B).

3.2 Windowing

Axial slices in both soft tissue window setting (window width, WW = 400 HU; window level, WL = 30 to 40 HU) and pulmonary parenchyma window setting (WW = 1500 HU; WL = -800 to -600 HU) represent the base for diagnostic interpretation. When only fixed standard soft tissue window settings are used, especially in combination with a high iodine injection rate, small PE may be obscured by the dense contrast medium and may be consequently missed. Therefore, the use of a modified relatively wide soft tissue window (WW = 700 HU; WL = 100 HU) has been proposed by some authors. Alternatively, an individual adaptation of the window setting can be applied that is flexibly adapted to the degree of vascular enhancement and vascular size: the WW is set slightly lower than twice the mean attenuation in the pulmonary trunk and the WL is set at about half of the mean attenuation of the pulmonary trunk (53).

A poor vascular enhancement is more difficult to overcome as the density difference between the opacified vessel and the thrombus is decreased. In this case, narrowing the window width and lowering window level settings may help to obtain a more confident diagnosis.

Although soft tissue window settings are necessary to provide direct visualization of intravascular contrast defects and thus provide the base for diagnosis, pulmonary window settings are also indispensable for the assessment of movement artefacts, which result in endovascular contrast inhomogeneities which may mimic pulmonary thrombi. The pulmonary parenchyma window setting is also important to differentiate pulmonary arteries from mucus filled bronchi and from venous structures that may not be opacified in an early scan phase (no accompanying bronchial structure).

The simultaneous assessment of either standard or adapted soft tissue window setting and pulmonary parenchyma window setting (e.g., on two monitors side to side or by toggling) will shorten the interpretation time and will potentially reduce false positive findings.

3.3 Image interpretation

An interactive cine mode interpretation on either a dedicated work station or using the PACS workstation is warranted to assess the large number of slices, usually 300-450 slices for a multi-detector CTA. The magnitude of the dataset is determined by the slice thickness and the reconstruction index and not by the number of CT detectors. Therefore, the number of images does not necessarily increase with the use of CT systems with more detectors. Scrolling through the dataset is helpful to identify and follow the pulmonary arteries, to identify pulmonary emboli and to differentiate between pulmonary arteries and other pulmonary structures. Thorough knowledge of the anatomy of the pulmonary arterial tree and the hilar structures and a systematic approach are essential for optimal interpretation. One possible and in our view useful and practical approach is to start with the pulmonary trunk and follow per lobe every artery from its origin to the periphery.

3.4 Multiplanar and curved reformats

With MDCT isotropic 3D datasets are obtained that allow for reconstruction in different directions without distortion or step-artefacts that are inherent to non-isotropic datasets obtained with SDCT or MDCT scanners below 16 detector rows.

While axial slices represent the base to evaluate a CTPA examination, additional reconstructions such as MPR's or curved planar reformats (CPR's), i.e., along the long axis of the vessel of interest and perpendicular to its lumen, are used as problem-solving tools: these reconstructions are helpful for the assessment of pulmonary arteries that are oriented oblique or parallel to the imaging plane, to distinguish central clots from perivascular lymphatic tissue, and to differentiate pulsation artefacts from real thrombi. Findings at MPR or other processing techniques should always be verified and correlated with findings in the axial plane.

MPR's represent the simplest and most frequently used processing technique. To obtain a good quality MPR, the slice thickness is usually 2 mm. MPR's can be reconstructed in any direction and the optimal direction is dependent on the patient's vascular anatomy and the individual findings and therefore should be done individually and not in a standardized way. Some vendors offer point-related MPR's in all three directions on demand: given a focal intravascular inhomogeneity that requires further attention, this particular area of interest will be automatically displayed in all three directions on demand allowing for analysis of the vascular inhomogeneity in the long as well as short axis of the vessel.

3.5 Maximum intensity projections

Maximum intensity projections (MIP's) are an excellent tool to obtain angiography-like images. As MPR's they can also be reconstructed in every direction. Since MIPs use 3D information, they show in opposite to MPRs the vessel to a longer extent. Sliding thin slab MIP's (3-5 mm thickness, with a maximum of 10 mm) were found to improve delineation of small peripheral vessels. Small peripheral thrombi will appear as less enhanced vessel segments with a lower density as compared to neighboring vessels with the same size. The use of MIP's is therefore recommended in every patient in which the initial standard axial reconstructions did not reveal PE.

The most important pitfall using MIP reconstructions refers to small hypodense structures (i.e., endovascular thrombi) that might be obscured by surrounding hyperdense structures (dense contrast-enhanced vessels). This occurs when MIP's slab thickness is too high or the display window is too narrow resulting in a too small contrast range. Choosing sufficiently thin slabs and adapting the window settings is therefore important.

Also MIPs represent an instantaneous feature on all dedicated and in our days most PACS workstations. MIP thickness and direction can be adapted on-line.

3.6 Computer aided diagnosis

The meticulous review of up to 300-500 axial images per CTPA study is a rather time-consuming task that requires a high level of attentiveness of the readers. While the majority of scans is made to exclude PE, the chance of missing small emboli increases with time pressure, anatomic and technical complexity and decreasing readers' experience (54).

CAD algorithms (figure 5) have been therefore developed to improve the detection performance of observers, to decrease interobserver variability and eventually to decrease reading time. None of the CAD algorithms for the detection of PE is currently FDA approved, and experience so far is therefore limited to scientific evaluation and study results.

Publications report an improved detection rate of small segmental and subsegmental emboli.

While CAD seems to be of no use in patients with multiple, central and rather obvious emboli, it may help especially inexperienced readers to detect small peripheral emboli which are seen in only a subset of patients and whose clinical relevance is still under debate. The number of false positive calls by the CAD algorithm is strongly related to image quality (figure 5) and may increase to more than 30 false positive calls in patients with a low enhancement or serious movement artefacts which undoubtedly is unpractical (55, 56). The majority of scans however have less than 5 false positive calls, which are quite easy to dismiss and therefore do not cause diagnostic problems. Use of CAD as "second reader" - meaning that CAD results are only used as additional information after having analyzed the scan first without CAD - inevitably leads to further increase of reading time. It is still under evaluation whether CAD may be used more efficiently as "concurrent reader" meaning that already the initial reading process is supported by CAD candidates. In the future the automatic detection of vascular emboli may be also used for the quantification of thrombus load (57).

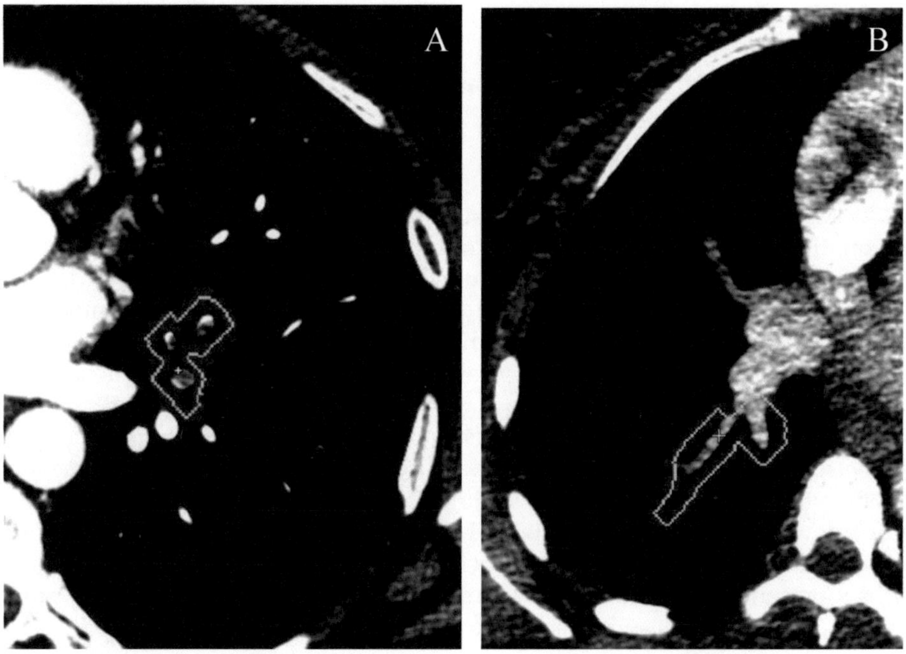

True positive candidate **False positive candidate**

Fig. 5. Automatic detection of pulmonary emboli using a CAD prototype (Philips Healthcare, the Netherlands): (A) example of true positive candidates, and (B) false positive candidates in badly opacified pulmonary arteries.

4. Imaging characteristics of PE

For correct interpretation of a CTPA study, every single artery from the main PA to the subsegmental branches has to be examined for signs of acute or chronic PE. Not only knowledge of the direct and indirect imaging characteristics of PE is essential, also familiarity with the pitfalls of the interpretation of the scan is required. Therefore the imaging characteristics of both acute and chronic PE will be outlined first followed by an overview of pitfalls related to technique, anatomy and patient.

4.1 Findings in acute PE

Direct signs of acute PE (figures 1, 4, 6-8) adapted and modified from the original description by Sinner (58), can be identified as:

a. a complete intraluminal filling defect caused by thrombus occluding the entire vessel lumen, potentially leading to a diameter enlargement of the affected artery compared to other pulmonary arteries of the same order of branching,

b. a partial filling defect centrally located in the vessel lumen caused by a clot surrounded by contrast medium: the finding is also named 'polo mint sign' when seen in cross section or 'railway track sign' when imaged along the long axis of the vessel, or
c. an eccentric partial filling defect that makes an acute angle with the PA wall caused by a mural thrombus that is outlined by contrast material (59-62).

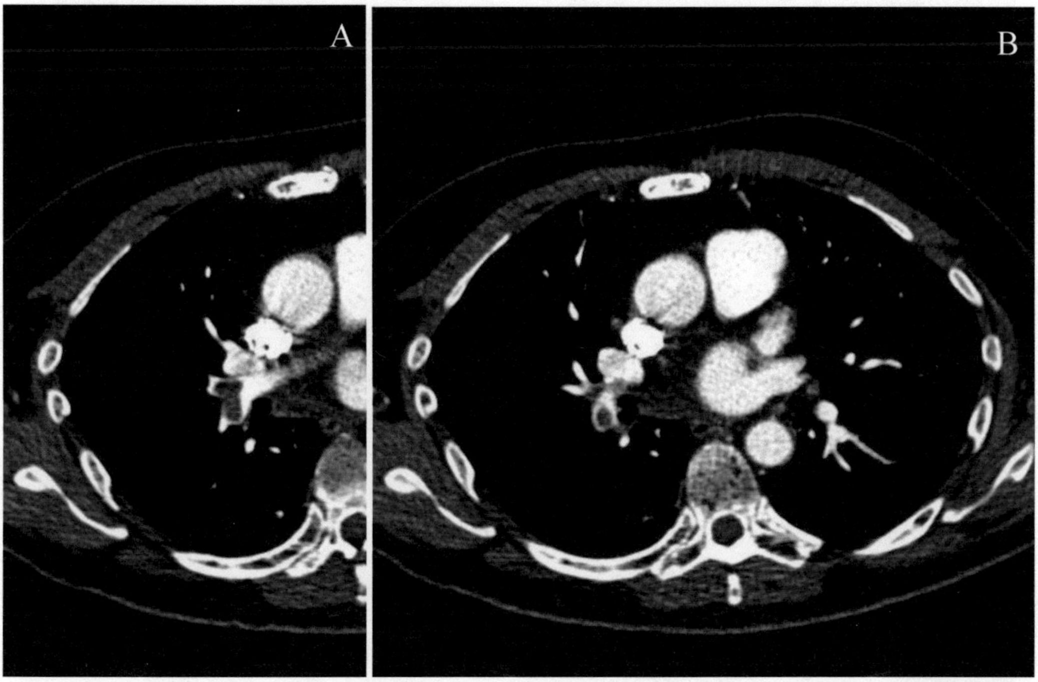

Fig. 6. Examples of direct and indirect signs of acute PE: centrally located non-obstructing thrombus, branching over the bifurcation of a pulmonary vessel, with acute angles to the vessel wall (A); centrally located partial filling defect ('doughnut or polo mint sign') with diameter enlargement as compared to the opposite side (B).

Several ancillary findings can be seen in patients with PE, but most of these are non-specific as they are seen also in other conditions. Wedge-shaped pleural-based consolidations and linear bands have shown to be statistically significantly related to PE (63). A peripheral wegde-shaped consolidation, typically without an air bronchogram, is likely to represent pulmonary infarction (figure 7) potentially with secondary haemorrhage. This is rarely encountered in healthy individuals because the bronchial artery collateral circulation will take over the blood flow to the embolized area. Other indirect findings include pleural effusions (figure 7) and atelectasis that are usually small, both quite frequently seen but non-specific signs. A mosaic perfusion pattern, caused by focal areas of hypoperfusion due to acute obstruction of blood flow through one or more pulmonary arteries, is more often seen on angiography than on computed tomography pulmonary angiography (CTPA) (64).
Although these indirect findings are considered to be of limited diagnostic value, they may suggest further investigations in case of an inconclusive CTPA.

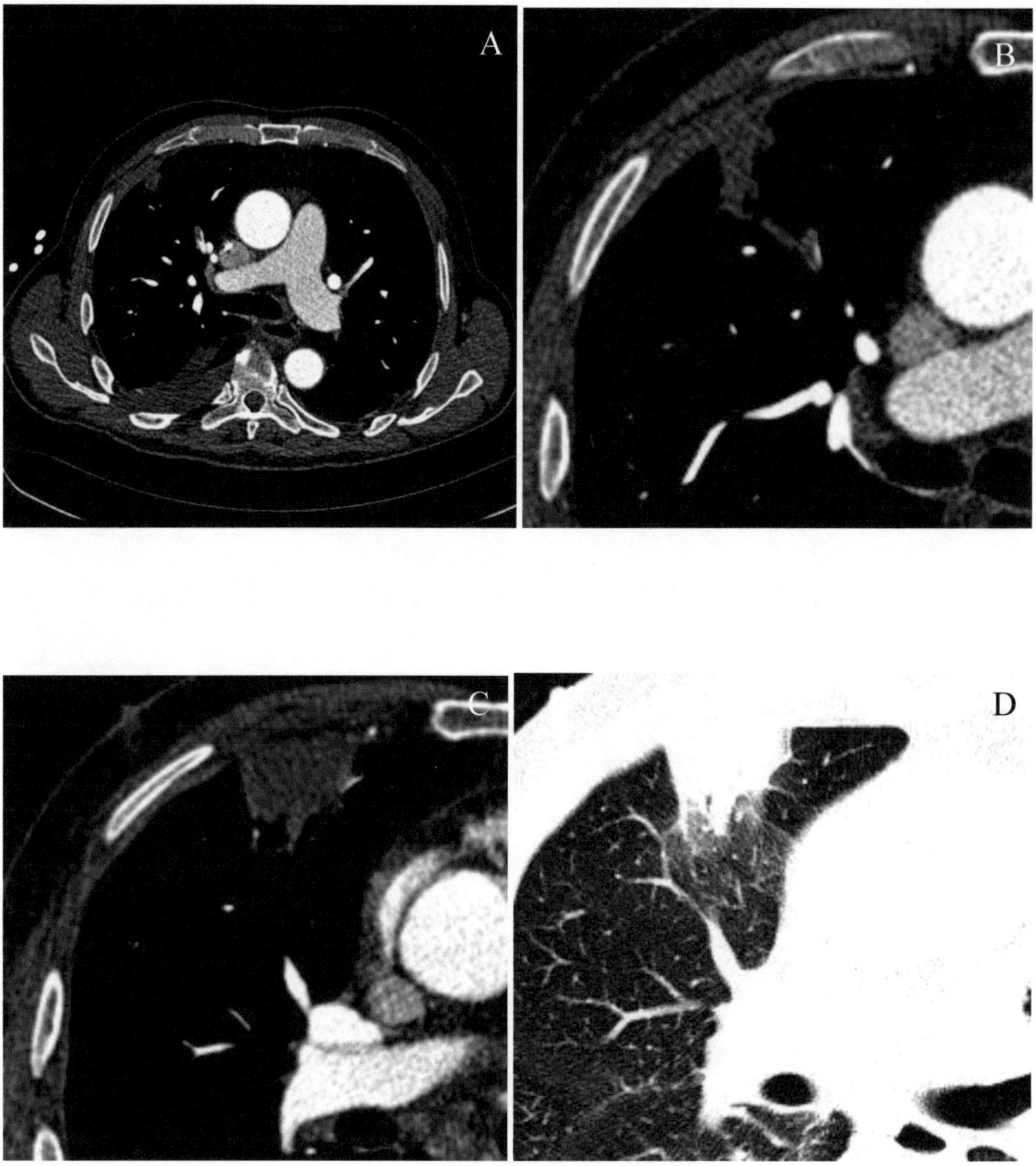

Fig. 7. Complete obstruction of a subsegmental pulmonary artery (A-C) with a wedge-shaped pleural-based consolidation (D) indicating a pulmonary infarction. A small pleural effusion is also present.

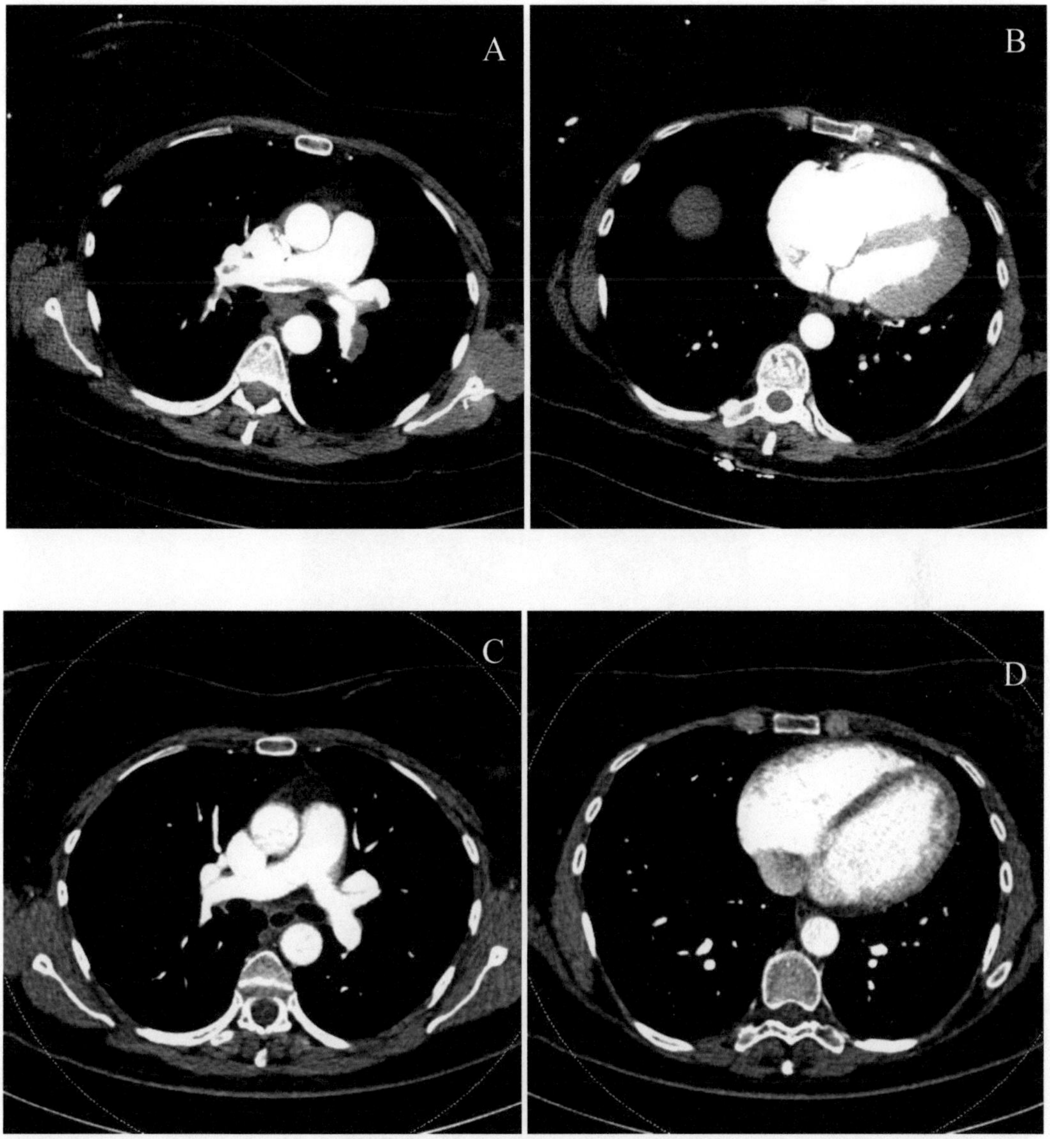

Fig. 8. CTPA of a 42-year-old female patient who presented with acute chest pain and hypotension revealed extensive central pulmonary emboli in combination with dilatation of the main PA (A) and the right ventricle (B). A follow-up scan after thrombolysis and 6 months of anticoagulant treatment revealed diameter normalization of the main PA (C) and the right ventricle (D). No residual thrombus was found.

4.2 Findings in chronic PE

Chronic PE has several imaging characteristics on a CTPA (figures 9-12), which correspond to imaging findings known from conventional pulmonary angiography. It can be identified as:

a. a complete intraluminal filling defect of a PA that is *smaller* than the adjacent patent pulmonary arteries,

b. an eccentrically located partial intraluminal filling defect that makes an obtuse angle with the PA wall,
c. an abrupt vessel narrowing often due to recanalization after complete occlusion by thrombus,
d. an apparently thick-walled artery, sometimes with irregular contours with irregularly narrowed lumen after recanalization
e. webs or bands visible in the arterial lumen,
f. partial or complete obstruction organizing with a concave configuration, with or without the appearance of distal pulmonary arteries on sequential scanning (65)
g. an intraluminal filling defect with the morphology of an acute PE present for more than 3 months (64, 66-68).

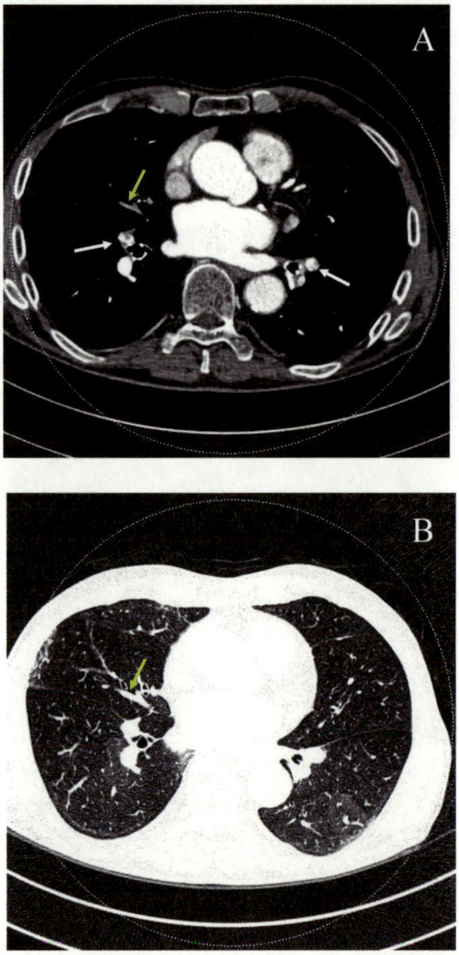

Fig. 9. Chronic PE in a 72-year-old male patient. CTPA with 1-mm axial reconstruction demonstrating bilateral eccentric thrombi with both acute and obtuse angles to the vessel wall (A, white arrows). A non-opacified vessel on the right side was (green arrow) found not to be accompanied by a bronchus on the pulmonary window setting (B), which is in agreement with a pulmonary vein. In addition, mosaic perfusion is present due to the chronic PE.

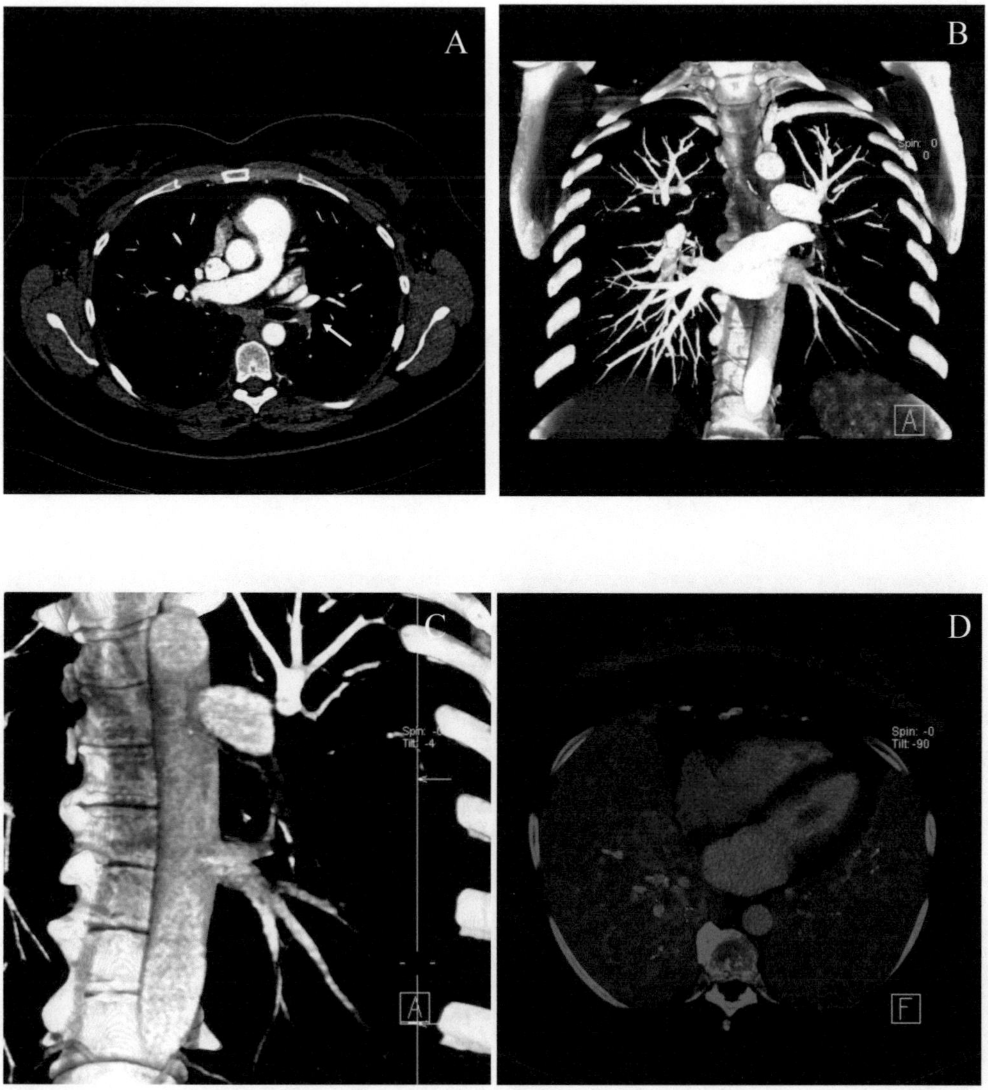

Fig. 10. Fifty-year-old female patient with complete obstruction of the left lower lobe PA due to chronic PE. Several CTPA scans were obtained for both follow-up and recurrent dyspnea. Complete obliteration and decreased diameter of the left lower lobe PA is demonstrated at 1-mm axial reconstruction performed using a single-source CT scanner (A, white arrow) and at additional coronal thin MIP reconstructions (B and C, detail). A fused color-coded and virtual 120 kV axial image demonstrates decreased perfusion in the left lower lobe (D, black area).

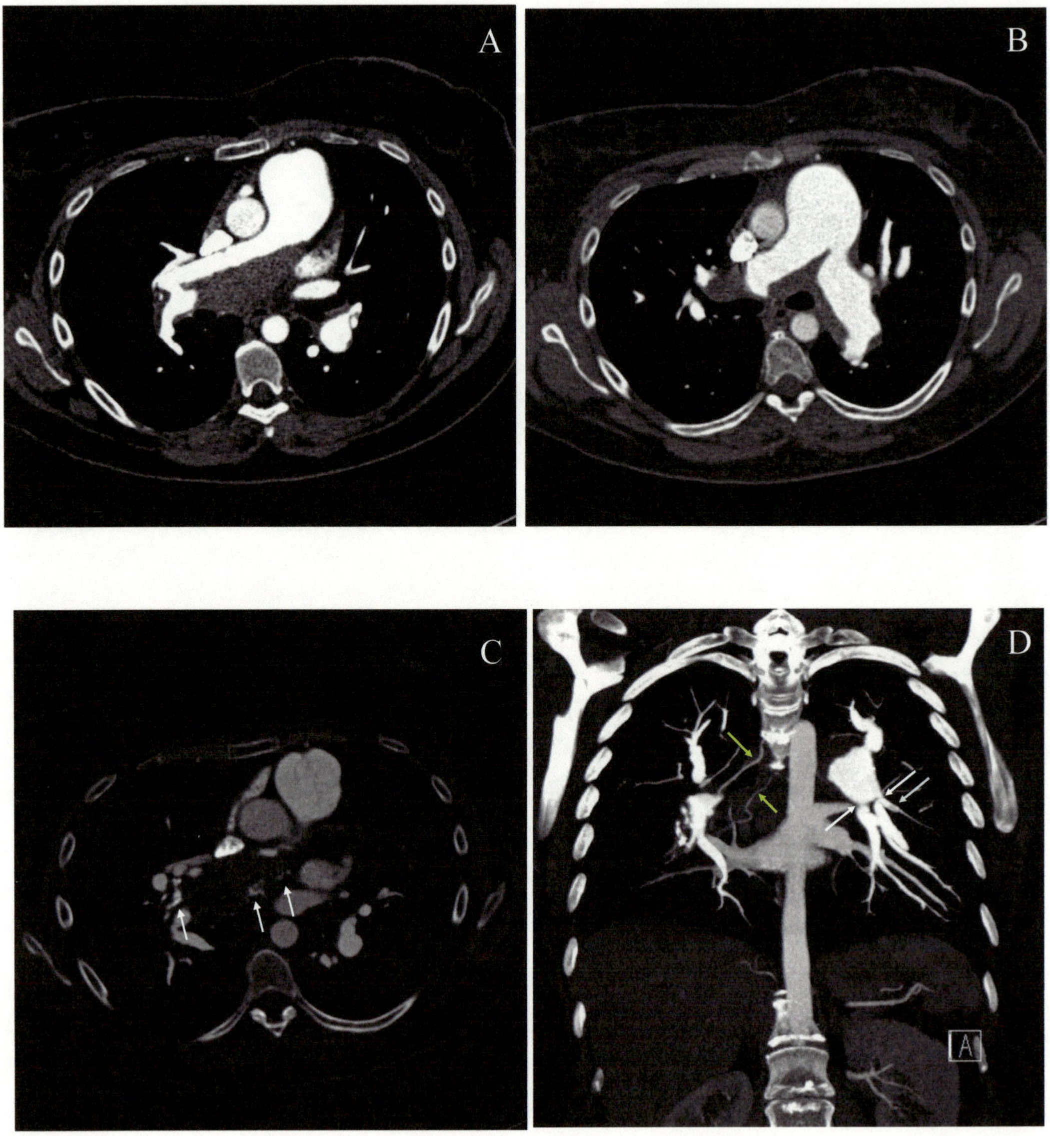

Fig. 11. Forty-year-old female patient with chronic thrombo-embolic PH. CTPA shows extensive eccentric thrombus with irregular contours of the inner surface in the right (A) and left (B) PA resembling a thick-walled PA. Calcifications (white arrows) in the thrombus are demonstrated with adaptation of the window settings (C). Coronal MIP reconstruction (D) demonstrates webs (white arrows), a small intraluminal filling defect (blue arrow) and dilatation of the bronchial arteries (green arrows) secondary to the chronic PE. The marked increase in diameter of the central pulmonary arteries (A and B) and the tortuosity of the pulmonary arteries (C) are indicative of PH.

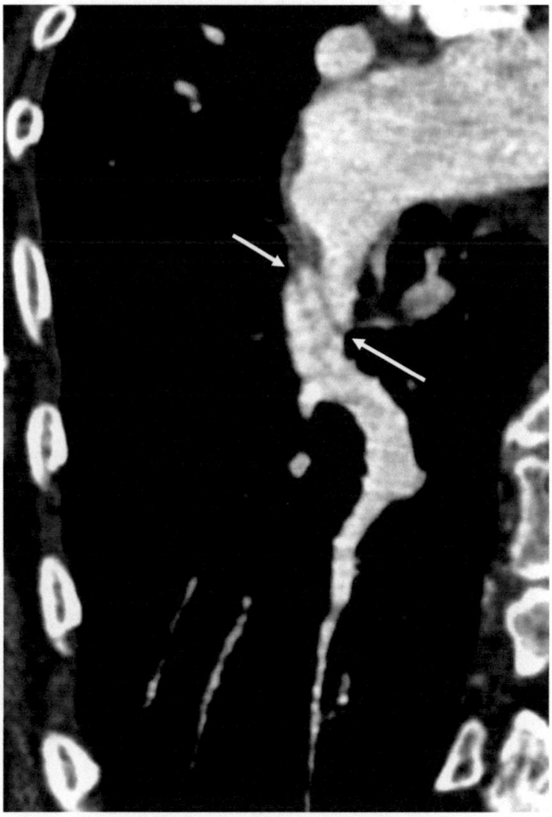

Fig. 12. Curved planar reformat of the right lower lobe PA in a patient with chronic PE demonstrates an intrapulmonary web (arrows).

At conventional pulmonary angiography, post-stenotic dilatation or aneurysm has been described in the setting of chronic PE in combination with the above findings (65).
Calcifications can be seen within the chronic thrombi in a small number of patients though it requires adaptation (widening) of the window settings in such a way that the calcifications are not obscured by the contrast material. Calcified thrombi in the subsegmental or smaller branches are often indistinguishable from small lung parenchymal calcifications, however their microtubular shape and position at the site of arterial branching may be helpful in the differential diagnosis (67).
A relatively common and serious complication of chronic PE is secondary PH, having an incidence of approximately 4 percent in the first two years after the first episode of PE (69). Therefore specific attention has to be paid to CT signs related to PH such as dilatation of the main PA (diameter more than 29 mm) (70), tortuous pulmonary vessels (71), hypertrophic bronchial arteries (72) a mosaic pattern and of lung attenuation due to variable perfusion. Mosaic pattern and the presence of systemic collateral supply are helpful signs to differentiate primary from secondary PH which has therapeutic implications (72, 73). In patients with recurrent PE, both chronic and acute PE can be present (figure 13).

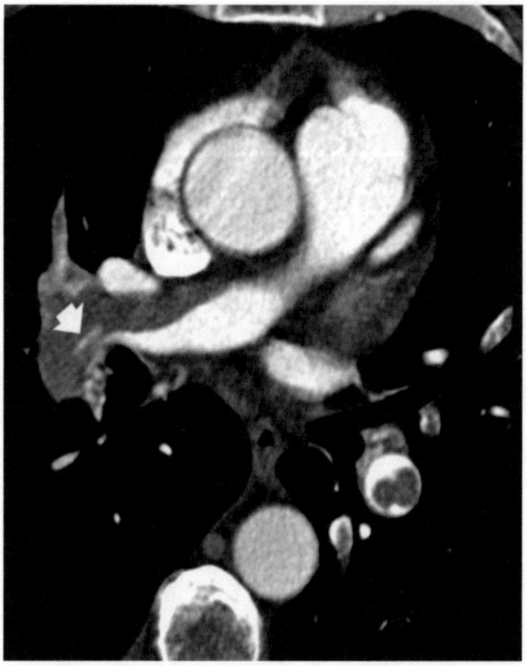

Fig. 13. Axial 1-mm thin slice demonstrating acute PE on the left side whereas on the right side a large centrally located eccentric thrombus is present with contrast in the thrombus as a result of recanalization (white arrow).

5. Pitfalls

To obtain an adequate interpretation of a CTPA the radiologist should be familiar with the various diagnostic pitfalls that can occur. Pitfalls can be divided into three groups dependant on their underlying cause we differentiate pitfalls related to technique, anatomy or patient factors (table 4).

Technique	Motion artefact Suboptimal contrast injection technique Partial volume effect Image noise Window settings Lung algorithm artefact Stair-step artefact
Anatomy	Pulmonary veins Hilar lymph nodes
Patient	Vascular abnormalities Mucus plugs PA sarcoma PA stump in situ thrombosis

Table 4. Pitfalls in the interpretation of CT of the pulmonary arteries.

5.1 Technique related pitfalls

5.1.1 Motion artefacts

One of the most common technique related pitfall is motion artefact, which is the major cause of an indeterminate CTPA (2). Respiratory and cardiac motion give rise to volume averaging of the vessel and surrounding lung parenchyma and can mimic a PE (figures 3 and 14) (62, 67). In addition, breathing can also result in inhomogeneous opacification of pulmonary arteries due to variations in the blood flow between inspiration and expiration, simulating an intraluminal filling defect (74).

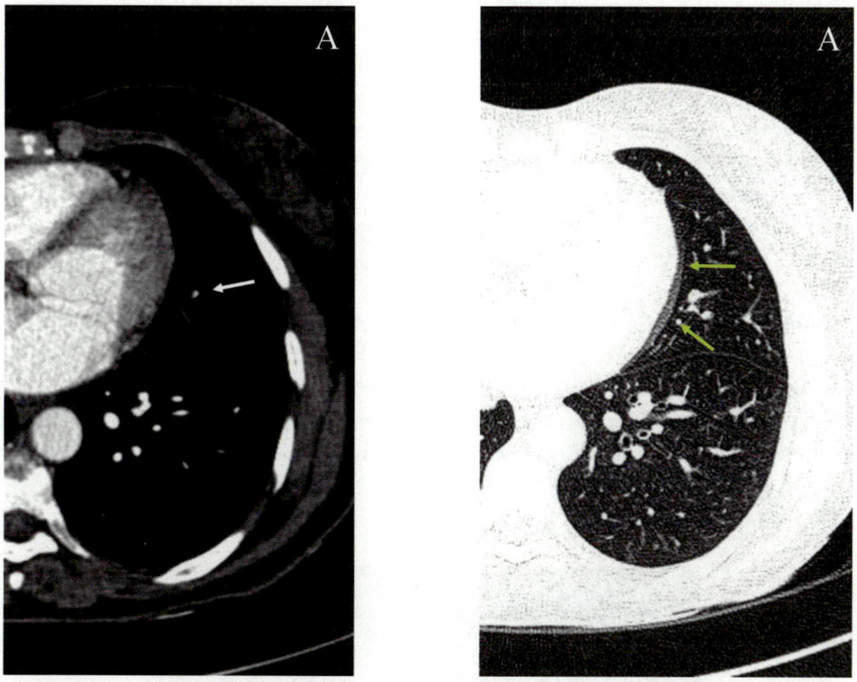

Fig. 14. Axial 1-mm slice showing a very small hypodense area in a small PA in the lingula (A, white arrow), which was due to a pulsation artefact as shown on the pulmonary window setting (B, green arrows).

Obvious motion can easily be detected by a rapid change in position and diameter on contiguous images or by observing the chest wall for respiratory motion during cine viewing of the images. When subtle, motion artifacts may be difficult to see on the mediastinal window settings, but can be clearly recognized on the lung window settings showing composite images of the vessels ('seagull sign') (62).

The rate of indeterminate studies due to motion artefacts has diminished with the introduction of multislice CT, since scanning times are reduced from 30 to 5-10 s, therefore requiring shorter breath holds. In a heavily dyspnoeic patient, image quality may be improved by limiting the scan range in z-direction e.g., to the range between superior contour of the aortic arch to the level of the inferior pulmonary veins, or by letting the patient gently breath during scan acquisition (59). A possibly artefact-free CTPA in an intubated patient can be achieved by suspending the ventilation in deep inspiration for the duration of the scan, which is possible in most sedated patients.

A disadvantage of the fast multislice CT scanners is that once a patient starts breathing during data acquisition, a relatively large scan volume might render indeterminate. Therefore gentle breathing during scanning may be preferred to deep inspiration in some patients, even though under these circumstances visualization and thus evaluation of peripheral small arteries is limited.

5.1.2 Suboptimal contrast injection technique

Another common pitfall related to scan technique is suboptimal contrast enhancement of the pulmonary arteries, due to inappropriate scan delay, flow rate or iodine concentration (22, 75, 76). Artefacts caused by improper scan delay are easily recognized because they typically result in appropriate vascular enhancement in the cranial or caudal part of the scan volume. Dependent on the extent of inappropriate vascular enhancement, a repeat examination with special focus on the suboptimally displayed anatomic area may be required.
A low flow rate can lead to poorly opacified pulmonary arteries especially at the level of the (sub)segmental arteries. The quality of enhancement of the small segmental and subsegmental arteries can be improved by using contrast material with a high iodine concentration. The disadvantage of high-contrast concentration, however, is streak artefacts at the level of the SVC (figure 15). Although these artefacts are readily identified by their radiating, poorly defined nature, as well as their usually non-anatomic configuration, they may create pseudo-filling defects in the right pulmonary and upper lobe arteries and may therefore render this part of the examination indeterminate.
Nowadays, to obtain optimal contrast enhancement in the pulmonary arteries high flow (4-6 ml/s) and high concentration (370-400 mg of iodine/ml) protocols are used in combination with a saline bolus injected immediately after the contrast bolus to reduce streak artefacts (19) (see also under 'injection protocol').

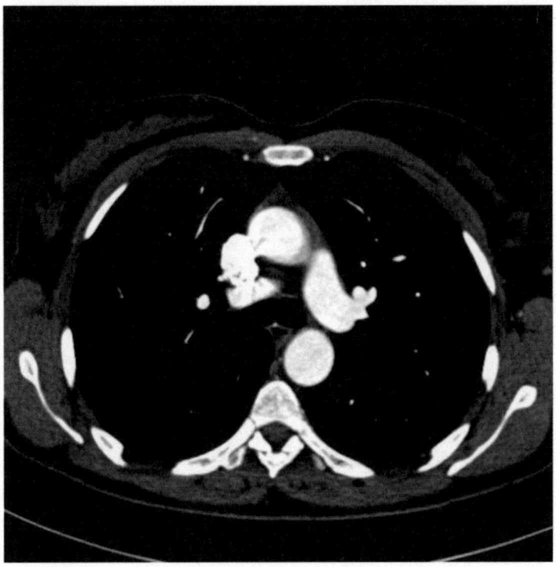

Fig. 15. CTPA of a 42-year-old male patient with acute chest pain 2 weeks after surgery revealing streak artefacts at the level of the right PA due to dense contrast in the SVC. No PE was found.

5.1.3 Partial volume effects

Small vessels that run parallel to the axis of the scan plane may simulate a PE by volume averaging with the surrounding lung parenchyma or adjacent bronchus (60, 62, 77). The arteries of the lingua and medial and lateral segments of the right middle lobe are particularly prone to such a volume averaging artefact. By using a thin collimation (< 2 mm) and multiplanar reformations the effects of volume averaging can be overcome enabling accurate analysis also of these vascular structures and thereby reducing false positive results.

5.1.4 Image noise

Especially in obese patients, image noise may substantially degrade image quality, and make the evaluation of the small segmental and subsegmental arteries very difficult if not even indeterminate. Although increasing the reconstruction width to 2.5 mm helps to decrease image noise and thereby improve signal-to-noise ratio and thus scan quality, it also decreases the sensitivity for detecting small pulmonary emboli (62, 78).

5.1.5 Window settings

The standard mediastinal window settings (window width 300-450, window level 30-50) may not always be adequate in the detection of PE, because the dense contrast material may obscure an intravascular thrombus (77). Therefore a more individual window setting is preferred (see under 'windowing'). The use of these settings in combination with the standard mediastinal and lung parenchym window settings will help to improve diagnostic accuracy.

5.1.6 Lung algorithm artefact

When the pulmonary arteries are visualized with images that are calculated using a high spatial frequency reconstruction convolution kernel used to improve the depiction of pulmonary vessels, bronchi and interstitium with the lung window, a high attenuation rim around vertically orientated vessels may be observed, potentially mimicking a PE. Interpretation of these vessels with the soft tissue reconstruction algorithm is crucial as these will no longer reveal the intraluminal filling defect (59, 62).

5.1.7 Stair-step artefact

The stair-step artefact is defined as the presence of surface irregularity artefacts along the margins of the pulmonary vessels ranging from a minimal indentation of the vessel margin to an appearance that mimics a pair of steps when viewed in profile (79). On the axial images, particularly in the vessels that run perpendicular to the scan plane, it may simulate a filling defect on one single slice, while neither the previous nor the next slice show abnormalities (80). However, on coronal and sagittal reformatted images stair-step artefacts are typically seen as horizontal high and low attenuation lines crossing the PA. Factors that can reduce this artefact are a narrow collimation and overlapping reconstruction intervals. Moreover, the use of multidetector CT has significantly reduced these artefacts.

5.2 Anatomy related pitfalls

5.2.1 Normal bronchovascular anatomy

Familiarity with the normal bronchovascular anatomy is essential in the diagnosis of PE. Pulmonary arteries run adjacent to their accompanying bronchus, with the exception of the apical posterior segment of the left upper lobe and the lingular arteries, which may course

separately for a short distance before rejoining with their bronchus. Pulmonary veins course in the interlobular septa, are not accompanied by a bronchus (figure 9) and can be followed towards the left atrium. By verifying their position and following their course on contiguous sections, a true arterial embolus can easily be distinguished from a pseudofilling defect in a pulmonary vein, the latter mostly due to flow artefacts or slow flow.
A vascular bifurcation can be misinterpreted as a web or band on the axial images. Coronal and sagittal reconstructions are helpful to reveal the true nature of this linear filling defect.

5.2.2 Hilar lymph nodes

The normal hilar lymph nodes are small, usually less than 3 mm, hypoattenuating, triangular or linear structures that follow the borders of the bronchovascular interstitium and are thus located in close proximity to the pulmonary arteries and bronchi (81). They can be divided into four groups in the right lung (i.e. the upper lobe, interlobar, middle and lower lobe groups) and four groups in the left lung (i.e. the culminal, interlobar, lingular and lower lobe groups) (81, 82). Knowledge of their size and location is important as they are a potential cause of a false positive diagnosis of PE. A small detector width and coronal and sagittal reconstructions can help distinguish them from a thrombus, showing their extramural location and the preservation of the smooth contour of the contrast-filled artery.

5.3 Patient related pitfalls

5.3.1 Vascular abnormalities

Asymmetric opacification of the pulmonary arteries can be caused by a unilateral increase in pulmonary vascular pressure, for example due to consolidation, atelectasis or pleural fluid, resulting in decreased flow in the ipsilateral arteries. Furthermore, absent or faint enhancement can be the result from unilateral obstruction of a main PA, or from unilateral shunting of blood from the systemic into the pulmonary circulation (74, 77). Left-to-right shunts can be due to the presence of intracardiac shunts, but most commonly they are encountered in patients with acquired disorders, particularly in chronic inflammatory diseases like bronchiectasis, in which a prominent bronchopulmonary circulation may exist. Retrograde flow of unopacified systemic blood from the bronchial arteries into the enhanced pulmonary arteries may potentially simulate a PE. Right-to-left shunting can arise in patients with a patent foramen ovale (PFO) if the pressure in the right atrium exceeds the left atrial pressure. This is a transient physiologic response during deep inspiration, Valsalva manoeuvre or coughing, but is a more persistent situation in cases of PE or PH (83). During CTPA this frequently leads to insufficient attenuation of the pulmonary arteries in combination with early and strong enhancement of the aorta, thereby limiting the diagnosis of PE.

5.3.2 Mucus plugs

Bronchi impacted with mucoid can be misinterpreted by an inexperienced reader as a PE. However, the observation of the contrast enhanced artery immediately adjacent to the apparent filling defect and the visualisation of normal bronchus proximally or distally on contiguous images on the lung window settings will easily reveal the nature of the tubular structure as a bronchus (62).

5.3.3 PA sarcoma

A sarcoma arising from the PA is a very rare lesion, which can be difficult to differentiate from acute or chronic PE. Knowledge of some distinguishing features is therefore important

(84, 85). In PA sarcoma the filling defect frequently spans the entire luminal diameter of the main or proximal PA, a finding which is unusual in PE. Moreover, vascular distension of the involved PA and local extravascular spread are other imaging characteristics that favour the diagnosis of a sarcoma. Late heterogeneous enhancement of the mass, due to neovascularity, necrosis, haemorrhage and occasionally calcifications, are sometimes observed. If a patient who was initially diagnosed as having a PE fails to respond to anticoagulant therapy, a PA sarcoma – though a rare occasion - should be considered.

5.3.4 PA stump in situ thrombosis

The incidence of PA stump thrombosis in patients who underwent pneumonectomy is approximately 12% (86, 87). Although local trauma of the vessel or the hypercoagulable state of blood in patients with a malignancy might contribute to the formation of the clot, the most important factor seems to be the stasis of blood flow, since the clot appears to be related to the length of the stump (86). Moreover, as it is often discovered as an incidental finding on routine follow-up CT and rarely shows other PA thrombi remote from the stump site, it is mostly considered a benign entity and not related to PE (87).

6. Summary

Since the introduction of spiral CT for the detection of PE, the continuous development of multi-detector technique and faster scanning lead to considerable improvement of image quality and visualization especially of smaller peripheral vascular structures. Though the overall percentage of non-diagnostic scans could be substantially improved, optimization of scan protocols, contrast administration and patient instruction remain crucial in order to obtain good quality scans. Inadequate vascular enhancement is still one of the most important causes for a non-diagnostic scan result. With scanning times of less than 5 s, a proper patient instruction has become even more important to avoid a Valsalva maneuver and breathing artefacts. Furthermore, the intravascular contrast can be optimized by lowering the kV and/or increasing the amount of iodine injected per s. With the development of the newer generation scanners the radiation dose can be substantially decreased. Further dose reduction is possible by reducing the scan range, reducing the kVp and using weight-adapted scan parameters. Special adaptations of the scan and contrast injection protocol are recommended in young patients and in pregnant women. In addition to the direct visualization of intravascular clots, indirect signs of acute PE may be helpful when image quality is suboptimal. An increased RV/LV ratio correlates well with PE severity and has been shown to be an independent predictor of an adverse outcome. The role of other CT parameters such as thrombus load as an independent predictor of outcome still needs to be determined.

With a DSCT scanner, lung perfusion can be directly visualized with potential additional functional information. CAD software packages have been developed in order to increase and harmonize diagnostic performance and decrease reading time. Though these new techniques are very promising, their value within the diagnostic algorithm for acute PE is not yet determined.

7. References

[1] Remy Jardin M, Remy J, Wattinne L, Giraud F. Central pulmonary thromboembolism: diagnosis with spiral volumetric CT with the single-breath-hold technique--comparison with pulmonary angiography. Radiology 1992; 185:381-387.

[2] Jones SE, Wittram C. The Indeterminate CT Pulmonary Angiogram: Imaging Characteristics and Patient Clinical Outcome. Radiology 2005; 237:329-337.
[3] Stein PD, Fowler SE, Goodman LR, et al. Multidetector Computed Tomography for Acute Pulmonary Embolism. N Engl J Med 2006; 354:2317-2327.
[4] Matsuoka S, Hunsaker AR, Gill RR, et al. Vascular Enhancement and Image Quality of MDCT Pulmonary Angiography in 400 Cases: Comparison of Standard and Low Kilovoltage Settings. Am. J. Roentgenol. 2009; 192:1651-1656.
[5] Szucs-Farkas Z, Kurmann L, Strautz T, Patak M, Vock P, ST. S. Patient exposure and image quality of low-dose pulmonary computed tomography angiography. Comparison of 100- and 80-kVp protocols. Invest Radiol 2008; 43:871-876.
[6] Heyer CM, Mohr PS, Lemburg SP, Peters SA, Nicolas V. Image Quality and Radiation Exposure at Pulmonary CT Angiography with 100- or 120-kVp Protocol: Prospective Randomized Study1. Radiology 2007; 245:577-583.
[7] Sigal-Cinqualbre AB, Hennequin R, Abada HT, Chen X, Paul J-Fo. Low-kilovoltage multi-detector row chest CT in adults: feasibility and effect on image quality and iodine dose. Radiology 2004; 231:169-174.
[8] Schueller-Weidekamm C, Schaefer-Prokop CM, Weber M, Herold CJ, Prokop M. CT Angiography of Pulmonary Arteries to Detect Pulmonary Embolism: Improvement of Vascular Enhancement with Low Kilovoltage Settings1. Radiology 2006; 241:899-907.
[9] Greess H, Wolf H, Baum U, et al. Dose reduction in computed tomography by attenuation-based online modulation of tube current: evaluation of six anatomical regions. Eur Radiol 2000; 10:391-394.
[10] Mastora I, Remy-Jardin M, Suess C, Scherf C, Guillot JP, Remy J. Dose reduction in spiral CT angiography of thoracic outlet syndrome by anatomically adapted tube current modulation. Eur.Radiol. 2001; 11:590-596.
[11] The 2007 roecommendations of the International Commission on Radiological Protection. ICRP publication 103. . Ann ICRP 2007; 37:1-332.
[12] European guidelines on quality criteria for computed tomography. Eur 16262 EN. . http://www.drs.dk/guidelines/ct/quality/htmlindex.htm
[13] Tack D, De Maertelaer V, Petit W, et al. Multi-Detector Row CT Pulmonary Angiography: Comparison of Standard-Dose and Simulated Low-Dose Techniques. Radiology 2005; 236:318-325.
[14] Schaefer Prokop C, Bankier A, Janata K, al. E. Complete chest CTA versus limited range CTA for the diagnosis of PE: what do we miss? ECR (abstract) 2005.
[15] Marten K, Engelke C, Obenauer S, Baum F, Grabbe E, Funke M. Diagnostic performance of retrospectively ECG-gated multislice CT of acute pulmonary embolism. [Diagnostischer Stellenwert der retrospektiven EKG-Triggerung in der mehrschicht-spiral-CT der akuten Lungenembolie]. Fortschr R"ntgenstr 2003; 175 1490-1495.
[16] White CS, Kuo D, Kelemen M, et al. Chest Pain Evaluation in the Emergency Department: Can MDCT Provide a Comprehensive Evaluation? American Journal of Roentgenology 2005; 185:533-540.
[17] Bae KT. Optimization of contrast enhancement in thoracic MDCT. Radiol.Clin.North Am. 2010; 48:9-29.
[18] Prokop M. Multislice CT angiography. Eur.J.Radiol. 2000; 36:86-96.
[19] Schoellnast H, Deutschmann HA, Fritz GA, Stessel U, Schaffler GJ, Tillich M. MDCT Angiography of the Pulmonary Arteries: Influence of Iodine Flow Concentration on

Vessel Attenuation and Visualization. American Journal of Roentgenology 2005; 184:1935-1939.

[20] Schoellnast H, Deutschmann HA, Berghold A, Fritz GA, Schaffler GJ, Tillich M. MDCT Angiography of the Pulmonary Arteries: Influence of Body Weight, Body Mass Index, and Scan Length on Arterial Enhancement at Different Iodine Flow Rates. In, 2006; 1074-1078.

[21] Bae KT, Tao C, GÃ¼rel S, et al. Effect of Patient Weight and Scanning Duration on Contrast Enhancement during Pulmonary Multidetector CT Angiography1. Radiology 2007; 242:582-589.

[22] Wittram C. How I Do It: CT Pulmonary Angiography. AJR Am.J.Roentgenol. 2007; 188:1255-1261.

[23] Haage P, Schmitz-Rode T, Hubner D, Piroth W, Gunther RW. Reduction of Contrast Material Dose and Artifacts by a Saline Flush Using a Double Power Injector in Helical CT of the Thorax. American Journal of Roentgenology 2000; 174:1049-1053.

[24] Coche EE, Hammer FD, Goffette PP. Demonstration of pulmonary embolism with dynamic gadolinium-enhanced spiral CT. Eur.Radiol. 2001; 11:2306-2309.

[25] Remy-Jardin M, Bahepar J, Lafitte J-J, et al. Multi-Detector Row CT Angiography of Pulmonary Circulation with Gadolinium-based Contrast Agents: Prospective Evaluation in 60 Patients1. Radiology 2006; 238:1022-1035.

[26] Gosselin MV, Rassner UA, Thieszen SL, Phillips J, Oki A. Contrast dynamics during CT pulmonary angiogram. J.Thorac.Imaging 2004; 19:1-7.

[27] Pontana F, Faivre J-B, Remy-Jardin M, et al. Lung Perfusion with Dual-energy Multidetector-row CT (MDCT): Feasibility for the Evaluation of Acute Pulmonary Embolism in 117 Consecutive Patients. Academic Radiology 2008; 15:1494-1504.

[28] Thieme SF, Johnson TRC, Lee C, et al. Dual-Energy CT for the Assessment of Contrast Material Distribution in the Pulmonary Parenchyma. Am. J. Roentgenol. 2009; 193:144-149.

[29] Fink C, Johnson TR, Michaely HJ, et al. Dual-Energy CT Angiography of the Lung in Patients with Suspected Pulmonary Embolism: Initial Results. Dual-Energy-CT-Angiografie der Lunge bei Patienten mit Verdacht auf Lungenembolie: Erste Ergebnisse 2008; 180:879-883.

[30] Zhang L-J, Chai X, Wu S-Y, et al. Detection of pulmonary embolism by dual energy CT: correlation with perfusion scintigraphy and histopathological findings in rabbits. European Radiology 2009; 19:2844-2854.

[31] Remy-Jardin M, Faivre J-B, Pontana F, et al. Thoracic Applications of Dual Energy. Radiologic clinics of North America; 48:193-205.

[32] Kerl JM, Bauer RW, Renker M, et al. Triphasic contrast injection improves evaluation of dual energy lung perfusion in pulmonary CT angiography. European Journal of Radiology 2010; In Press, Corrected Proof.

[33] Lu GM, Wu SY, Yeh BM, Zhang LJ. Dual-energy computed tomography in pulmonary embolism. Br J Radiol 2010; 83:707-718.

[34] Thieme SF, Becker CR, Hacker M, Nikolaou K, Reiser MF, Johnson TRC. Dual energy CT for the assessment of lung perfusion--Correlation to scintigraphy. European Journal of Radiology 2008; 68:369-374.

[35] Thieme SF, Graute V, Nikolaou K, et al. Dual Energy CT lung perfusion imaging--Correlation with SPECT/CT. European Journal of Radiology; In Press, Corrected Proof.

[36] Krissak R, Henzler T, Reichert M, Krauss B, Schoenberg SO, Fink C. Enhanced Visualization of Lung Vessels for Diagnosis of Pulmonary Embolism Using Dual Energy CT Angiography. Investigative Radiology 2010; 45:341-346.

[37] Remy-Jardin M, Pistolesi M, Goodman LR, et al. Management of Suspected Acute Pulmonary Embolism in the Era of CT Angiography: A Statement from the Fleischner Society1. Radiology 2007; 245:315-329.

[38] Matthews S. Imaging pulmonary embolism in pregnancy: what is the most appropriate imaging protocol? In, 2006; 441-444.

[39] Schuster ME, Fishman JE, Copeland JF, Hatabu H, Boiselle PM. Pulmonary Embolism in Pregnant Patients: A Survey of Practices and Policies for CT Pulmonary Angiography. In, 2003; 1495-1498.

[40] Boiselle PM, Reddy SS, Villas PA, Liu A, Seibyl JP. Pulmonary embolus in pregnant patients: survey of ventilation-perfusion imaging policies and practices. In, 1998; 201-206.

[41] van Beek EJR, Wild JM, Fink C, Moody AR, Kauczor H-U, Oudkerk M. MRI for the diagnosis of pulmonary embolism. Journal of Magnetic Resonance Imaging 2003; 18:627-640.

[42] International commission on radiological protection publication 84: pregnancy and medical radiation. Ann ICRP 2000; 30.

[43] Mallick S, Petkova D. Investigating suspected pulmonary embolism during pregnancy. Respiratory Medicine 2006; 100:1682-1687.

[44] Balan KK, Critchley M, Vedavathy KK, Smith ML, Vinjamuri S. The value of ventilation-perfusion imaging in pregnancy. In, 1997; 338-340.

[45] Nijkeuter M, Geleijns J, De Roos A, Meinders AE, Huisman MV. Diagnosing pulmonary embolism in pregnancy: rationalizing fetal radiation exposure in radiological procedures. Journal of Thrombosis and Haemostasis 2004; 2:1857-1858.

[46] Remy-Jardin M, Remy J. Spiral CT angiography of the pulmonary circulation. Radiology 1999; 212:615-636.

[47] Mabie W, DiSessa T, Crocker L, BM. S, KL. A. A longitudinal study of cardiac output in normal human pregnancy. Am J Obstet Gynecol 1994; 170:849-856.

[48] Wood KE. Major pulmonary embolism : review of a pathophysiologic approach to the golden hour of hemodynamically significant pulmonary embolism. Chest 2002; 121:877-905.

[49] Gibson N, Sohne M, Buller H. Prognostic value of echocardiography and spiral computed tomography in patients with pulmonary embolism. Current Opinion in Pulmonary Medicine 2005; 11:380-384.

[50] Bankier AA, Janata K, Fleischmann D, et al. Severity assessment of acute pulmonary embolism with spiral CT: evaluation of two modified angiographic scores and comparison with clinical data. J.Thorac.Imaging 1997; 12:150-158.

[51] Mastora I, Remy-Jardin M, Masson P, et al. Severity of acute pulmonary embolism: evaluation of a new spiral CT angiographic score in correlation with echocardiographic data. European Radiology 2003; 13:29-35.

[52] Qanadli SD, Hajjam ME, Vieillard-Baron A, et al. New CT index to quantify arterial obstruction in pulmonary embolism: comparison with angiographic index and echocardiography. AJR Am.J.Roentgenol. 2001; 176:1415-1420.

[53] Bae KT, Mody GN, Balfe DM, et al. CT Depiction of Pulmonary Emboli: Display Window Settings. Radiology 2005; 236:677-684.

[54] van Rossum AB, van Erkel AR, van Persijn van Meerten EL, Ton ER, Rebergen SA, Pattynama PMT. Accuracy of helical CT for acute pulmonary embolism: ROC analysis of observer performance related to clinical experience. Eur.Radiol. 1998; 8:1160-1164.
[55] Wittenberg R, Peters JF, Sonnemans JJ, Bipat S, Prokop M, Schaefer-Prokop CM. Impact of Image Quality on the Performance of Computer-Aided Detection of Pulmonary Embolism. In; 95-101.
[56] Dewailly M, Rémy-Jardin M, Duhamel A, et al. Computer-Aided Detection of Acute Pulmonary Embolism With 64-Slice Multi-Detector Row Computed Tomography: Impact of the Scanning Conditions and Overall Image Quality in the Detection of Peripheral Clots. Journal of Computer Assisted Tomography 2010; 34:23-30.
[57] Engelke C, Schmidt S, Auer F, Rummeny EJ, Marten K. Does computer-assisted detection of pulmonary emboli enhance severity assessment and risk stratification in acute pulmonary embolism? Clinical Radiology 2010; 65:137-144.
[58] Sinner W. Computed tomographic patterns of pulmonary thromboembolism and infarction. Journal of Computed Assisted Tomography 1978; 2:395-399.
[59] Ghaye B, Remy J, Remy-Jardin M. Non-traumatic thoracic emergencies: CT diagnosis of acute pulmonary embolism: the first 10 years. European Radiology 2002; 12:1886-1905.
[60] Kuzo RS, Goodman LR. CT evaluation of pulmonary embolism: technique and interpretation. AJR.Am.J.Roentgenol. 1997; 169:959-965.
[61] Remy-Jardin M, Remy J, Artaud D, Deschildre F, Fribourg M, Beregi J. Spiral CT of pulmonary embolism: technical considerations and interpretive pitfalls. Journal of Thoracic Imaging 1997; 12:103-117.
[62] Wittram C, Maher MM, Yoo AJ, Kalra MK, Shepard J-AO, McLoud TC. CT angiography of pulmonary embolism: diagnostic criteria and causes of misdiagnosis. Radiographics 2004; 24:1219-1238.
[63] Coche EE, MÃ¼ller NL, Kim KI, Wiggs BR, Mayo JR. Acute pulmonary embolism: ancillary findings at spiral CT. Radiology 1998; 207:753-758.
[64] Wittram C, Kalra MK, Maher MM, Greenfield A, McLoud TC, Shepard J-AO. Acute and Chronic Pulmonary Emboli: Angiography-CT Correlation. Am. J. Roentgenol. 2006; 186:S421-429.
[65] Auger WR, Fedullo PF, Moser KM, Buchbinder M, Peterson KL. Chronic major-vessel thromboembolic pulmonary artery obstruction: appearance at angiography. Radiology 1992; 182:393-398.
[66] Gottschalk A, Stein PD, Goodman LR, Sostman HD. Overview of prospective investigation of pulmonary embolism diagnosis II. Seminars in Nuclear Medicine 2002; 32:173-182.
[67] Remy-Jardin M, Mastora I, Remy J. Pulmonary embolus imaging with multislice CT. Radiologic Clinics of North America 2003; 41:507-519.
[68] Wittram C, Maher MM, Halpern EF, Shepard J-AO. Attenuation of Acute and Chronic Pulmonary Emboli1. Radiology 2005; 235:1050-1054.
[69] Pengo V, Lensing AWA, Prins MH, et al. Incidence of Chronic Thromboembolic Pulmonary Hypertension after Pulmonary Embolism. New England Journal of Medicine 2004; 350:2257-2264.
[70] Tan RT, Kuzo R, Goodman LR, Siegel R, Haasler GB, Presberg KW. Utility of CT Scan Evaluation for Predicting Pulmonary Hypertension in Patients With Parenchymal Lung Disease. Chest 1998; 113:1250-1256.

[71] Tardivon A, Musset D, Maitre S, et al. Role of CT in chronic pulmonary embolism: comparison with pulmonary angiography. Journal of Computed Assisted Tomography 1993; 17:345-351.

[72] Remy-Jardin M, Duhamel A, Deken Vr, Bouaziz Nb, Dumont P, Remy J. Systemic Collateral Supply in Patients with Chronic Thromboembolic and Primary Pulmonary Hypertension: Assessment with Multiâ€"Detector Row Helical CT Angiography1. In, 2005; 274-281.

[73] Grosse C, Grosse A. CT Findings in Diseases Associated with Pulmonary Hypertension: A Current Review. Radiographics 2010; 30:1753-1777.

[74] Remy-Jardin M, Remy J, Artaud D, Fribourg M, Beregi J. Spiral CT of pulmonary embolism: diagnostic approach, interpretive pitfalls and current indications. European Radiology 1998; 8:1376-1390.

[75] Hansell DM. Spiral computed tomography and pulmonary embolism: current state. Clin.Radiol. 1997; 52:575-581.

[76] Remy Jardin M, Remy J, Artaud D, Deschildre F, Fribourg M, Beregi JP. Spiral CT of pulmonary embolism: technical considerations and interpretive pitfalls. J.Thorac.Imaging 1997; 12:103-117.

[77] Gotway MB, Patel RA, Webb WR. Helical CT for the evaluation of suspected acute pulmonary embolism: diagnostic pitfalls. J.Comput.Assist.Tomogr. 2000; 24:267-273.

[78] Schoepf UJ, Holzknecht N, Helmberger TK, et al. Subsegmental Pulmonary Emboli: Improved Detection with Thin-Collimation Multi--Detector Row Spiral CT. Radiology 2002; 222:483-490.

[79] Boiselle PM, Hasegawa I, Nishino M, Raptopoulos V, Hatabu H. Comparison of artifacts on coronal reformation and axial CT pulmonary angiography images using single-detector and 4- and 8-detector multidetector-row helical CT scanners. Acad.Radiol. 2005; 12:602-607.

[80] Aviram G, Levy G, Fishman JE, Blank A, Graif M. Pitfalls in the diagnosis of acute pulmonary embolism on spiral computer tomography. Current Problems in Diagnostic Radiology 2004; 33:74-84.

[81] Remy-Jardin M, Duyck P, Remy J, et al. Hilar lymph nodes: identification with spiral CT and histologic correlation. Radiology 1995; 196:387-394.

[82] Sone S, Higashihara T, Morimoto S, et al. CT anatomy of hilar lymphadenopathy. Am. J. Roentgenol. 1983; 140:887-892.

[83] Henk CB, Grampp S, Linnau KF, et al. Suspected Pulmonary Embolism: Enhancement of Pulmonary Arteries at Deep-Inspiration CT Angiographyâ€"Influence of Patent Foramen Ovale and Atrial-Septal Defect1. Radiology 2003; 226:749-755.

[84] Cox CE, et al. Pulmonary artery sarcomas: a review of clinical and radiologic features. Journal of Computed Assisted Tomography 1997; 21:750-755.

[85] Yi C, Lee K, Choe Y, Han D, Kwon O, Kim S. Computed tomography in pulmonary artery sarcoma: distinguishing features from pulmonary embolic disease. Journal of Computed Assisted Tomography 2004; 28:34-39.

[86] Kim SY, Seo JB, Chae EJ, et al. Filling Defect in a Pulmonary Arterial Stump on CT After Pneumonectomy: Radiologic and Clinical Significance. Am. J. Roentgenol. 2005; 185:985-988.

[87] Kwek BH, Wittram C. Postpneumonectomy Pulmonary Artery Stump Thrombosis: CT Features and Imaging Follow-up1. Radiology 2005; 237:338-341.

2

Application of Optical CT Scanning in Three-Dimensional Radiation Dosimetry

Andy Y. Xu and C. S. Wuu
Department of Radiation Oncology, Columbia University
New York, NY,
USA

1. Introduction

There has been much research effort in the development of an accurate and reliable three-dimensional dose verification system, prompted by the advances of technologies in radiation treatment of cancer patients. New radiotherapy techniques such as intensity modulated radiation therapy (IMRT), stereotactic radiosurgery (SRS) and high dose rate (HDR) brachytherapy are aimed at dose deliveries that are highly localized within the tumor volumes. The dose distributions from these treatment methods are typically characterized with high dose gradients around the boundaries of the targets, which present certain challenges for one or two-dimensional dosimeters such as film, TLD, and ion chamber (Webb, 2001).

In recent years, gel dosimeter has emerged as a promising candidate for 3D dosimetry (Baldock et al, 2010). Extensive studies have been done on the development of different types of gel formulas (Maryanski et al, 1996; Baldock et al, 1998; Pappas et al, 1999; Fong et al, 2001; Adamovics and Maryanski, 2006). Between the two classes of gel dosimeters that have been studied so far, the radiochromic Fricke gel is easier to make and handle than the polymer gel, but it suffers from a major error of diffusion. The blurring of the dose distribution image within time as short as an hour makes it inconvenient to be implemented into clinics. The polymer gel has the advantage of preserving the spatial accuracy of the dose distribution, but is sensitive to oxygen contamination and thus needs to be made freshly before each measurement. Furthermore, both types of gels suffer from a long-term drift of the baseline optical density, either due to self-oxidation of the ferrous ions in the Fricke gel or polymerization initiated by the redox reactions in the polymer gel.

The readout of gel dosimeters was initially conducted by magnetic-resonance imaging (MRI) (Gore et al, 1984; Maryanski et al, 1993; Audet and Schreiner 1997; De Deene et al, 1998; Low et al, 1999; Lepage et al, 2002) and subsequently extended to other imaging modalities such as optical computed tomography (CT) (Gore et al, 1996; Kelly et al, 1998; Doran et al, 2001; Xu et al, 2003), X-ray CT (Hilts et al, 2000) and ultrasound (Mather and Baldock, 2003). The idea of optical CT was first introduced to gel dosimetry in 1996 (Gore et al, 1996) together with a new tissue equivalent polymer gel dosimeter (Maryanski et al, 1996). Since then, optical CT scanners in a variety of forms have been built for imaging gel phantoms irradiated with photon, electron, proton beams as well as brachytherapy radiation sources (Islam et al, 2003; Wuu et al, 2003; Oldham and Kim, 2004; Xu et al, 2004; Doran et al, 2006; DeJean et al, 2006;

Krstajic and Doran, 2006; Sakhalkar and Oldham, 2008; Olding et al, 2010). Currently, the advantage of the optical CT approach over other dose readout methods for gel dosimetry is commonly acknowledged (Oldham et al, 2001; Lopatiuk-Tirpak et al, 2008). It has been postulated that gel dosimetry using a bench-top optical CT scanner will be a valuable tool for patient specific treatment dose verification, periodic quality assurance of radiation therapy units, and commissioning of new treatment techniques and machines.

The purpose of this paper is to give a brief summary of the challenges that are unique in optical CT-based 3D radiation dosimetry. The structure of the chapter is as follows: section 2 describes the two classes of optical CT scanners that have been developed so far; section 3 addresses the use of refractive index matching liquid for minimizing the multiple reflection and refraction at the boundary of a dosimeter; section 4 discusses the dynamic range problem associated with three-dimensional optical CT; section 5 summaries the effects of light scattering on the reconstructed dose distribution in optical CT; section 6 gives the results from 3D dosimeters irradiated with three representative radiation treatment plans.

2. Speed and accuracy of optical CT scanning

When radiation is delivered to a gel phantom, the physical properties (density or color) of the gel material inside the phantom will change according to the dose distribution deposited. Optical computed tomography can be used to generate a three-dimensional optical density map to reproduce the recorded dose distribution. Optical CT is a technique analogous to x-ray CT, except utilizing visible light instead of x-rays. The designing of optical CT scanners for gel dosimetry has been driven by two major considerations. First, unlike X-ray CT, the reconstructed images from optical CT need to be quantitatively accurate to within a few percent. This imposes certain limitations on the implementation of the existing technologies from X-ray CT in gel dosimetry. Second, acquisition of a complete set of 3D images from a gel dosimeter should be done reasonably fast rendering the dosimetric verification system practical for routine clinical practice. As such, two groups of optical CT scanners have been built. One is based on a single laser source coupled to a single photodiode detector and the other uses an incoherent broad light source and a large area detector such as a CCD camera.

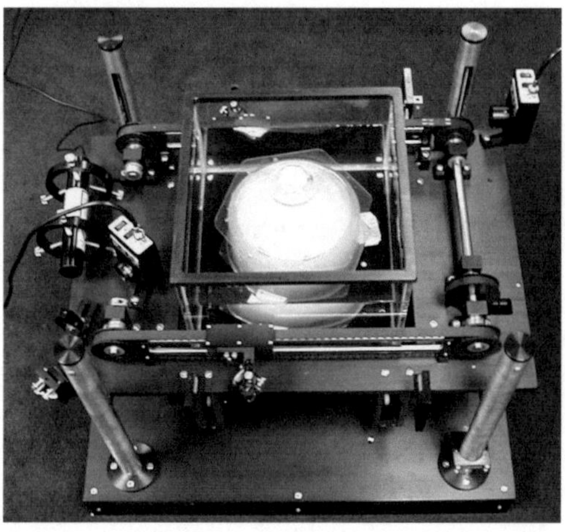

Fig. 1. Top view of the OCT-OPUS™ research scanner (MGS Research, Inc., Madison, CT, USA) with a Barex gel cylinder mounted in the scanning tank.

Figure 1 is a picture of the OCT-OPUS™ optical CT scanner (MGS Research, Inc., Madison, CT, USA) with a gel cylinder mounted for scanning. The basic running principle and the prototype configuration of this scanner can be summarized as the following (Gore et al, 1996; Xu et al, 2004). A single He-Ne laser beam (633-nm wavelength) is guided by a stepper motor and a series of mirrors and lenses to scan across a rectangular water tank repeatedly with a fixed field of view. The light transmitted through the tank is collected by a photodiode during each cycle of translational motions as single projection data. The laser output can be monitored by a reference photodiode through measurement of the light reflected from a beam-splitter. The photodiode voltage signals are fed into two different channels of a 16-bit plug-in PCI data acquisition board. The gel to be scanned is mounted on a turntable at the bottom of the scanner's tank. The tank is otherwise filled with a liquid mixture of water, glycerol and a blue dye, to minimize the effect of reflection and refraction around the container wall. The turntable rotates 360 degrees at a selected angular increment to collect projection data for a planar image.

Three dimensional CT scanning is realized based on the motion of 3 stepper motors. Motor #1 is mounted on the scanning platform to move the scanning mirror to generate parallel scanning laser beams. Motor #2 is connected to the turntable within the water tank to position the imaged dosimeters at different rotation angles. Motor #3 is used to drive the scanning platform up and down relative to the water tank for slice selection.

Data acquisition is synchronized with the motion of the scanning mirror. A pixel is defined as the distance traveled by the scanning mirror while 100 data points are sampled. The signal for each pixel is taken as the average of these 100 points. The data acquisition rate, the pixel size, the pixel numbers per projection and the number of projections per slice are controlled by the user. The whole process of scanning and data acquisition is controlled by a computer program written with TESTPOINT.

The unit-length optical density distribution for a transverse slice is reconstructed from the projection data using filtered back projection with the Shepp-Logan filter. The reconstructed images can be viewed and analyzed by the ImageJ software (http://rsb.info.nih.gov/ij) or imported into a computer program for isodose analysis in the transverse, coronal and sagittal directions.

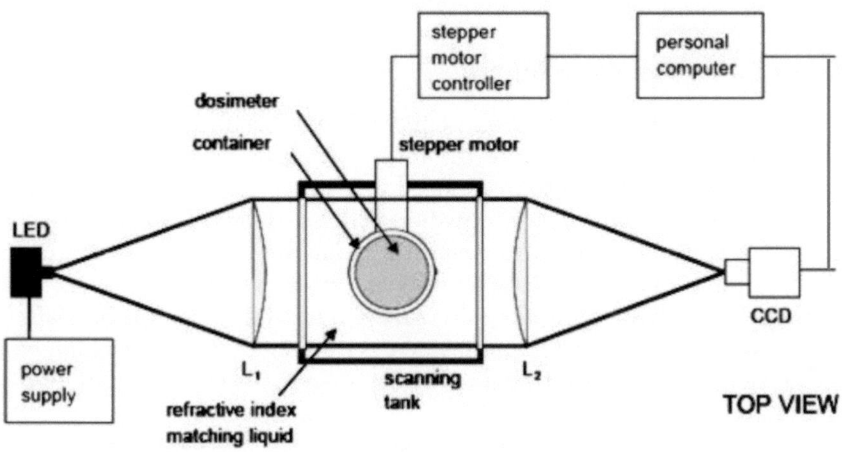

Fig. 2. Schematic diagram of a CCD-camera based optical tomography scanner.

Figure 2 is a schematic picture of an optical CT scanner using a broad, collimated beam and a charge coupled detector (CCD) (Krstajic and Doran, 2006). To summarize, a LED light source sits behind a circular pinhole of 1 mm diameter. The pinhole is placed on the focal point of collimating lens L1, creating a parallel beam. The parallel beam passes through the water tank and gets focused by lens L2 on to a CCD lens. The CCD lens focuses the incoming light rays further onto a CCD chip inside the camera. The scanned dosimeter is placed on a rotation stage driven by a stepper motor. The stepper motor rotates the dosimeter while the CCD takes images via a PC frame-grabber card in a 'stop and shoot' protocol. Data acquisition and rotation control are synchronized via an in-house develop computer program.

CCD-based optical CT scanners can also be designed using cone-beam configuration. This was first proposed by Wolodzko et al (1999) and a similar device is marketed as a research tool by Modus Medical devices Inc. (London, Ontario, Canada) under the name *Vista*.

Optical CT scanners using broad light sources are inherently fast. There is no technical difficulty in acquiring all the raw data points from an irradiated gel via a CCD camera within a few minutes. However, the use of broad light sources and large area detectors presents certain challenges for separating the useful signal from various other signal contributions. In particular, the deviation of the light rays from straight line passages caused by various inhomogeneities within the imaged objects will be difficult to model and ultimately limit the accuracy of the approach. This problem could be more severe than that in X-ray CT and megavoltage portal dosimetry considering the high penetrating power of the X-ray beams and the quantitative accuracy requirement from gel dosimetry.

The scanners using a point laser beam and a single photodiode detector do not suffer from the intrinsic light "entanglement" problem but have the limitation of long scanning time. For instance, it could take up to 10 hours for the first generation of the OCTOPUS™ scanner (MGS Research Inc., Madison, CT, USA) to perform a 3D scan on a dosimeter of regular size with 1 mm resolution in three dimensions. Therefore, the scanner has been used only for research purpose so far even though it is accurate and stable enough for clinical use.

Development of clinically applicable optical CT scanners has been moving in two directions: to increase the speed of the scanners using single laser sources; and to improve the accuracy of the scanners using broad beam illumination.

3. Refractive index matching liquid

In conventional x-ray CT, the refraction of the primary beam at the interface of different materials was never a concern because the refractive index of X-rays in most of media is close to one. So deflection of the primary beam only occurs at very small angles and does not cause any difficulties to the data acquisition process. In optical CT-based gel dosimetry, the bending of the visible light rays resulting from the refractive index change at the boundaries of the scanned dosimeters presents certain challenges. As is schematically shown in figure 3a, when the central region of a cylindrical dosimeter is optically scanned, a straight line passage of the incident light ray across the dosimeter can be obtained. When the incident laser beam is in the peripheral region, deviation from straight line passage is expected because of the multiple reflection and refraction around the boundary of the dosimeter. This phenomenon is more pronounced for dosimeters with containers of different refractive, and with increasing thickness of the containers (Gore et al, 1996).

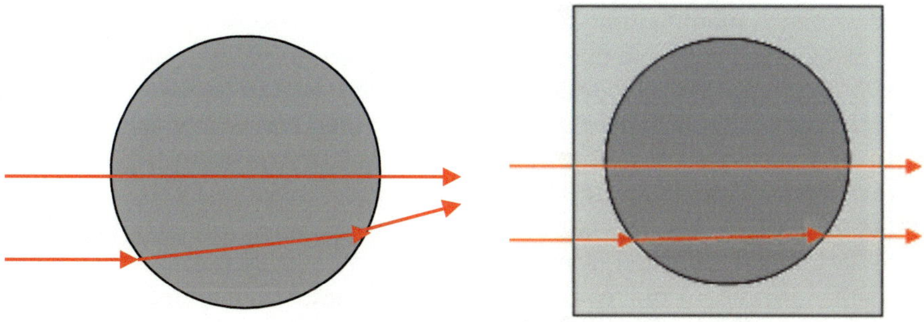

a) b)

Fig. 3. Illustration of the laser path problem in optical CT: a) bending of the laser path because of the refraction at the surface of the cylindrical dosimeter; b) the use of refractive index matching liquid to maintain straight line laser passage.

The spatial and angular deflections of the light rays at the boundaries of the scanned dosimeters could cause practical difficulties to the data acquisition in optical CT. For scanners using a small area detector whose position is fixed relative to the scanning mirror, missing of the primary signal is possible depending on the degree of the deviation of the laser beam (Gore et al, 1996; Kelly et al, 1998; Xu et al, 2004). For scanners using a broad beam and a large area detector, the deflection could cause all or part of the optical density drop from a specific laser path to be wrongly assigned (Doran 2009).

One solution to this problem is to immerse the scanned dosimeter into a refractive index matching liquid during optical CT scanning (see figure 3b). The refractive matching liquid is normally housed in a rectangular tank with transparent walls. Computer simulation can be used to determine the optimal refractive index of the matching liquid for the diameter of the imaged dosimeter, the thickness of the container wall and the refractive indices of these two materials.

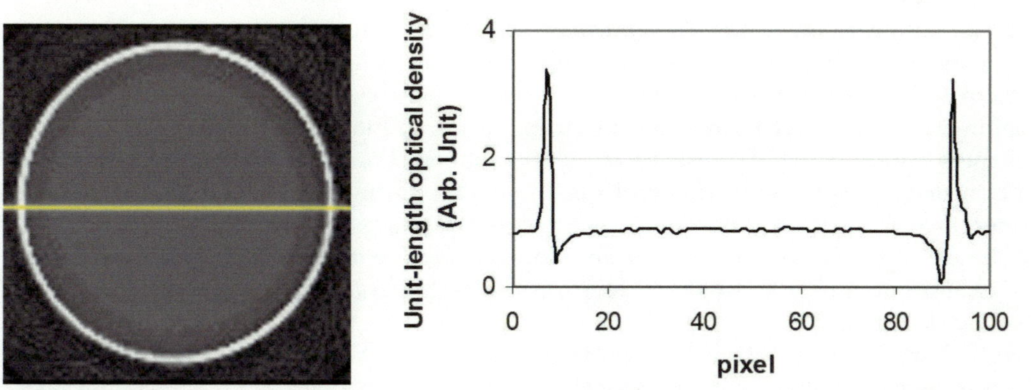

a) b)

Fig. 4. Results from scanning a BANG gel cylinder filled with non-irradiated gel using an OCT-OPUS™ optical CT scanner: a) reconstructed image of a transverse slice; b) line profile along the line shown in a).

Ideally, a perfect match would eliminate the effect of beam deflection completely and permit acquisition of data over the whole diameter of a dosimeter. In practice, it is not an easy task to make a matching liquid with the exact refractive index from calculation. Furthermore, the reflection of the beam at the interface can not be eliminated simultaneously. Figure 4 shows a line profile on a reconstructed transverse slice of an un-irradiated BANG gel phantom (Barex container with 17 cm diameter and 1 mm thickness) from the OCTOPUS™ optical CT scanner (Xu et al, 2004). When the laser beam hits the container wall from outside, part of the beam is reflected and deflected from the forward direction. This causes a sudden drop in the signal. As the laser beam moves further, more light gets transmitted and collected, but the structure of the signal becomes complicated by the multiple refraction and reflections along the container wall. It is only when the laser is sufficiently far away (about 2cm) from the inner side of the container wall that the signal flattens out to within 3 to 4%.

The effect of light reflection and refraction on optical-CT based 3D dosimetry is at least twofold: first, most of the dosimetric phantoms have been made as cylinders so far, to make the effect of multiple refraction and reflection easy to model. Second, the useable region of a dosimeter is usually limited, excluding a region that is a few millimeters or a few centimeters from the surface of the dosimeter.

4. Dynamic ranges of optical CT scanners

The dynamic range of an optical CT scanner is an important factor in the designing and operation of optical CT-based 3D dose verification systems. As an irradiated gel dosimeter is optically scanned in three dimensions, the net optical density function usually changes in a much wider range than it does in 2D study of the same plan using film dosimeters. This phenomenon is caused by the longer and varying path lengths of the laser beams associated with 3D CT scan. Therefore, development of methods for adjusting gel formation and reducing noise level in optical CT scanner is necessary for optimal image contrast.

The usable dynamic range of a scanner is usually limited by several aspects of the configuration of the scanner, including the noise level in the signals collected and the performance of the image reconstruction algorithm that processes the signals. For instance, a scanner with a 16-bit A/D data acquisition board has a fundamental digitization noise of 2^{-16}, thereby limiting the dynamic range of the scanner to less than 4.8 (Xu et al, 2003). The effective dynamic range of the scanner is further narrowed by the signal-to-noise requirement and the electronic and mechanic noises in the scanner. Therefore, when such scanners are used for 3D dose verification, cautions should be taken to ensure that the optical density increments along all possible paths during scanning of an irradiated gel never exceed a certain maximum. On the other hand, the maximum optical density increment across an irradiated gel is desired to be as close to the effective dynamic range of the scanner as possible, in order to maintain high signal-to-noise ratio and thus high dosimetric accuracy.

Figure 5 demonstrates the effect of over-dosing by comparing the reconstructed images for transverse slices with maximum optical density increments of 2.5, 2.8 and 3. The images were obtained from a BANG gel phantom irradiated with a 6MV, 6 cm x 6 cm square field using an OCTOPUS™ optical CT scanner with an effective dynamic range of 2.5 (Xu et al 2003). The depths of the transverse slices are 6 cm, 4 cm and 3 cm from the bottom of the dosimeter respectively). As can be seen from figure 5 (b) and (c), when the optical density increment (ODI) is larger than 2.5, an artifact arises in addition to the expected large uncertainty and becomes more pronounced with increasing ODI. The dark stripes along the diagonal of the squares indicate that the signals in these regions were larger than their actual values. Also, the reconstruction artifact in these regions will be systematically propagated across the entire image as seen in Figure 5(c).

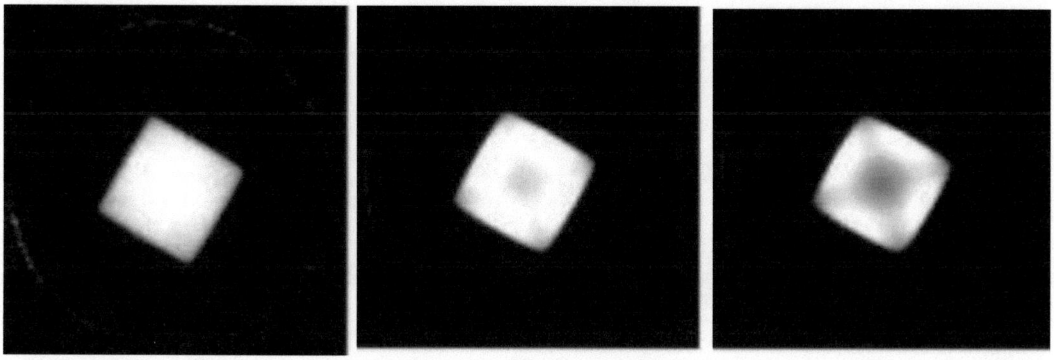

a) b) c)

Fig. 5. Reconstructed image for 3 transverse slices (depth 6, 4, 3cm) of a 6MV, 6cm x 6cm single field using an optical CT scanner of 2.5 dynamic range; the maximum optical density increments for these planes are 2.48, 2.8 and 3.1 respectively.

The distortions of the images in figure 5 (b) and 5(c) can be attributed primarily to the significant contribution from scattered photons at high ODI. In polymer gels, optical attenuation is caused by the Rayleigh/Mie scattering of light on polymer particles. Therefore, collection of some of the scattered photons at the detector's aperture is inevitable but normally does not cause any detectable error in the reconstructed image. With increasing optical density increments, the number of scattered photons produced increases whereas the intensity of the transmitted primary beam decreases. The fraction of the scattered light in the signals collected will increase and eventually become a significant source of error. The image reconstruction algorithm interprets the overestimated signals as less attenuation near the diagonals of the square field and produce less dose in these regions.

The optical density increments across an irradiated polymer gel depend on the dose response property of the gel material and the dose distribution delivered to the gel. To meet the requirement of the effective dynamic range of a scanner, it is necessary to predict theoretically the maximum optical density increment across an irradiated polymer gel first before actual dose delivery and optical scanning. Adjustment to gel formulation can be made in advance to get optimal scanning results.

The optical density for a given path *s* across an irradiated gel is the line integral of the unit-length optical density function along the path:

$$OD(s)=\int(A_0+kD(r)))dr \tag{1}$$

where A_0 is a constant characterizing the unit length opacity of the non-irradiated gel, k is the slope of the calibration function (or gel sensitivity), and $D(r)$ is the dose at point r. The sensitivity k of BANG® gels can be chemically modified by the manufacturer. The net optical density increment (*ODI*) along the path *s* across the irradiated gel is:

$$ODI = \int A(r)dr - A_0\int dr = k\int D(r)dr \quad (2)$$

since the maximum ODI_{max} across an irradiated gel is constrained by the usable dynamic range of the scanner, the optimal sensitivity factor k for study of a treatment plan can be determined by finding the maximum value $max\{\int D(r)dr\}$ from among all line integrals of dose across all projections in all axial slices of the dose distribution to be delivered. The sensitivity factor can then be determined from:

$$k = ODI_{max} \Big/ max\{\int D(r)dr\} \quad (3)$$

Figure 6a shows a schematic picture of the computer program for the calculation of the maximum optical density increment on the plane of optical CT scanning. The dotted line in Figure 6b is the laser path with maximum optical density increment for a transverse slice of an IMRT plan. The maximum optical density increment during the process of scanning a gel phantom can be obtained by comparing all the maximum values on different transverse slices.

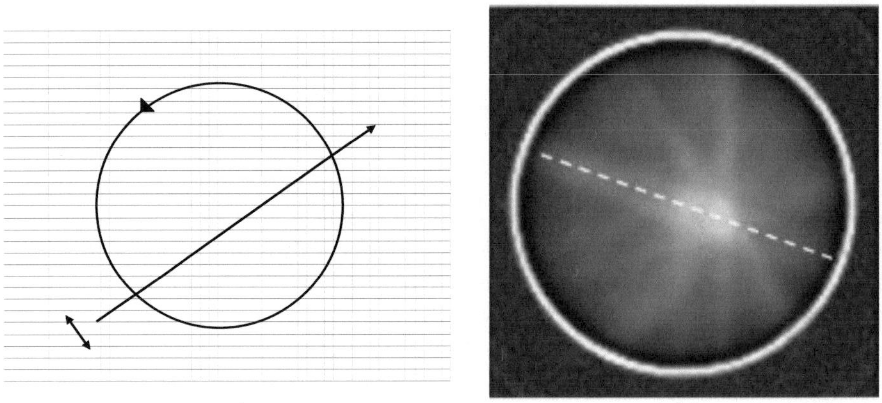

a) b)

Fig. 6. a) schematic picture for calculation of the maximum optical density increment in the plane of scanning: circle, boundary of the gel container and the integration region; little square, pixel; long arrow, laser beam. The computer program simulates the translation of the laser beam and the rotation of the container as indicated by the short arrows; b) a transverse slice of a 5-field IMRT irradiation; the white dashed line indicates the laser path with maximum optical density increment for the slice.

5. Light scattering in optical CT

Light scattering is also an important concern in optical CT-based gel dosimetry. In theory, only the portion of the incoming laser beam that survives the multiple Rayleigh-Mie scattering and/or light absorption in the forward direction should be used for image reconstruction. But collection of scattered photons in the detector apertures is inevitable in all optical CT scanners. Artifacts caused by the scattered light in optical CT could be more difficult to deal with than those in conventional X-ray CT considering the high penetrating power of X-ray beams (Olding et al, 2010).

To quantitatively estimate the intensity of the scattered light in regions where light signals might be collected for image reconstruction in optical CT-based 3D dosimetry, a Thorlabs PM100D optical power meter (Thorlabs Inc, Newton, NJ, USA) with an optical sensor of 1 mm diameter sensitive area was used (Xu et al, 2010b). The dosimetry phantom to be measured was put into the scanning tank of an OCTOPUS™ optical CT scanner (MGS Research Inc, Madison, CT, USA) filled with a refractive index matching liquid. A laser diode was positioned at one side of the water tank to generate a stationary laser beam of 0.8 mm width. On the other side of the tank, an in-house manufactured positioning system was used to move the optical sensor in the direction perpendicular to the outgoing laser beam from the dosimeters at an increment of 1 mm.

To compare the light scattering effect in different types of dosimeters, a BANG gel phantom and a Presage phantom were made as cylinders of 15.2 cm diameter and 10 cm height. Both dosimeters were irradiated with 6 MV photons using a Varian Clinac 2100EX. The irradiations were given such that the maximum optical density drops across the dosimeters are close to the dynamic range of the OCTOPUS™ optical CT scanner (about 2.5).

Figure 7 plots the relative intensities of the scattered light as a function of the off-axis distance for the matching liquid only and for those with a dosimeter in place. The relative intensities are normalized to the intensities of the primary beam at the center position (about 1500 milli-watts, 5 milli-watts and 5 milli-watts respectively). The intensities of the scattered light from both dosimeters were found to be more than 1% of the primary light signal within 2 mm from the laser beam but decreases sharply with increasing off-axis distance. The amount of scattered photons from the Presage dosimeter is more than an order of magnitude larger than that from the same position of the refractive index matching liquid. The amount of scattered photons from the BANG gel dosimeter is approximately an order of magnitude larger than that from the Presage dosimeter.

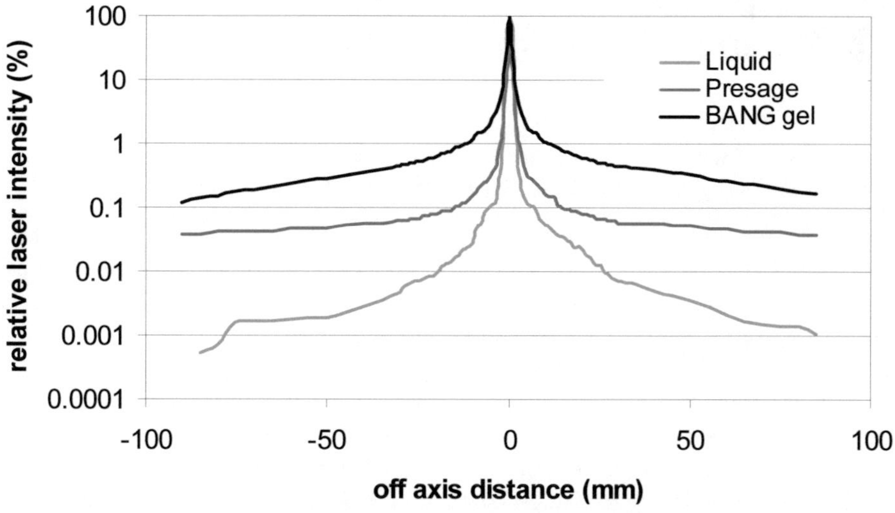

Fig. 7. Comparison of the scattered light intensity distributions from the BANG gel dosimeter, the Presage dosimeter and the matching liquid. Both dosimeters were irradiated to have a maximum optical density drop of 2.5.

The result shown in figure 7 is consistent with the fact that BANG gel is a scattering media and Presage is an absorbing media (Baldock et al, 2010). In theory, artifacts caused by the scattered light in optical CT scanners using a single laser source can be eliminated by reducing the detector apertures. In CCD-based optical CT scanners, telecentric lens can be used to select parallel beams from the scanned dosimeters (Krstajic and Doran, 2006; Sakhalkar and Oldham, 2008), thus minimizing the collection of the scattered light in the camera apertures.

6. Results

The ultimate goal of optical CT-based gel dosimetry is to verify radiation dose distribution in 3D. The major challenge in gel dosimetry is to achieve a spatial and dose accuracy and precision that satisfy the requirements for 3D dose verification of radiation treatments that are performed in the radiation hospital. Extensive study has been done on the development of a fast, accurate optical CT scanner and a stable gel manufacture system. A clinically applicable 3D dose verification system is not available at present time but results obtained so far are promising.

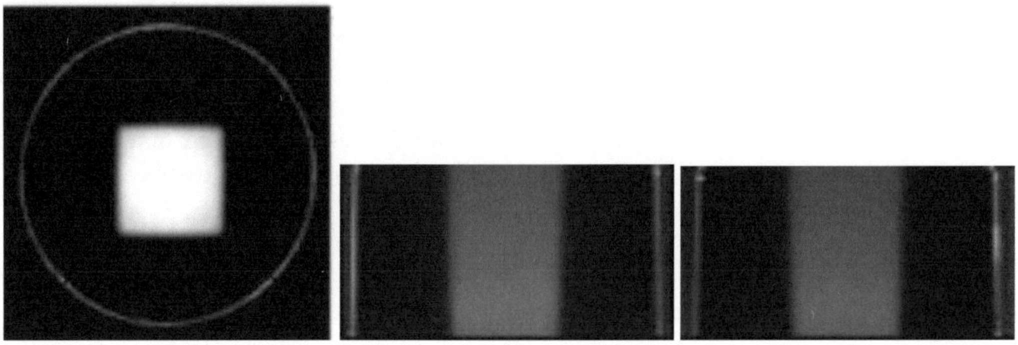

a) b) c)

Fig. 8. Reconstructed images from scanning a cylindrical BANG gel phantom irradiated with a 6cm x 6cm, 6MV single field: a) transverse slice at 8cm depth; b) coronal slice passing through the central axis; c) sagittal slice passing through the central axis.

Figure 8 shows the grayscale images for one slice in each direction from scanning a cylindrical BANG gel phantom irradiated with a 6 cm x 6 cm, 6MV radiation field (Xu et al, 2004). The coronal and sagittal images were obtained by re-slicing the reconstructed transverse slices from optical CT using the ImageJ software. The positions of the container wall and the main features of the square field are reproduced well in these images.

Figure 9 compares the absolute dose distributions from the gel measurement and the Eclipse planning system for one transverse and one coronal slice of a BANG gel phantom irradiated with a 6 cm x 6 cm, 12 MeV electron field. The 3-D gel dose distributions were obtained using the dose response curve extracted from the percent depth dose curve of a 16 MeV, 6 cm x 6 cm single field irradiation (Xu et al, 2010a). The BANG gel phantoms used in this study were 17 cm diameter x 12 cm high cylinders thermoformed from 1 mm-thick Barex plastic sheet. The irradiated gel phantoms were scanned using an OCTOPUS™ optical CT scanner. The scans were done with 1 mm pixel size, 200 pixels per projection, 300 projections per slice (for a total rotation angle of 180) and a slice separation of 1 mm. The slice thickness was about 0.6 mm (diameter of the laser beam). The phantoms were scanned within 4 days after the irradiations, with a scanning time of about 10 hours for each phantom (100 slices). All the features of the planned dose distributions were well reproduced in the gel experiment.

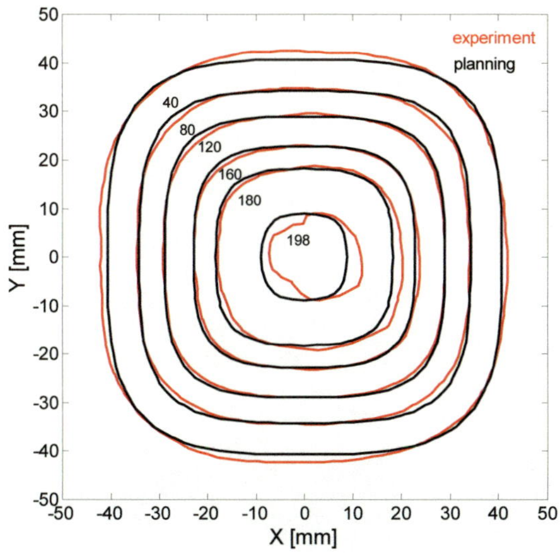

a)

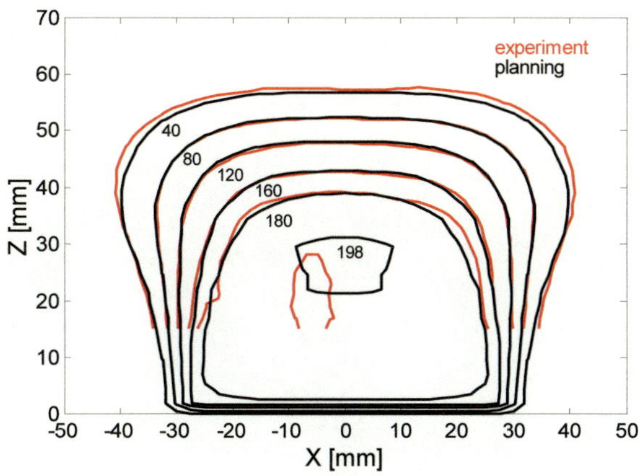

b)

Fig. 9. Comparison of the isodose lines (198, 180, 160, 120, 80 and 40 cGy) from the gel measurement (red lines) and the treatment plan (black lines) for a 12 MeV, 6 cm x 6 cm electron field: a) transverse slice at 3.5 cm depth; b) coronal slice that passes through the isocenter.

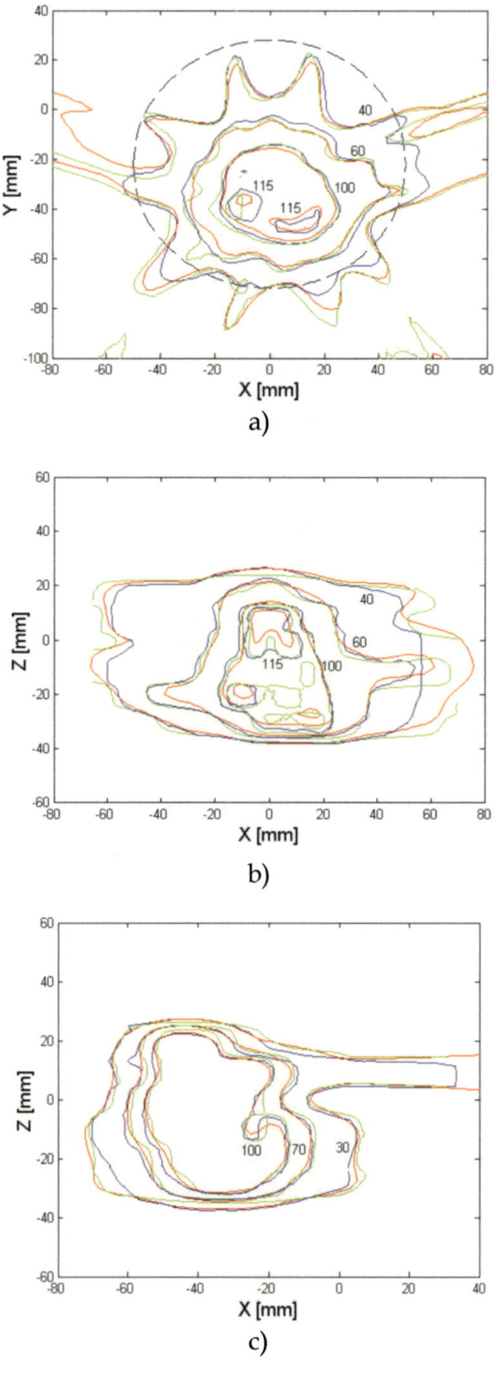

Fig. 10. Comparison of isodose dose distributions from treatment planning calculations (red), gel measurement (blue), and EDR2 measurements (green) for a 5 field IMRT plan: a) transverse slice; b) coronal slice; c) sagittal slice. All slices passes through the isocenter.

Figure 10 shows comparison of the isodose dose distributions from the gel measurement (blue lines), the film measurement (green lines) and the Eclipse-Helios treatment planning system (red lines) for a 5 field IMRT irradiation (Wuu and Xu, 2006). The IMRT plan used in this study was a real treatment plan for a patient with a small brain tumor (19.8 cc) generated by the Helios inverse planning system (Varian Corporation, Palo Alto, CA, USA). The plan delivered 180 cGy to the 100% isodose, with maximum dose around 218 cGy. The leaf sequence files and monitor units for the patient plan were used to generate a hybrid phantom plan, which was delivered in a 24x24x20 cm phantom. This phantom geometry was used for gel and film measurements. For comparative dosimetry the cylindrical gel phantom was immersed in a 24x24x20 cm water tank during IMRT irradiation. The gel phantom used was also a BANG gel cylinder with 17 cm diameter and 12 cm height. The gel irradiation was performed under the same set-up geometry as used in the hybrid phantom plan. The set-up geometry of the gel measurement was verified with the source-to-surface distance from irradiation.

The irradiated gel phantom was scanned using an OCTOPUS™ optical CT scanner (MGS Research, Inc., Madison, CT, USA) with 1 mm resolution. The reconstructed transverse images were normalize to two selected points of the treatment plan along the central axis, one at 98% dose and the other at 70% dose, to obtain the 3D relative dose distribution inside the irradiated gel. The results show good agreement among all three methods in all the three directions. The dose distribution in the axial direction from gel measurement is valid only in the regions marked by the dotted circle. The limited useful volume (in the central region with 75% of the diameter of the gel container) in the gel is due to the erroneous optical density values caused by the reflection and refraction of the laser rays at the interface between the gel and the container (Xu et al, 2004). This study demonstrates the feasibility of using a gel phantom to perform 3D dose verification of a complex radiation treatment plan.

7. Conclusions

Optical CT-based gel dosimetry is a promising technique that could have wide applications in radiation therapy physics. Extensive studies have been done on the development of different types of gel formulas, implementation of various optical CT scanners for gel dosimetry, and technical advantages and difficulties associated with 3-D dosimetry. The framework for optical CT-based 3D dosimetry is well established. The properties of the BANG gel polymer dosimeter and the Presage dosimeter have been intensively studied. The speed and the accuracy of the optical CT scanning process have improved significantly over the past 15 year. In particular, scanners with broad beam illustrations have been designed based on both parallel beam and cone beam geometry. Three dimensional dose measurements have been performed on various radiation treatment delivery units and compared with those from treatment planning systems and other dose measurement tools. The 3D gel dosimetry has been demonstrated to be comparable to the existing dose measurement tools in terms of dosimetric accuracy and spatial resolution. The challenge remained is to develop a fast, accurate, and robust 3D dose verification system that satisfies the requirements from routine clinical practice of radiation therapy physics. Development of software tools for the display and the quantitative evaluation of 3D dose distributions is also an area to explore.

8. References

Adamovics, J. & Maryanski, M. J. (2006). Characterization of PRESAGE: a new 3-D radiochromic solid polymer dosimeter for ionizing radiation *Radiat. Prot. Dosim.* 120 107–12

Audet, C. & Schreiner, L. J. (1997). Multiple-site fast exchange model for spin-lattice relaxation in the Fricke-gelatin dosimeter *Med. Phys.* 24 201-209

Baldock, C., Burford, R. P., Billingham, N., Wagner, G. S., Patval, S., Badawi, R. D. & Keevil, S. F. 1998 Experimental procedure for the manufacture and calibration of polyacrylamide gel (PAG) for magnetic resonance imaging (MRI) radiation dosimetry *Phys. Med. Biol.* 43 695–702

Baldock, C., De Deene, Y., Doran, S., Ibbott, G., Jirasek, A., Lepage, M., McAuley, K. B., Oldham, M., & Schreiner, L. J. (2010). Polymer gel dosimetry *Phys. Med. Biol.* 55 R1-R63

De Deene, Y., De Wagter, C., Van Duyse, B., Derycke, S., De Neve, W. & Achten, E. (1998). Three dimensional dosimetry using polymer gel and magnetic resonance imaging applied to the verification of conformal radiation therapy in head and neck cancer *Radiol. Oncol.* 48 283-291

DeJean, P., Senden, R., McAuley, K. B., Rogers, M. & Schreiner, L. J. (2006). Initial experience with a commercial cone beam optical CT unit for polymer gel dosimetry II: Clinical potential *J. Phys. Conf. Ser.* 56 183–186

Doran, S. J., Koerkamp, K. K., Bero, M. A., Jenneson, P., Morton, E. J. & Gilboy, W. B. (2001). A CCD-based optical CT scanner for high-resolution 3D imaging of radiation dose distributions: equipment specifications, optical simulations and preliminary results *Phys. Med. Biol.* 46 3191-3213

Doran, S. J., Nowais, S., Krstajic, N., Adamovics, J., Kacperek, A. & Brunt, J. (2006). True-3D scans using PRESAGE™ and Optical-CT: A case study in proton therapy *J. Phys. Conf. Ser.* 56 231–234

Doran, S. J. (2009). The history and principles of optical computed tomography for scanning 3-D radiation dosimeters: 2008 update *J. Phys. Conf. Ser.* 164 012020

Fong, P. M., Keil, D. C., Does, M. D. & Gore, J. C. (2001). Polymer gels for magnetic resonance imaging of radiation dose distributions at normal room atmosphere *Phys. Med. Biol.* 46 3105–13

Gore, J. C., Kang, Y. S. & Schulz, R. J. (1984). Measurement of radiation dose distributions by nuclear magnetic resonance (NMR) imaging *Phys. Med. Biol.* 29 1189-97

Gore, J. C., Ranade, M., Maryanski, M. J. & Schulz, R. J. (1996). Radiation dose distributions in three dimensions from tomographic optical density scanning of polymer gels: I. Development of an optical scanner *Phys. Med. Biol.* 41 2695-2704

Hilts, M., Audet, C., Duzenli, C. & Jirasek, A. (2000). Polymer gel dosimetry using x-ray computer tomography: A feasibility study *Phys. Med. Biol.* 45 2559-2571

Islam, K. T. S., Dempsey, J. F., Ranade, M. K., Maryanski, M. J. & Low, D. A. (2003). Initial evaluation of commercial optical CT-based 3D gel dosimeter *Med. Phys.* 30 2159-2168

Kelly, R. G., Jordan, K. J. & Battista, J. J. (1998). Optical CT reconstruction of 3D dose distributions using the ferrous-benzoic-xylenol (FBX) gel dosimeter *Med. Phys.* 25 1741-50

Krstajic, N. & Doran, S. J. (2006). Focusing optics of a parallel beam CCD optical tomography apparatus for 3D radiation gel dosimetry *Phys. Med. Biol.* 51 2055-2075

Lepage, M., McMahon, K., Galloway, G. J., De Deene, Y., Back, S. A. & Baldock, C, (2002). Magnetization transfer imaging for polymer gel dosimetry *Phys. Med. Biol.* 47 1881-90

Lopatiuk-Tirpak, O., Langen, K. M., Meeks, S. L., Kupelian, P. A., Zeidan, O. A. & Maryanski, M. J. (2008). Performance evaluation of an improved optical computer tomography polymer gel dosimeter system for 3D dose verification of static and dynamic deliveries *Med. Phys.* 35 3847-3859

Low, D. A., Dempsey, J. F., Venkatesan, R., Mutic, S., Markman, J., MarkHaacke, E. & Purdy, J. A. (1999). Evaluation of polymer gels and MRI as a 3D dosimeter for intensity-modulated radiation therapy *Med. Phys.* 26 1542-51

Maryanski, M. J., Gore, J. C., Kennan, R. P. & Schulz, R. J. (1993). NMR relaxation enhancement in gels polymerized and cross-linked by ionizing radiation: a new approach to 3D dosimetry by MRI *Magn. Reson. Imaging* 11 253-258

Maryanski, M. J., Zastavker, Y. Z. & Gore, J. C. (1996). Radiation dose distributions in three dimensions from tomographic optical density scanning of polymer gels: II. Optical properties of the BANG polymer gel *Phys. Med. Biol.* 41 2705-2717

Mather, M. L. & Baldock, C. (2003). Ultrasound tomography imaging of radiation dose distributions in polymer gel dosimeters: Preliminary study *Med. Phys.* 30 2140-2148

Oldham, M., Siewerdsen, J. H., Shetty, A. S. & Jaffray, D. A. (2001). High resolution gel-dosimetry by optical-CT and MR scanning *Med. Phys.* 28 1436-1444

Oldham, M. & Kim, L. (2004). Optical-CT gel-dosimetry II: Optical artifacts and geometrical distortion *Med. Phys.* 31 1093-1104

Olding, T., Holmes, O. & Schreiner, L. J. (2010) Cone beam optical computed tomography for gel dosimetry I: scanner characterization *Phys. Med. Biol.* 55 2819-2840

Pappas, E., Maris, T. G., Angelopoulos, A., Paparigopoulou, M., Sakelliou, L., Sandilos, P., Voyiatzi, S. & Vlachos, L. (1999). A new polymer gel for magnetic resonance imaging (MRI) radiation dosimetry *Phys. Med. Biol.* 44 2677–84

Sakhalkar, S. & Oldham, M. (2008). High-resolution 3D dosimetry utilizing a novel optical-CT scanner incorporating tertiary telecentric collimation *Med. Phys.* 35 101-111

Webb, S. (2001). Verification of 3D Dose Distribution, in: *Intensity Modulated Radiation Therapy*, Institute of Physics Publishing, ISBN 0750306998, 2001.

Wolodzko, J. G., Marsden, C. & Appleby, A. (1999). CCD imaging for optical tomography of gel radiation dosimeters *Med. Phys.* 26 2508–13

Wuu, C. S., Schiff, P. B., Maryanski, M. J., Liu, T., Borzillary, S. & Weinberger, J. (2003). 3D dosimetry study of Re-188 liquid balloon for intravascular brachytherapy using bang polymer gel dosimeters *Med. Phys.* 30 132-137

Wuu, C. S., & Xu Y. (2006). Three-dimensional dose verification for intensity modulated radiation therapy using optical CT based polymer gel dosimetry *Med. Phys.* 33 1412-1419

Xu, Y., Wuu, C. S. & Maryanski, M. J. (2003). Determining optimal gel sensitivity in optical CT scanning of polymer gels *Med. Phys.* 30 2257-2263

Xu, Y., Wuu, C. S. & Maryanski, M. J. (2004). Performance of optical CT scanning of polymer gels as a tool for 3D dose verification *Med. Phys.* 31 3024-3030

Xu, Y., Wuu, C. S. & Maryanski, M. J. (2010a). Sensitivity calibration procedures in optical CT scanning of BANG polymer gel dosimeters *Med. Phys.* 37 861-868

Xu Y., Adamovics J., Cheeseborough J., Chao K. S. & Wuu C. S. (2010b). Light scattering in optical CT scanning of Presage dosimeters *Journal of Physics: Conference series* 250, 012063

3

PET/CT

Joshua D. Schaefferkoetter, Eric R. Carlson and Amy K. LeBlanc
University of Tennessee Medical Center
United States

1. Introduction

Clinical imaging exists for the noninvasive, *in vivo* study of disease in the body. Modalities such as computed tomography (CT) and magnetic resonance imaging (MRI) do this by providing information about patient anatomy, so physicians can identify physical abnormalities in the tissue morphology. In contrast, molecular imaging modalities like positron emission tomography (PET) do not describe the anatomy directly, but rather track specific biological processes. This enables the investigation of bodily function, allowing the identification of abnormalities in tissue physiology.

Central to molecular imaging is the molecule, or more specifically, the radiopharmaceutical. PET is used to study many processes including blood flow, tissue perfusion, neurological function, cellular proliferation, and tumor metabolism, and each application uses a unique radiotracer that has been engineered to track a specific molecule or biochemical process. For example, the most common radiopharmaceutical used in PET today is 2-deoxy-2-(^{18}F)fluoro-D-glucose or ^{18}F-FDG. In this tracer, ^{18}F (a radioactive isotope of Fluorine) is substituted in place of the 2' hydroxyl group in the glucose molecule. FDG is chemically similar to glucose, and so it begins to follow the same metabolic pathway. The accumulation of FDG is subsequently used as an index of tissue metabolism. PET forms an image by measuring (estimating) the spatiotemporal distribution of the biomarker.

Information about cellular metabolism proves especially useful in oncology, as rapidly growing tumors have increased energy demands. (Warburg, Posener et al. 1931) In the clinical setting, PET provides physicians with a standardized tool for the assessment, diagnosis, and treatment planning of neoplastic diseases. Many developments have facilitated its integration into the clinic, but few as rapidly as the addition of the CT modality, and now the hybrid PET/CT.

In modern PET/CT, the CT transmission scan is integral to important calculations in the processing of the PET data. Additionally, this configuration provides information about anatomy as well as physiology. The influence of the combined modality provides an unsurpassed level of patient care. Physicians are able to better diagnose disease and plan and monitor response to treatment more effectively.

2. Background

Before exploring the benefit of adding CT to PET, it is worthwhile to review some basic principles of positron emission tomography. As expected, PET scanners measure the energy released as the result of a positron emission. When an unstable isotope randomly decays, it can do so in a number of ways. In the case of proton-heavy isotopes like Fluorine-18, the process is positive beta (β^+) decay,[1] where a proton is converted into a neutron, emitting a positron and neutrino.

The positron is the anti-matter counterpart of the electron, namely it has the same mass and spin as the electron, but with the opposite charge. When the ejected positron encounters a nearby electron, the pair self-annihilates, and is converted to pure energy according to Einstein's theory of relativity. This energy is released as two 511keV (the rest mass of the electron and positron) photons, propagating in opposite directions, thus conserving momentum.[2]

The fundamental job of the PET tomograph is to detect these annihilation photons and identify pairs arising from the same event. Modern PET scanners consist of multiple rings of detectors and use a detection acceptance timing window of a few nanoseconds, enough time needed for a photon to traverse the full diameter of the transaxial field of view (FOV). When a photon is detected, the timing window is triggered. If another photon is detected within this window, the two are assumed to be from the same annihilation and are registered as a prompt event. The imaginary line connecting the two detectors, along which the event occurred, is termed the line-of-response (LOR) and is recorded for each prompt.

If a second photon is not detected within the timing window, the original detected photon is recorded as a single event and does not have an LOR associated with it. The singles rate is typically a few orders of magnitude greater than the prompts. Additionally, multiple photons can hit the detectors within the timing window, giving rise to multiple events. These are rejected since no LOR can be assigned.

In a routine scan, millions of prompt events are recorded each second, and each LOR has its own prompt count-rate frequency. This frequency is directly related to the total activity contained within a 'tube' connecting the detector faces along the LOR. Thus, PET is a quantitative tool, in that it is possible to measure the activity concentration in a small unit volume in an absolute sense. However, it is important to remember that a PET scanner does not measure the activity distribution directly, but only as linear sums through the distribution, meaning some information is lost. The acquisition data are grouped as sums along parallel LORs, which define angular 'projections', which are then arranged in rows for each successive angle to form sinograms. The estimation of the original object from this projection data is a daunting task that receives ever-increasing attention. (Barrett and Myers 2004)

3. Gantry design

A modern PET scanner consists of a horizontal bed which passes through a circular bore encasing multiple rings of detectors. The port diameter size of a typical gantry is 70-80 cm with an axial field of view (FOV) around 20 cm. The subject is positioned appropriately, and each bed position is scanned for 2-3 minutes.[3]

---

[1] F-18 has a branching fraction of 0.97 which means there is a 3% chance that it will decay via electron capture, (Shapiro 2002) where an innermost orbital electron combines with a nuclear proton to create a nuclear neutron, releasing only a neutrino.

[2] The relative alignment of the initial particle spins and the positron's kinetic energy at the time of annihilation may affect the number and direction of the emitted photons; however, these effects are usually considered negligible in practice. (Valk 2003)

[3] A routine whole-body scan (from the cranial orbits to mid-thigh) typically includes 4-6 bed positions. Melanoma scans of the entire body use as many as twelve.

Today's PET detection systems are scintillation-based; once a 511keV photon strikes a detector crystal, it is converted into light. This light is collected by a system of coupled photomultiplier tubes (PMTs), which then output an electrical pulse. [4] The strength of this pulse determines the initial energy deposited in the crystal and can be used to reject (scatter) events that do not satisfy the energy threshold. The Biograph TruePoint TrueV PET/CT scanner (Siemens Molecular Imaging) employs four rings of 48 detector blocks, each containing an array of 13 x 13 crystals. (Jakoby, Bercier et al.)
The first PET/CT images came from individual systems operated independently from each other. The CT data was manipulated for use in the PET corrections, and the images were registered manually. Modern tomographs contain the PET and CT components within the same gantry, separated by 80 cm axially. (Townsend, Beyer et al. 2003) Software now automates both acquisition processes, as well as data correction, reconstruction, and co-registration of the final images. (Barrett and Myers 2004)

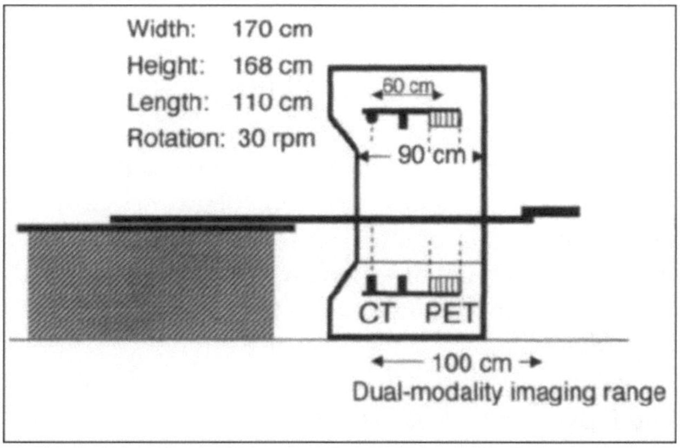

Fig. 1. Schematic diagram of early PET/CT concept. Centers of fields-of-view of PET and CT are 60 cm apart. Combined PET/CT gantry is 110 cm deep, 170 cm high, and 168 cm wide. (Beyer, Townsend et al. 2000)

4. PET Errors

Most reconstruction algorithms treat the data as if they are free of noise or error, but in reality, the PET acquisition process is far from perfect. There are many physical effects that can corrupt the integrity of the data, including photon attenuation, random registration, scattered coincidences, varying detector sensitivity profiles, and gantry geometry. These errors degrade image quality by adding noise to the PET data and must typically be corrected prior to reconstruction for accurate image quantization. It is common in modern PET to perform these data corrections based on large-scale, statistical models of these effects. Every registered prompt event is not the result of a true coincident pair of photons. In fact, each acquired prompt can belong to one of three groups, trues, randoms or scatter. Both randoms and scatter cause the system to associate incorrect LORs to their events and therefore must be corrected.

[4] The PMTs are arranged in a light-sharing configuration (four PMTs per detector block) to reduce cost and packing fraction. (Casey and Nutt 1986)

4.1 Randoms

Random coincidences happen when two photons from different events randomly hit two detectors within the same timing window. These events contain no useful information about the tracer distribution and, because they are random in nature, add smooth background noise to the data. The random coincidence rate is related to the size of the timing window and the singles rates on the detectors.

A few methods have been proposed to model the randoms distribution, including detector singles-based calculations and tail-fitted, Gaussian estimations. (Valk 2003) Currently however, the most commonly implemented technique is the delayed channel method. Here, a timing window is delayed (a few times the timing window length) to acquire a duplicate data stream in parallel to the prompts. The delayed timing window guarantees that any recorded coincident photon pair did *not* belong to the same annihilation event. These delayed data provide accurate representation of the prompt randoms rate and can usually be stored independently, allowing post-processing the randoms data to reduce noise.

4.2 Scatter

Scattered events occur when at least one photon of the coincident pair is Compton scattered, deflecting it before hitting the detector ring. Scattering decreases the energy of a photon, so this effect is addressed by acquiring only the photons lying within the photopeak energies. This is accomplished with an appropriate energy-acceptance window (typically 450-650 keV for LSO-based scanners). However, a photon can scatter through a relatively large angle and still have enough energy to be accepted, so many scattered events are not rejected by the energy discriminator. These prompt scatter events are generally treated as a nuisance to the data which should be removed.

In the early years of PET, 2D acquisition was commonly used; disks of lead shielding were positioned between each detector ring to "shadow" the activity arising outside of the direct plane. This decreased the number of randoms and scatter events and simplified the reconstruction process. Now however, 3D, or septaless, acquisition has almost completely replaced its 2D counterpart, due to its increased sensitivity. This change was due to sophisticated correction methods and faster reconstruction algorithms.

Many techniques have been developed to handle scatter correction. Empirical schemes have been used that measure auxiliary data, such as the coincidence rates below 511keV, under the assumption that these lower energy photons must be the result of scattering. By employing multiple energy windows, this auxiliary data is scaled and subtracted from the data in the photopeak window. (Grootoonk, Spinks et al. 1996) Scatter correction based on multiple energy measurements has the advantage of accounting for scatter arising from activity outside of the field of view. However, the auxiliary data are noisy and their processing requires more computing power. Another technique is to estimate the scatter distribution from prompt counts registered at places known to contain no activity. Scatter has a low frequency, broad distribution with tails that extend beyond the boundaries of the object. These tails can be used to fit a smooth Gaussian function to the scatter distribution. (Stearns 1995) This model performs reasonably well in brain studies, but can lead to errors in whole-body scans where the thorax occupies a larger portion of the FOV, resulting in relatively small scatter tails to fit.

Some approaches used in 2D PET (with inter-ring septa) are convolution-based integral transformations of the projections. (Bergström, Eriksson et al. 1983) In this method, the scatter distribution is estimated through the convolution of a spatially dependent scatter "kernel" with the linear projections of the prompt photopeak data. The resulting distribution profiles are then subtracted from the projections to yield scatter-free estimates of the data. It works well in regions of relatively homogeneous density like the brain. This method was developed for 2D PET but has been extended to 3D systems. (Bailey and Meikle 1994)

Modern 3D PET algorithms, however, most commonly use theoretical simulation techniques to correct for scatter. They are arguably the most accurate scatter corrections, in that they attempt to realistically simulate the scattering process. Scatter simulations model the distribution based on the underlying physics of Compton scattering. With an initial estimate of the emitter distribution and a coefficient map of the attenuating material, Klein-Nishina calculations are used to accurately compute the scatter distribution. (Ollinger 1996)

4.3 Attenuation

In addition to the noise in the prompt counts, PET data is also degraded by other effects including attenuation. Compton scattering (in combination with photoelectric absorption) contributes to photon attenuation along each LOR. It is directly related to the amount of matter (tissue) lying in the small tube centered along the LOR, so attenuation is a bigger problem in larger patients.

This loss of count data results in reduced image contrast and detail for internal features, especially those lying deep inside the subject. For a given scan, any volume contains a finite amount of attenuating material, and a coefficient of total linear attenuation can thus be associated to each LOR. These coefficients are ordered and arranged in sinograms, similar to the PET projections, to yield an attenuation coefficient factor (ACF) map. In the simplest sense, attenuation correction is the multiplication of the PET projection data with the ACF map.

Before the introduction of hybrid PET/CT, ACF maps were generated using a 511keV photon transmission scan of the subject prior to the emission measurement. This typically involved rotating a line source of annihilation photons (usually ^{68}Ge) around the patient to provide information about tissue density. Sinogram windowing and data from the subsequent emission measurement were used to remove most of the emission counts from the transmission data. Furthermore, FDG studies have relatively low count rates, and there is little increase in noise in the correction due to emission activity. (Carson, Daube-Witherspoon et al. 1988) These methods produced accurate ACF maps, but required increased patient time in the scanner.

4.4 Normalization

Reconstruction algorithms generally assume the same sensitivity for all LORs, but this is not the case. Differences in crystal elements and photomultiplier tubes, as well as scanner geometry and detector block gaps, all contribute to varying sensitivities for different LORs. As a result, quality control must be performed regularly to assure that the PET scanner is operating optimally and that the sensitivity profiles are known for all LOR projections. This is usually accomplished by scanning a uniform source; since all LORs are illuminated by the same activity concentration, they should yield consistent projections. The (inverse of the) projection data is used to calculate the normalization, i.e. those with higher relative sensitivity appear hotter and will be weighted less in the routine clinical reconstructions.

Noisy data is not the only drawback to emission tomography. With regards to spatial resolution, nuclear imaging modalities are inferior to conventional anatomical imaging. For example, a typical PET image has an average spatial resolution of 4 mm but that of a typical CT image can be 0.5 mm. This is due to many factors, including the finite size of detector elements, positron range, Compton scatter, and photon non-collinearity.

PET is a complex procedure that is susceptible to many errors. Compared to most other imaging modalities, emission tomography is a relatively noisy process; the amount of available data is fundamentally count-limited by the ethically allowed dose of the radiotracer and convenient patient time inside the scanner. Furthermore, the acquired data are degraded by the many physical distortions previously mentioned. Modern correction techniques are very sophisticated and evolved through innovations in technology and methodology. One of the most significant of these developments was the addition of CT to the PET system.

5. Hybrid PET/CT

The PET/CT scanner, invented by Dr. Ron Nutt and Dr. David Townsend, was originally built at the University of Pittsburgh in 1998. (Townsend, Beyer et al. 1998) CT-based PET corrections had been investigated (Beyer, Kinahan et al. 1994) and the idea to co-register images from different modalities had been proposed for brain studies, (Pelizzari, Chen et al. 1989; Pietrzyk, Herholz et al. 1996) but the hybrid prototype was the first time multiple medical imaging modalities had been combined into a single gantry. This new tool offered improved clinical diagnoses and patient management; it also increased patient comfort and scanner throughput. (Kluetz, Meltzer et al. 2000) The PET/CT scanner was named invention of the year in 2000 by Time Magazine.

5.1 Attenuation

In the past, the data for the PET attenuation correction came from a 10-15 min 511keV transmission scan that was usually administered for each bed position, prior to the emission scan. With the combination of PET and CT, it was possible to generate an ACF map using the CT transmission scan. It is no longer necessary to include PET transmission components with the scanners, eliminating their initial costs as well as those associated with the periodic replacement of decayed sources. The high flux of X-rays leads to lower statistical noise in the ACF measurement and shorter transmission scan leaves longer times for emission scan, further lowering statistical noise for the total scan duration.

The attenuation coefficients are not constant between CT and PET energies. Attenuation is a combination of photon scatter and absorption, and the ratio of these effects is not necessarily the same for different photon energies and material densities. The ACFs found at CT energies, from 40-140 keV, (Shreve and Townsend 2008) require scaling if they are to be used to correct emission data at the 511keV PET energy.

It has been shown that linear scaling methods produce proper ACFs when Compton interactions dominate the attenuation. However they yield poor estimates when photoelectric contributions dominate, as they do at lower CT energies, especially in high-density regions like bone. (Kinahan, Townsend et al. 1998) Thus, accurate attenuation coefficients cannot be rigorously estimated through simple linear scaling. For this reason, density segmentation of different tissue regions has been used successfully, but, just as linear scaling methods have errors caused by the different ratio of attenuation coefficients for bone, segmentation methods produce errors in regions where there are variations in density, such as the lung. (Beyer, Kinahan et al. 1994)

CT-based PET attenuation factors are typically computed through a hybrid combination of both methods. The ratios of attenuation coefficients at CT and PET energies are roughly equal for all tissue except bone (Hubbell and Standards 1969), so current methods segment regions above 300 Hounsfield units as bone tissue and below 300 as soft tissue, respectively. The respective CT-to-PET ACF scaling is 2.26 and 1.90. (Shreve and Townsend 2008) This bi-linear scaling has shown excellent results that perform superior to 511keV transmission methods with lower noise. (Kinahan, Townsend et al. 1998)

5.2 Scatter

Scatter is a major problem in 3D PET (Cherry, Dahlbom et al. 1991); a 511 keV photon traveling in water (or human tissue) has a 50% chance of being scattered by an electron. Consequently, in a clinical scan, 40-60% of the data may be from scattered photon events. Today, the most commonly used correction methods in quantitative clinical 3D PET are based on scatter simulations, which require a coefficient map of the attenuation to realistically model the scattering process. The 511keV ACF scaled from the CT transmission scan is an excellent source of this information.

Monte Carlo simulation is widely used to model scatter and provides the most complete realization of the physical effects associated with it. This technique is used for both evaluation and for the correction itself, but it is currently too slow to be used clinically and is limited to research applications. Instead of accounting for all scattering interactions, the model can be simplified by considering only single scatter events, i.e. events where just one photon of the pair is scattered only once. (Watson, Newport et al. 1996) This simplification is reasonable since it has been shown that 75-80% of scattered coincidences are due to these single scatter events. (Barney, Rogers et al. 1991) It is further justified by the fact that multiple scatter has little effect on the total distribution.

The single scatter simulation (SSS) calculation relies on a volume integral of a scattering kernel over the body, using the relationship between an initial estimate of the activity distribution volume,[5] the reconstructed attenuation volume, and Compton scattering cross-sections calculated from the Klein-Nishina formula. The scatter contribution is calculated for every LOR across all possible scattering points in the FOV. A faster method has been proposed that is better suited to clinical application. (Watson 2000) With this method, fewer LORs are used in the calculation and continuity is replaced by discrete sampling of the volume data. The sample points are relative to the transaxial FOV (not the patient) and, since the scatter distribution is relatively smooth, the sampling can be fairly coarse (around 2 cm) without much loss of accuracy. This coarse-scatter sinogram is then interpolated to account for the missing data. Speed is further improved by reusing computed ray sums through the object since scatter calculations in multiple LORs may involve the same photon travel paths. (Mumcuoglu, Leahy et al. 1996) Accuracy is further improved by iterating the scatter calculation, i.e. with each iteration, the previously corrected emission is used in the calculation.

5.3 Reconstruction

In addition to data corrections, the CT information is used in the actual reconstruction process. Modern reconstruction algorithms do not produce images by directly inverting the

[5] different methods have been employed for initial estimates of the emission volume distribution; Watson et al. used 3d reconstructions of the projection data, which include scatter. (Watson, Newport et al. 1996)

projection data, as they did in the past. Instead, they are based on sequential, iterative estimates that converge to an image that best represents the original object. These algorithms are termed expectation maximization (EM) and are well suited to emission tomography because they are less sensitive to noise in the data.

Iterative reconstruction involves the forward and back-projection of simulated data in the attempt to match the measured data as closely as possible. Integral to this method is the system matrix which models the characteristics of the scanning process. It essentially defines the individual probabilities that each projection bin contributes to each image pixel, and vice versa. Ideally, the system matrix accounts for all physical effects of scanner geometry and performance. Attenuation-weighted (AW) algorithms incorporate the attenuation map from the CT scan into the system matrix, and the forward projector is better able to realistically simulate the acquisition process. This increases the accuracy of the physical model unique to the individual scan.

CT data can also be used in the reconstruction scheme as prior information. Prior distributions are sometimes used to regularize the algorithm, enforcing smoothness in the image. Images with high frequency noise (large differences between neighboring pixels) are assigned a lower probability, i.e. they are penalized by the prior. The CT image can be used to segment the image into regions in which uniform tracer concentration is expected. These segmented boundaries are incorporated in a prior so that smoothness is only imposed in regions belonging to the same anatomical region. The use of anatomical images as prior information in *maximum a posteriori* (MAP) reconstructions has yielded improved reconstructions in mathematical phantom simulations. (Gindi, Lee et al. 1991) However this approach is typically not used clinically since anatomical information is readily available to be visually interpreted in the fused images.

6. Clinical impact

PET/CT has revolutionized healthcare, and it continues to expand its utility to a wide array of applications. This is illustrated by the growing number of world-wide scanner sales. In 2002, only a couple years after its introduction, PET/CT systems accounted for nearly half of the total PET scanner sales, with the other half belonging to that of dedicated PET scanners. By 2005, PET/CT systems had almost completely overtaken the market. Today, nearly all commercial systems are PET/CT.

The first PET scans were conducted in the 70's at Washington University in St. Louis by Michael Phelps, et al. (Phelps, Hoffman et al. 1975; Phelps, Hoffman et al. 1976) With the development of FDG later that decade, PET gained more attention for its potential clinical value; but due to the difficulties of the imaging process and the high costs of the radiopharmaceuticals, PET was strictly used for research. However, as more PET studies were performed, its clinical utility began to emerge, specifically in the evaluation of disorders of the heart and brain. This led to the first reimbursement of PET in 1995, for myocardial perfusion imaging using Rubidium-82. (Workman and Coleman 2006) The first Medicare reimbursement of FDG-PET scans in oncology came in January of 1998 for the initial staging of non small-cell lung cancer and the characterization of single pulmonary nodules. (Bietendorf 2004) Coverage for colorectal cancer, lymphoma, melanoma, and many others followed in the next few years.

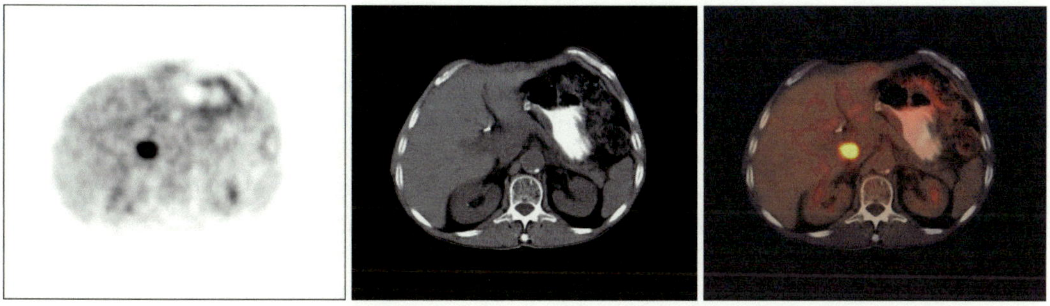

Fig. 2. Transaxial PET, CT, and fused images taken from a 68 year-old male diagnosed with cholangiocarcinoma. The combined modality provides physiological information as well as anatomical location. The disease is not obvious in the CT image alone but the PET scan shows an intense focus of metabolic activity medial to the hepatic caudate lobe likely compatible with recurrent malignancy.

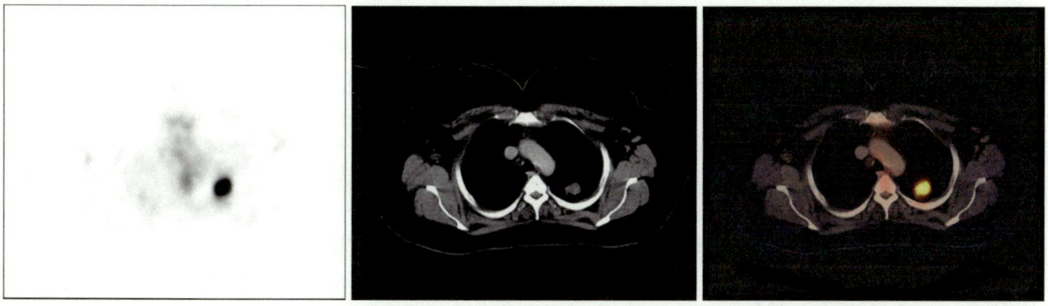

Fig. 3. Transaxial PET, CT, and fused images of a 40 year-old female with a history of heavy smoking. The intense metabolic uptake illustrated by the PET scan is accompanied by a 2.2 x 2.8 cm upper lobe mass on the CT image, which was later diagnosed as non-small cell carcinoma.

Today, Medicare provides reimbursement of PET for the diagnoses and monitoring of nearly every form of cancer. Furthermore, PET is also reimbursed for non-cancerous diseases including myocardial perfusion and viability, dementia, neurodegenerative disease, and pre-surgical evaluation of patients with refractory seizures. (Evaluations and Pain).

6.1 Applications in humans

The staging, preoperative assessment and surgical planning of several human cancers realizes theoretical advantages in the use of PET/CT scanning rather than conventional imaging with CT. One such cancer is oral/head and neck cancer. In 2010 the American Cancer Society estimated that 36,540 cases of cancer of the oral cavity and pharynx would be diagnosed among a total of 1,529,560 (2.4%) cancer diagnoses during the same year. (Jemal, Siegel et al. 2010) While most cancers of the oral cavity and pharynx are squamous cell carcinomas, and therefore mucosal in origin and readily detectable on self-examination, the five year survival rate of such cancers has remained relatively dismal over the past 50 years at 50%. Early detection of the primary cancer and regional lymphatic spread to the cervical lymph nodes might be a means to improving the survival of patients with this disease. To this end, clinical examination of at risk patients and anatomic imaging with ultrasound (Gor, Langer et al. 2006), computed tomography (Coughlin and Resto 2010), or magnetic resonance imaging (Coughlin and Resto 2010) could possibly represent a means for early detection of cancer of the oral cavity and pharynx, and their regional lymph nodes, thereby leading to more expedient treatment of these cancers with the possibility of a more favorable prognosis. In oncologic terms, a patient with no signs of cervical lymph node involvement is labeled N0, while the patient with palpable cervical lymph node disease is labeled N+. The designation of the neck in the TNM classification (tumor size, neck lymph nodes, metastasis) represents one of the more important aspects of staging of patients with cancer of the oral cavity and pharynx. Specifically, the removal of cervical lymph nodes that identify occult histologic disease has survival benefits to patients, rather than adopting the wait and watch approach to the cervical lymph nodes and resorting to a neck dissection only when clinically palpable lymph nodes are present. Studies have been carried out regarding the imaging criteria that would permit prediction of metastatic disease in the cervical lymph nodes, particularly those that are equivocal in their size and clinical character. Nonetheless, most studies have shown that imaging studies are of limited value for the accurate staging of cervical lymph nodes. (van den Brekel 2000) Owing to the anatomic and physiologic assessment inherent in PET/CT scanning, investigators have looked towards this modality of imaging to determine if increased sensitivity and specificity can be realized when applying this technology to the assessment of the cervical lymph nodes in patients with oral cavity cancers. Such reports have shown that PET/CT is effective for the diagnosis, staging, and restaging of malignancies of the head and neck region. (Myers, Wax et al. 1998; Blodgett, Fukui et al. 2005; Fukui, Blodgett et al. 2005) There was a reported sensitivity of 70-90% and specificity of 80-95% for the patients in whom their cervical lymph nodes are determined to be clinically positive (N+). (Mukherji and Bradford 2006)

In 2007 our molecular imaging research center investigated the role of 18F-FDG PET/CT in the preoperative prediction of the presence and extent of neck disease in patients with oral/head and neck cancer. (Nahmias, Carlson et al. 2007) Seventy patients were enrolled in the study, 47 of whom had a clinically negative neck (N0), 19 of whom had a clinically positive unilateral neck (N+), and 4 of whom had a negative neck on one side and positive on the other. Each patient underwent a PET/CT study prior to undergoing selective neck dissection for N0 disease or modified radical neck dissection for N+ disease. Eighty-three neck dissections were performed in the 70 patients. The neck dissections were oriented as to oncologic levels for the pathologist processing and interpreting the tissues so as to permit correlation between histopathologic findings and the imaging results. One hundred ninety-two (11.4%) of the 1,678 lymph nodes recovered were histologically positive for metastatic disease. The sensitivity and specificity of the PET/CT procedure were 79% and 82% for the N0 neck, and 95% and 25% for the N+ neck. In patients with clinically negative necks, therefore, a negative PET/CT result would not help the oncologic surgeon in the management of the patient due to the rate of false-negative results, but a positive PET/CT result can diagnose metastatic deposits with a high positive predictive value. In patients with clinically positive necks, a positive test will confirm the presence of disease, although false-negative lymph nodes were additionally identified in these clinically positive necks. With respect to the lymph nodes, the sensitivity of the imaging procedure is such that the results could not assist the surgeon in deciding whether the patients with N0 necks benefit by a prophylactic neck dissection. This realization reinforces the 21st century practice of prophylactic neck dissections in patients with N0 staging associated with cancer of the oral cavity.

In 2009 our molecular imaging research center investigated the use of PET/CT in patients with oral/head and neck cancer with an assessment of the cervical lymph nodes according to time points. In this study, patients underwent a dynamic PET/CT scan consisting of nine time points over 60-115 minutes post-injection. Sixty patients underwent 64 neck dissections whereby 2,170 lymph nodes were evaluated by a static 90 minute study and 118 lymph nodes were studied by time points. A mean SUV (standard uptake value) of hypermetabolic lymph nodes was plotted as a function of time. A lymph node with greater than 10% change was designated as metastatic. The time point data showed a sensitivity and specificity of 58% and 71% respectively.

6.2 Applications in animals

PET/CT is considered novel as a diagnostic technique in clinical veterinary medicine although its use in live animal research endeavors is well recognized. Lack of available equipment and high cost of PET radiopharmaceuticals have limited the use of PET as a clinical diagnostic tool in veterinary medicine, and the few reports available to date have focused on ^{18}FDG PET and PET/CT in veterinary oncology. (Page, Garg et al. 1994; Matwichuk, Daniel et al. 1999; Bassett, Daniel et al. 2002; Bruehlmeier, Kaser Hotz et al. 2005; Ballegeer, Forrest et al. 2006; LeBlanc, Jakoby et al. 2009) Currently, the availability of PET for staging and evaluation of response to therapy in clinical veterinary patients is limited to a few locations in the United States. Applications in veterinary oncology will increase as this technology becomes more widely available, aided considerably by regional cyclotron distribution networks for radiopharmaceutical sales.

Both dogs and cats have been used in research settings for novel PET tracer validation studies for many years as their physical size permits serial blood sampling and *in vivo* imaging procedures, in addition to their comparable metabolic and physiologic characteristics. (Larson, Weiden et al. 1981; Larson, Weiden et al. 1981; Page, Garg et al. 1994; Cook, Carnes et al. 2007) To date, the majority of radiopharmaceuticals employed for clinical PET in companion animals are commercially available ^{18}F-labelled molecules such as ^{18}FDG and ^{18}FLT. The majority of these studies have been performed in animals with known or suspected malignancies for the purposes of lesion characterization, tumor staging or for monitoring response to anticancer therapy.

Special considerations for veterinary species undergoing PET/CT imaging center on the necessary use of general anesthesia for patient positioning and immobilization for scanning procedures. PET/CT scans, similar to other cross-sectional imaging techniques such as CT or MRI, are uniformly performed with widely used sedative and anesthetic drugs in veterinary patients. Risks associated with general anesthesia may preclude the use of this diagnostic technique in sick or debilitated animals. There are no standardized recommendations regarding ^{18}FDG dose, but ranges of 0.1 - 0.2 mCi per kg body weight have been reported. (LeBlanc, Jakoby et al. 2008; Lawrence, Vanderhoek et al. 2009; LeBlanc, Jakoby et al. 2009; LeBlanc, Wall et al. 2009) Veterinary patients require 12 hours' fast and use of sedative premedications with cage confinement after ^{18}FDG injection to minimize aberrant uptake of ^{18}FDG in skeletal muscle during the tracer uptake period. Some imaging sites also use general anesthesia for the tracer uptake period for radiation safety considerations, as it is difficult to control spontaneous urination and/or defecation of radioactive waste in companion animals. Following the tracer uptake period, animals are placed under general anesthesia and the CT and PET data collected as for a human patient scan. (LeBlanc, Jakoby et al. 2008; LeBlanc, Jakoby et al. 2009; LeBlanc, Wall et al. 2009)

Reports of clinical PET and PET/CT in companion animals are sparse in the veterinary literature. Recent studies of whole-body PET and PET/CT in normal dogs and cats demonstrate patterns of ^{18}FDG distribution and SUVs for parenchymal organs to assist in lesion interpretation in disease states. (LeBlanc, Jakoby et al. 2008; LeBlanc, Wall et al. 2009)

A recent investigation of whole-body PET as a staging tool demonstrated the avidity of canine cutaneous mast cell tumor and lymphoma for ^{18}FDG. (LeBlanc, Jakoby et al. 2009)

Newer studies have documented ^{18}FDG uptake using PET/CT fusion in specific malignancies, inflammatory brain disease, and have investigated the impact of different anesthesia protocols on physiologic brain uptake of ^{18}FDG. (Lee, Lee et al. ; Lawrence, Vanderhoek et al. 2009; Kang, Kim et al. 2010; Lee, Lee et al. 2010; Lee, Ko et al. 2010)

As studies are published that fully validate its use as a non-invasive whole-body staging method, PET using commercially-available tracers will become a useful and innovative tool in the management of veterinary patients. From a research perspective, companion animals represent robust and relevant models for the validation of new PET tracers in a variety of diseases that affect both humans and animals alike. (Lawrence, Rohren et al. 2010)

7. PET/CT: Today and tomorrow

Although a fairly young tool, PET/CT is already irreplaceable in many applications, and the continued improvement of scanner performance promises further clinical integration. However, its full potential remains unrealized largely due to the relative limited availability of useful radiotracers. As new tracers are developed and scanning protocols are further refined, the trend in patient care will become more personalized and tailored to specific disease, ultimately allowing doctors to provide the best possible care for their patients.

8. References

Bailey, D. and S. Meikle (1994). "A convolution-subtraction scatter correction method for 3D PET." Physics in Medicine and Biology 39: 411.

Ballegeer, E. A., L. J. Forrest, et al. (2006). "PET/CT Following Intensity Modulated Radiation Therapy for Primary Lung Tumor in a Dog." Veterinary Radiology & Ultrasound 47(2): 228-233.

Barney, J., J. Rogers, et al. (1991). "Object shape dependent scatter simulations for PET." Nuclear Science, IEEE Transactions on 38(2): 719-725.

Barrett, H. H. and K. J. Myers (2004). Foundations of image science. Hoboken, NJ, Wiley.

Bassett, C. L. M., G. B. Daniel, et al. (2002). "Characterization of Uptake of 2-Deoxy-2-[18F] Fluoro-D-Glucose by Fungal-Associated Inflammation:: The Standardized Uptake Value is Greater for Lesions of Blastomycosis than for Lymphoma in

Dogs with Naturally Occurring Disease." Molecular Imaging & Biology 4(3): 201-207.

Bergström, M., L. Eriksson, et al. (1983). "Correction for scattered radiation in a ring detector positron camera by integral transformation of the projections." Journal of Computer Assisted Tomography 7(1): 42.

Beyer, T., P. Kinahan, et al. (1994). The use of X-ray CT for attenuation correction of PET data, IEEE.

Bietendorf, J. (2004). "FDG PET Reimbursement." Journal of Nuclear Medicine Technology 32(1): 33.

Blodgett, T. M., M. B. Fukui, et al. (2005). "Combined PET-CT in the Head and Neck." Radiographics 25(4): 897.

Bruehlmeier, M., B. Kaser Hotz, et al. (2005). "Measurement of tumor hypoxia in spontaneous canine sarcomas." Veterinary Radiology & Ultrasound 46(4): 348-354.

Carson, R., M. Daube-Witherspoon, et al. (1988). "A method for postinjection PET transmission measurements with a rotating source." Journal of Nuclear Medicine 29(9): 1558.

Casey, M. and R. Nutt (1986). "A multicrystal two dimensional BGO detector system for positron emission tomography." IEEE Trans. Nucl. Sci 33(1): 460-463.

Cherry, S., M. Dahlbom, et al. (1991). "3D PET using a conventional multislice tomograph without septa." Journal of Computer Assisted Tomography 15(4): 655.

Cook, R. A. H., G. Carnes, et al. (2007). "Respiration-averaged CT for attenuation correction in canine cardiac PET/CT." Journal of Nuclear Medicine 48(5): 811.

Coughlin, A. and V. A. Resto (2010). "Oral Cavity Squamous Cell Carcinoma and the Clinically N0 Neck: The Past, Present, and Future of Sentinel Lymph Node Biopsy." Current oncology reports 12(2): 129-135.

Evaluations, A. P. and P. O. Pain "Medicare National Coverage Determinations Manual."

Fukui, M. B., T. M. Blodgett, et al. (2005). "Combined PET-CT in the Head and Neck." Radiographics 25(4): 913.

Gindi, G., M. Lee, et al. (1991). Bayesian reconstruction of functional images using registered anatomical images as priors, Springer.

Gor, D. M., J. E. Langer, et al. (2006). "Imaging of cervical lymph nodes in head and neck cancer: the basics." Radiologic Clinics of North America 44(1): 101-110.

Grootoonk, S., T. Spinks, et al. (1996). "Correction for scatter in 3D brain PET using a dual energy window method." Physics in Medicine and Biology 41: 2757.

Hubbell, J. and U. S. N. B. o. Standards (1969). Photon cross sections, attenuation coefficients, and energy absorption coefficients from 10 keV to 100 GeV, US National Bureau of Standards; for sale by the Supt. of Docs., US Govt. Print. Off.

Jakoby, B., Y. Bercier, et al. "Performance investigation of a time-of-flight PET/CT scanner."

Jemal, A., R. Siegel, et al. (2010). "Cancer statistics, 2010." CA: A Cancer Journal for Clinicians: caac. 20073v20071.

Kang, B. T., S. G. Kim, et al. (2010). "Correlation between fluorodeoxyglucose positron emission tomography and magnetic resonance imaging findings of non-suppurative meningoencephalitis in 5 dogs." The Canadian Veterinary Journal 51(9): 986.

Kinahan, P., D. Townsend, et al. (1998). "Attenuation correction for a combined 3D PET/CT scanner." Medical Physics 25: 2046.

Kluetz, P., C. Meltzer, et al. (2000). "Combined PET/CT Imaging in Oncology:: Impact on Patient Management." Clinical Positron Imaging 3(6): 223-230.

Larson, S. M., P. L. Weiden, et al. (1981). "Positron Imaging Feasibility Studies. II: Characteristics of 2-Deoxyglucose Uptake in Rodent and Canine Neoplasms: Concise Communication." J Nucl Med 22(10): 875-879.

Larson, S. M., P. L. Weiden, et al. (1981). "Positron Imaging Feasibility Studies. I: Characteristics of [3H]Thymidine Uptake in Rodent and Canine Neoplasms: Concise Communication." J Nucl Med 22(10): 869-874.

Lawrence, J., E. Rohren, et al. (2010). "PET/CT today and tomorrow in veterinary cancer diagnosis and monitoring: fundamentals, early results and future perspectives." Veterinary and Comparative Oncology 8(3): 163-187.

Lawrence, J., M. Vanderhoek, et al. (2009). "Use of 3-Deoxy-3-[18F]Fluorothymadine PET/CT for Evaluating Response to Cytotoxic Chemotherapy in Dogs with Non Hodgkin's Lymphoma." Veterinary Radiology & Ultrasound 50(6): 660-668.

LeBlanc, A. K., B. Jakoby, et al. (2008). "Thoracic and Abdominal Organ Uptake of 2-Deoxy-2-[18F]Fluoro-D-Glucose (18FDG) with Positron Emission Tomography in the Normal Dog." Veterinary Radiology & Ultrasound 49(2): 182-188.

LeBlanc, A. K., B. W. Jakoby, et al. (2009). "[18F]FDG PET Imaging in Canine Lymphoma and Cutaneous Mast Cell Tumor." Veterinary Radiology & Ultrasound 50(2): 215-223.

LeBlanc, A. K., J. S. Wall, et al. (2009). "Normal Thoracic and Abdominal Distribution of 2-Deoxy-2-[18F]Fluoro-D-Glucose (18FDG) in Adult Cats." Veterinary Radiology & Ultrasound 50(4): 436-441.

Lee, A., M. Lee, et al. (2010). "Imaging Diagnosis-FDG PET/CT of a Canine Splenic Plasma Cell Tumor." Veterinary Radiology & Ultrasound 51(2): 145-147.

Lee, M., J. Ko, et al. (2010). "Effects of Anesthetic Protocol on Normal Canine Brain Uptake of 18F-FDG Assessed by PET/CT." Veterinary Radiology & Ultrasound 51(2): 130-135.

Lee, M., A. Lee, et al. "Characterization of Physiologic 18F-FDG Uptake with PET/CT in Dogs." Veterinary Radiology & Ultrasound.

Matwichuk, C. L., G. B. Daniel, et al. (1999). "Fluorine-18 Fluorodeoxyglucose Accumulation in Blastomyces dermatitidis-Associated Inflammation in a Dog* 1." Clinical Positron Imaging 2(4): 217-221.

Mukherji, S. K. and C. R. Bradford (2006). "Controversies: Is There a Role for Positron-Emission Tomographic CT in the Initial Staging of Head and Neck Squamous Cell Carcinoma?" American Journal of Neuroradiology 27(2): 243.

Mumcuoglu, E., R. Leahy, et al. (1996). "Bayesian reconstruction of PET images: methodology and performance analysis." Physics in Medicine and Biology 41: 1777.

Myers, L. L., M. K. Wax, et al. (1998). "Positron Emission Tomography in the Evaluation of the N0 Neck." The Laryngoscope 108(2): 232-236.

Nahmias, C., E. Carlson, et al. (2007). "Positron Emission Tomography/Computerized Tomography (PET/CT) Scanning for Preoperative Staging of Patients With Oral/Head and Neck Cancer." Journal of Oral and Maxillofacial Surgery 65(12): 2524-2535.

Ollinger, J. (1996). "Model-based scatter correction for fully 3D PET." Physics in Medicine and Biology 41: 153.

Page, R. L., P. K. Garg, et al. (1994). "PET imaging of osteosarcoma in dogs using a fluorine-18-labeled monoclonal antibody Fab fragment." Journal of Nuclear Medicine 35(9): 1506.

Pelizzari, C., G. Chen, et al. (1989). "Accurate three-dimensional registration of CT, PET, and/or MR images of the brain." Journal of Computer Assisted Tomography 13(1): 20.

Phelps, M., E. Hoffman, et al. (1976). "Tomographic images of blood pool and perfusion in brain and heart." Journal of Nuclear Medicine 17(7): 603.

Phelps, M., E. Hoffman, et al. (1975). "Application of annihilation coincidence detection to transaxial reconstruction tomography." Journal of Nuclear Medicine 16(3): 210.

Pietrzyk, U., K. Herholz, et al. (1996). "Clinical applications of registration and fusion of multimodality brain images from PET, SPECT, CT, and MRI*." European journal of radiology 21(3): 174-182.

Shapiro, J. (2002). Radiation protection : a guide for scientists, regulators, and physicians. Cambridge, Mass. [u.a.], Harvard University Press.

Shreve, P. and D. W. Townsend (2008). Clinical PET-CT. New York; London, Springer.

Stearns, C. (1995). "Scatter correction method for 3D PET using 2D fitted Gaussian functions." J Nucl Med 36: 105.

Townsend, D., T. Beyer, et al. (2003). PET/CT scanners: a hardware approach to image fusion, Elsevier.

Townsend, D., T. Beyer, et al. (1998). The SMART scanner: a combined PET/CT tomograph for clinical oncology, IEEE.

Valk, P. E. (2003). Positron emission tomography : basic science and clinical practice. London; New York, Springer.

van den Brekel, M. W. M. (2000). "Lymph node metastases: CT and MRI." European journal of radiology 33(3): 230-238.

Warburg, O., K. Posener, et al. (1931). "The metabolism of the carcinoma cell." The Mechanism of Tumors: 129–169.

Watson, C. (2000). "New, faster, image-based scatter correction for 3D PET." Nuclear Science, IEEE Transactions on 47(4): 1587-1594.

Watson, C., D. Newport, et al. (1996). "A single scatter simulation technique for scatter correction in 3D PET." Three-Dimensional Image Reconstruction in Radiology and Nuclear Medicine 4: 255–268.

Workman, R. and R. Coleman (2006). PET/CT essentials for clinical practice, Springer.

4

CT Scan of Pediatric Liver Tumors

Qian Dong[1] and Jingjing Chen[2]
[1]*Department of pediatric surgery,*
[2]*Department of radiology The Affiliated Hospital of Medical College, Qing Dao University*
P.R.China

1. Introduction

Hepatic masses constitute only 5% to 6% of all intra-abdominal masses in children (Pobeil & Bisset, 1995) and primary hepatic neoplasms constitute only 0.5% to 2% of all pediatric malignancies (Davey & Cohen, 1996). Primary hepatic neoplasms are the third most common abdominal malignancy in childhood, after Wilms' tumor and neuroblastoma (Davey & Cohen, 1996). The majority of liver tumors in children are malignant. Only about one third of the liver tumors are benign (Jha et al., 2009).

Most children with benign or malignant liver masses present with a palpable mass on physical examination. Other presenting symptoms include pain, anorexia, jaundice, paraneoplastic syndromes, hemorrhage, or congestive heart failure. Although it is often obvious that these children have an upper abdominal mass, the organ of origin is often not clear without imaging.

Pediatricians and surgeons began to order more imaging studies because advances in imaging technology improved the diagnosis and management of disease. Imaging of pediatric hepatic masses has included multiple modalities, such as ultrasound, CT scan, MR imaging, angiography, and radionuclide techniques. Because surgical resection remains the mainstay of treatment for many of these lesions, detailed depiction of the extent of the mass and relationship to hepatic anatomy is essential. Ultrasound is usually the initial imaging modality in the evaluation of a child with a suspected abdominal mass. Ultrasound accurately excludes a mass when it is not present and identifies the organ of origin when a mass is present. Identifying the organ of origin helps determine the remainder of the child's imaging work-up. Ultrasound also evaluates whether a mass is cystic or solid and assesses vascular flow. When ultrasound confirms the lesion is in the liver, usually additional imaging is obtained with CT scan or MR imaging.

The advantage of CT requires less or no anesthesia due to faster scan times. So CT has always played a major role in the imaging of the liver. But at the same time pediatric patients present unique technical challenges for CT. Children are not simply small adults, and CT scan principles drawn from experience with adults can not accurately be extrapolated to the pediatric population. The methods of CT examination should be adjusted.

Whether CT scan or MR imaging is the modality of choice for definitive imaging of liver masses is a controversial issue. The choice is usually based on institutional experience and modality availability. Nevertheless, the development of multidetector row CT (MDCT) technology has helped CT to continue to excel in its already established indications (ie, hepatic lesion detection and characterization) and to add new clinical indications (ie, CT angiography for preprocedure mapping, liver perfusion). The fast pace of development challenged radiologists in terms of the cost of replacement of scanners, the optimization of CT protocols for existing indications, and the development of new protocols for the new applications introduced by the MDCT technology.

Hepatic tumors are classified into benign and malignant categories. Malignant hepatic neoplasms are twice as frequent as benign neoplasms and most of these are hepatoblastomas. Hepatocellular carcinoma, including the fibrolamellar variant, undifferentiated (embryonal) sarcoma, and angiosarcoma are less common malignant tumors. The common benign hepatic tumors are hemangioendothelioma, hemangioma, and mesenchymal hamartoma, with focal nodular hyperplasia and adenoma encountered less often (Kuhn et al., 2004; Helmberger et al., 1999; Emre & McKenna, 2004; Pobiel &, Bisset, 1995; Siegel et al., 2008).

2. Techniques of CT scan in children liver

Hepatic CT present significant technical challenges in children. There are several problems that are present in children but not present in adults. These include small patient size, lack of fat, and inability to suspend respiration or voluntary motion. With proper attention to technique, these problems can be minimized and can improve diagnostic quality .

The introduction of helical CT has greatly improved the capabilities of CT scanning. The subsecond scanning techniques eliminate respiratory misregistration, decrease the need for sedation, and enable scanning during arterial and venous phases of contrast administration. The helical data set also enables threedimensional imaging.

2.1 Preparation of children before the examination

To acquire an optimal CT examination adequate prescan patient preparation is as important as the optimization of the CT technique. Issues that should be addressed are (1) psychological preparation of children and parents (including the scanner environment), (2) the need for sedation or general anaesthesia, (3) oral contrast material preparation, and (4) intravenous (IV) contrast material preparation.

2.1.1 Psychological preparation before CT scanning

Adequate prescan patient preparation should include: (1)Age- and intellect-adapted information to the child and information for the parents about the CT examination (including written information, simulation, coaching or other forms of playing therapy). (2)Inviting one or both parents to stay with the child before, during and after the investigation.(3)Adaptation of the scanner environment to children (for instance by using a painted curtain covering the CT gantry, and (projection of) paintings on the wall or ceiling). This will help to reduce the anxiety of the child and positively influence their mood, increasing the success rate of the CT examination without the need for sedation or general anaesthesia.

2.1.2 Sedation

There has been a phenomenal increase in the number of diagnostic radiology procedures in the past decade. Consequently, the demand for fast, effective and safe sedation for children has grown exponentially as well. The parents expect an anxiety free experience for their children. The radiologists expect the child to be cooperative and not move (Krauss & Green, 2000; Shankar, 2008). In general, children 5 years of age and older will be able to undergo a CT examination without sedation after thorough patient instruction. However, there are still situations in which sedation or general anaesthesia will be required depending on the type of investigation, age and mental ability of the child and the clinical situation and question. The way sedation and general anaesthesia is organised depends largely on local agreements and legislations. The drugs most frequently used for sedation are oral chloral hydrate and intravenous pentobarbital sodium (American Society of Anesthesiologists Task Force,1996; Bisset & Ball,1991; Committee on Drugs,1992; Cote,1994; Frush et al,1996; Pereira et al,1993; Strain, 1988; Siegel, 1999; Nievelstein,2010).Oral chloral hydrate, 50 to 100 mg/kg, with a maximum dosage of 2000 mg, is the drug of choice for children younger than 18 months. Intravenous pentobarbital sodium, 6 mg/kg with a maximum dose of 200 mg, is advocated in children older than 18 months. It is injected slowly in fractions of one fourth the total dose and is titrated against the patient's response. This is an effective form of sedation with a failure rate of less than 5%.

Fentanyl citrate is in the class of narcotics and has the combined benefits of sedation and analgesia. Fentanyl is given for pain control. It is administered intravenously in a dose of 1.0 μg/kg. The drug is given slowly over 5 min. Maximum cumulative dose is 3 μg/kg. For those patients weighing over 25 kg, fentanyl is given in 25-μg aliquots until the desired analgesia is achieved. Onset is almost immediate, and duration of action is 30 to 60 min.

Regardless of the choice of drug, the use of parenteral sedation requires the facility and ability to resuscitate and maintain adequate cardiorespiratory support during and after the examination. After being sedated, the infant or child is placed on a blanket on the CT table. For the CT examination, the arms routinely are extended above the head to avoid streak artifacts and to provide an easily accessible route for intravenous injection. The upper arms can be restrained with sandbags, adhesive tape, or Velcro straps.

Patients who are to receive parenteral sedation should have no liquids by mouth for 3 hours and no solid foods for 6 hours prior to their examination.

2.1.3 Oral contrast material

As small children lack large amounts of intraabdominal fatty tissue, it is more difficult to interpretation of a CT of the abdomen in children than in adults. That is why we prefer US as the imaging modality of first choice for abdominal clinical problems in childhood. If CT of the abdomen is indicated, adequate oral contrast intake is often essential for the evaluation. Opacification of the small and large bowel is needed to determine the extent of extrahepatic disease (Siegel, 1998; Siegel, 1999; Siegel, 2001).A dilute (1–2%) solution of water-soluble, iodine-based oral contrast agent is given by mouth or through a nasogastric tube if necessary. A non-ionic iodinated oral contrast agent is often preferred because of the risk of aspiration. The oral contrast agent can be mixed with fruit juice if needed to mask the unpleasant taste. The gastrointestinal tract from the stomach to the terminal ileum usually can be well opacified if the contrast agent is given in two volumes, one is 45 to 60 min before the examination and the other is 15 min prior to scanning. The first volume should approximate that of an average feeding. The second volume should be approximately one half that of the first (Table 1).

Age	1st dose (ml) (±1h prior to CT)	2nd dose (ml) (15min prior to CT)
1-6 months	90-120	45-60
6 months-1 year	120-180	60-90
1-4 years	180-270	90-135
4-8 years	270-360	135-180
8-12 years	360-480	180-240
12-16 years	480-600	240-300

Table 1. Age-based amounts of oral CM for a biphasic preparation protocol, 1 h and 15 min prior to CT examination (Frush, 2008; Siegel, 2008; Nievelstein, 2010)

2.2 Intravenous contrast material

For the administration of intravenous (IV) contrast material, the use of a power injector instead of hand injection is preferred. Contrast is administered by a power injector if a 22-gauge or larger plastic cannula can be placed into an antecubital vein. (Siegel,1999a; Siegel,1999b; Roche,1996; Siegel,2001) The injection rate is determined by the caliber of the intravenous catheter. Contrast material is infused at 1.2 mL/sec for a 22-gauge catheter, at 1.5 mL/sec for a 20-gauge catheter, and at 2 mL/sec for an 18-gauge needle. A hand injection is needed if intravenous access is through a peripheral access line, a smaller caliber antecubital catheter or butterfly needle, or a central venous catheter.

The standard contrast material used for IV administration is a non-ionic, low-osmolar contrast agent with a concentration between 240 and 400 mg I/ml (most frequently 300 mg I/ml). Adjusting the iodine dose for body weight is particularly crucial in children because of the wide range of body sizes. The traditional dose of contrast medium administered in children is 2 mL/kg, with a maximum dose of 150 mL (Frush,1997). This scheme, which was based on use of low-concentration contrast media (240–300 mg I/mL), has been commonly practiced since early CT more than 30 years ago and is widely used even in the current era of fast MDCT and the general use of higher-concentration contrast media. Short scanning times offered by fast MDCT allow improved contrast enhancement and more efficient use of contrast media(Bae & Heiken,2005; Bae,2007; Bae ,2008).Some scholar indicated that to achieve consistent aortic or hepatic contrast enhancement in pediatric patients with abdominal 64-MDCT, the amount of contrast medium should be adjusted to the patient's body weight for all ages of pediatric patients: approximately 1.5 mL/kg, or 0.525 g I/kg, to yield 116 HU of hepatic attenuation or 50–55 HU of hepatic enhancement. (Bae ,2008)

In children the circulation time varies widely which makes adequate scan timing more difficult. Furthermore, the size, position and type of cannula will differ among different age groups, with as a consequence varying injection rates. In general, an injection rate of 2.0 ml/s suffices for most paediatric indications, especially when younger than 12 years of age. An empirically determined fixed delay time usually suffices for most routine indications, especially in the younger age group. However, the routine use of bolus tracking techniques is strongly recommended for most body indications, especially in case of a CT angiography (CTA) or arterial-phase CT (Bae & Heiken, 2005). An alternative for scan timing is the test bolus technique, although this technique is not suitable in very small children as the total volume of contrast material available is often too small. Both techniques share the disadvantage of additional (monitoring) scans, increasing the radiation dose for the child.

This additional dose should be weighed against the benefit of improved and individualized scan timing, and when applied the monitor scans should be obtained with a low-dose technique to limit this additional radiation dose.
Patients who are to receive intravenous contrast medium for the CT examination should be NPO (nothing per mouth) for 3 hours to minimize the likelihood of nausea or vomiting with possible aspiration during a bolus injection of intravenous contrast medium.

2.3 Selective organ shielding

The use of bismuth shielding of radiosensitive organs (e.g., breast, thyroid gland and eye lens) to reduce organ doses has been suggested. However, these shields may also reduce the amount of radiation reaching the detector ring in some projections and may add noise or artifacts to the images, especially if no standoff pads are used (Vollmar & Kalender, 2008). A fundamental study by Geleijns et al.(Geleijns et al,2006) showed that the reduction in organ dose can also be achieved more efficiently by lowering the tube current. In addition, these shields may complicate the use of dose modulation techniques with the risk of increasing radiation dose to the child. Therefore, it remains to be seen if selective organ shielding will be of any additional benefit if the CT protocols are already maximally optimised for children (Vollmar & Kalender, 2008; Geleijns et al., 2006; Leswick et al., 2008). We will therefore not advocate this method.

2.4 Scan and technical parameters

The CT protocol for evaluation of a possible liver mass is performed with a dual-phase spiral CT scan through the liver, with additional delayed scans obtained as needed (Aytekin et al,2005).A slice thickness of 5 mm is used with a pitch of 1 to 1.5, depending on patient size, and 3-mm reconstructions. For dual-phase imaging, the arterial dominant phase of liver enhancement should be initiated at 10 to 15 sec after the start of the contrast bolus. The portal venous phase is initiated as soon as possible after completion of the arterial phase of enhancement (interscan delay usually between 20 and 40 sec). In order to minimise the radiation dose to the child, some experts suggests that an empirically determined fixed-delay time of 50 s after initiation of the IV injection of contrast material usually suffices, resulting in a CT examination during the portal venous phase (Roebuck, 2009).
The scan field of view (FOV) should be tailored as much as possible to the size of the body region of interest. The major advantage of a smaller scan FOV is the higher spatial resolution, as the pixel size decreases with smaller FOV. The effect of the display FOV on resolution is often different—while some increase in resolution may result, after a certain threshold pixels are only blown up.
Due to the smaller size of children it is usually possible to lower the tube voltage with maintenance or even improvement of the diagnostic image quality and resulting in a significant dose reduction. In most children a tube voltage of 80–100 kVp will suffice, especially in children with a body weight <45 kg. In adolescents, a tube voltage of 120 kVp for the abdomen is usually sufficient. The tube current (mA) should be adapted to the size or weight of the child. Most modern MDCT scanners have tube rotation times between 0.3 and 0.5 s resulting in shorter scan times. In terms of image quality a rotation time of 0.5 s is often the best option. The tube current modulation techniques, available on almost all modern MDCT scanners, are increasingly used in paediatric MDCT (Nievelstein, 2010).

2.5 Techniques of CT reconstruction

State-of-the-art cross-sectional imaging techniques allow radiologists to visualize disease with greater certainty by subtracting the impact of overlying tissues, thus allowing separate evaluation of individual organs, which aids in the detection and characterization of pathology.

Radiologists discovered in the late 1970s that although diagnosis based on axial CT images alone was more sophisticated than with plain radiography, the lack of a third dimension (e.g. sagittal and coronal dimensions) was frequently frustrating. Many referring physicians with no basic training in cross-sectional imaging still encounter difficulties in appreciating normal anatomy and pathology on transverse CT images, being more familiar with anatomy depicted in the coronal plane.

Following the somewhat crude three-dimensional computer rendering algorithms initially developed in late 1970s, that allowed formation of images in the third dimension from data acquired in the axial plane(Fig.1d), the development of single-slice helical CT and more recently multidetector CT (MDCT) scanners has opened new chapters in 3D imaging. These advances were made possible by the rapid acquisition of volumetric data in the lower case z-axis using thin slices and improved rendering algorithms, which facilitate exquisite 3D reformats, devoid of degradation by respiration and other physiological movements. The pace of progress is being hastened with the rapid developments in MDCT technology (Aytekin et al, 2005; Maher, 2004). We describe 3D rendering techniques available for abdominal imaging including multiplanar reconstructions, surface rendering, virtual endoscopy, volume rendering and maximum intensity projections. These 3D reformats can show the feeding arteries and venous drainage of detected lesions better, In addition, they are preferred by surgeons for preoperative planning, because the relationship of the lesions to the blood vessels and bile ducts is better delineated (Sahani et al,2002)(Fig.cd). Multiplanar volume rendering and creation of maximum intensity projections from MDCT data allow evaluation of both parenchymal and vascular detail in real time, interactively.

Multiplanar reconstruction (MPR) provides efficient computation of images that lie along the non-acquired orthogonal orientations of the scanned volume by readdressing the order of voxels in the scanned volume. It is a fast and interactive algorithm that can represent several arbitrary planes at once and create multiplanar display in real-time. Generally, it is helpful whenever pathology cannot be accurately assessed on axial plane images alone(Fig.1 a).

Volume rendering (multiplanar volume rendering, MPVR) is the visualization and manipulation of objects represented as sampled data in three or more dimensions. The technique interpolates the entire data set rather than editing a single scan to generate 3D images directly from scanned volume data. Unlike other projection techniques such as SSD and MIP, MPVR does not distort objects in the reconstructed planes. It allows "quick view" of large MDCT scan data sets with comprehensive details of the anatomic orientation of lesion or structures of interest.

The maximum intensity projection (MIP) technique displays the pixels of greatest intensity along a predefined axis of the image. It is useful for the depiction of vascular anatomy when there is a large difference between attenuation values (Hounsfield value, HU) of vessels opacified by contrast agent, and the surrounding tissues(Fig.1b). MIP is useful for all types of CT angiography and has also been used for CT Urography (Caoili et al, 2002)(Cody,2002).

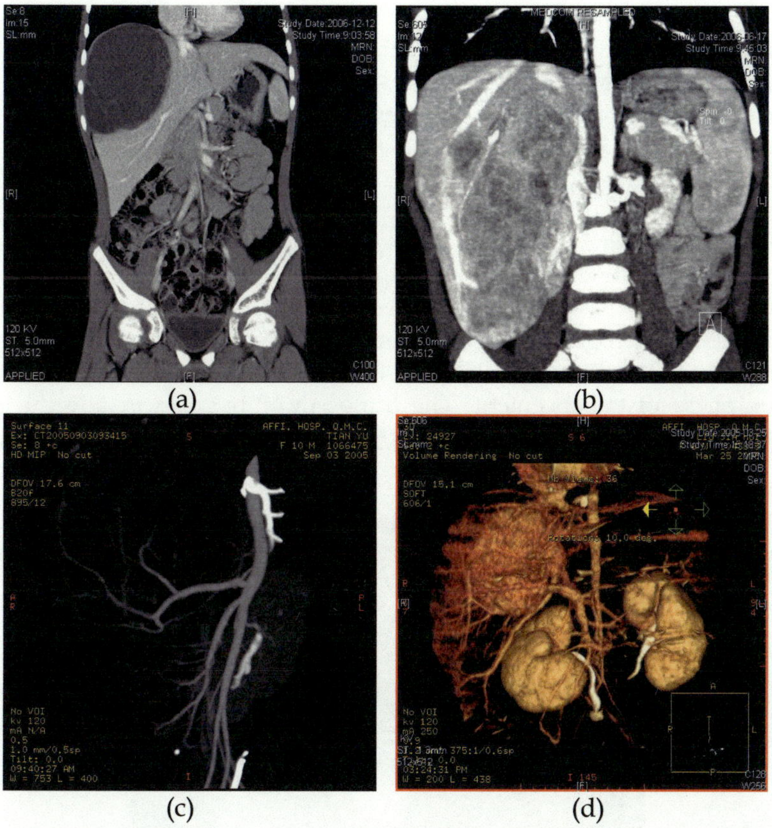

Fig. 1. a Coronal multiplanar reconstruction (MPR);b Maximum intensity projection (MIP) shows the elationship between the tumor and vein;c CT angiography(CTA);d 3D imaging.

3. Pathological characteristics and radiological features of primary liver tumors in children

The differential diagnosis for liver tumors in children includes benign and malignant neoplasms. Malignant neoplasms are usually hepatoblastomas or hepatocellular carcinomas (HCC) (Siegel,2001; Scuza & Narla,1992).Benign lesions are usually hemangioendotheliomas and less commonly mesenchymal hamartoma, cavernous hemangioma, focal nodular hyperplasia, and hepatic adenoma (Siegel,2001; Scuza & Narla,1992).Clinical information plays an important role in narrowing the differential diagnosis in cases where the imaging findings are nonspecific. Hemangioendothelioma is the most common mass in the first 6 months of life. Hepatoblastoma, mesenchymal hamartoma usually present in the first 3 years of life. HCC, focal nodular hyperplasia, and hepatic adenoma tend to occur in older children and adolescents. Certain liver tumors, such as hepatoblastoma and HCC, are associated with elevated serum alphafetoprotein levels (Greenberg & Filler, 1997; Siegel,2001).The clinical presentation also can suggest a specific diagnosis. Congestive heart failure in a neonate with a liver mass suggests the diagnosis of hemangioendothelioma. (Donnelly & Bisset, 1998) The role of imaging is to determine the organ of origin, character, and extent of the lesion. (Powers et al., 1994)

3.1 Malignant tumors

3.1.1 Hepatoblastoma

Hepatoblastomas are the most common primary liver tumors of the children with a peak presentation at 1–2 years of age and a male:female ratio of 2:1(Kuhn et al,2004; Helmberger et al,1999; Jha et al,2009). Less frequently, hepatoblastomas may also occur in older children, up to 15 years of age. Histologically, HB can be classified into an (a) epithelial, (b) mixed (epithelial/mesenchymal), or (c) anaplastic type. Epithelial HB is the most common type (60%). all HBs are large with an average diameter at diagnosis of 10±12 cm. Unenhanced CT typically shows a relatively well-defined, heterogeneous mass, slightly hypodense compared with liver tissue, with or without calcifications(Fig.2). On contrast-enhanced CT, the tumor reveals a heterogeneous enhancement (Fig. 3), The tumor enhances during the hepatic arterial phase of dynamic contrastenhanced CT and becomes hypoattenuating in the portal venous phase of enhancement. The tumor thrombus can invade the portal vein , spread along inferior vena cava(IVC) and encroach in the lumen of right atrium. Metastasis may be seen in lymph nodes and lung parenchyma, rarely in the bones and brain.

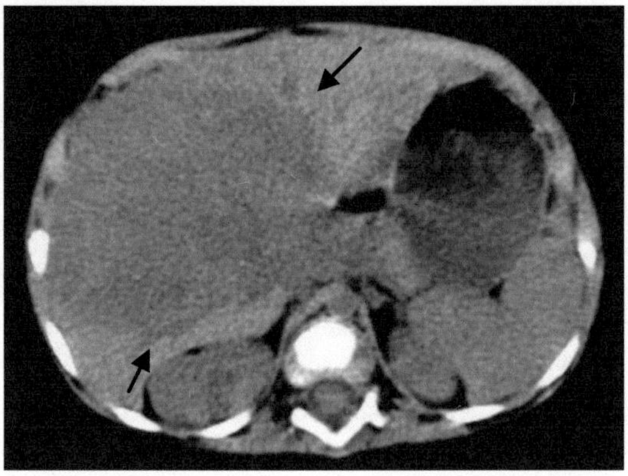

Fig. 2. A 5-year-old boy with hepatoblastoma. Unenhanced CT shows a relatively well-defined mass, slightly hypodense compared with liver tissue (arrowheads).

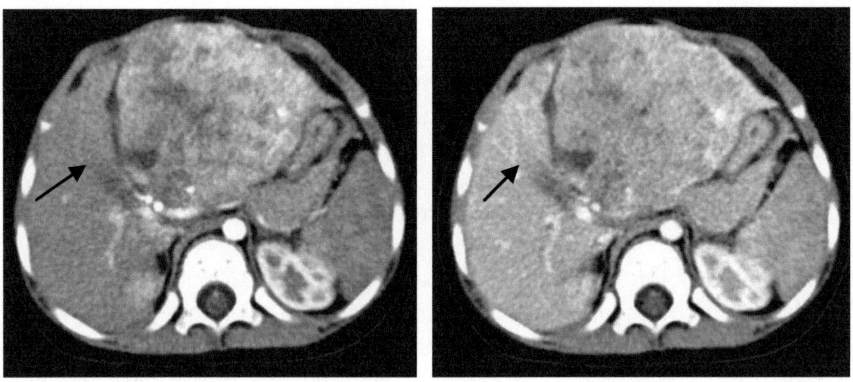

(a) (b)

Fig. 3. A 2-year-old boy with hepatoblastoma. Axial enhanced CT images of the abdomen demonstrate an ill-defined heterogeneous mass (arrowheads) with areas of necrosis appearing hypodense to the liver parenchyma

3.1.2 Hepatocellular carcinoma (HCC)

HCC is the second most common pediatric liver malignancy after hepatoblastoma. In the pediatric population, HCC has a median age of 12 years, with a range of 5 to 15 years, and is rare under 5 years (Greenberg & Filler, 1997;Davey & Cohen, 1996;Siegel, 2001). On CT, HCCs present with highly variable and non-characteristic features: the tumors may be homogeneous or heterogeneous, solitary or multifocal, well- or ill-defined. HCCs are typically isodense or slightly hypodense compared with liver parenchyma on unenhanced CT images and show an early arterial contrast enhancement and a rapid wash-out on enhanced CT (Fig. 4). Invasion of portal veins, hepatic veins, hepatic arteries and inferior vena cava may be seen. The diagnosis of an underlying cirrhosis may help in the differential diagnosis, but is rare in children. Diffuse involvement of the liver leads to a diffusely hypodense liver on CT. HCCs metastasize to lung, bone, skin and brain.

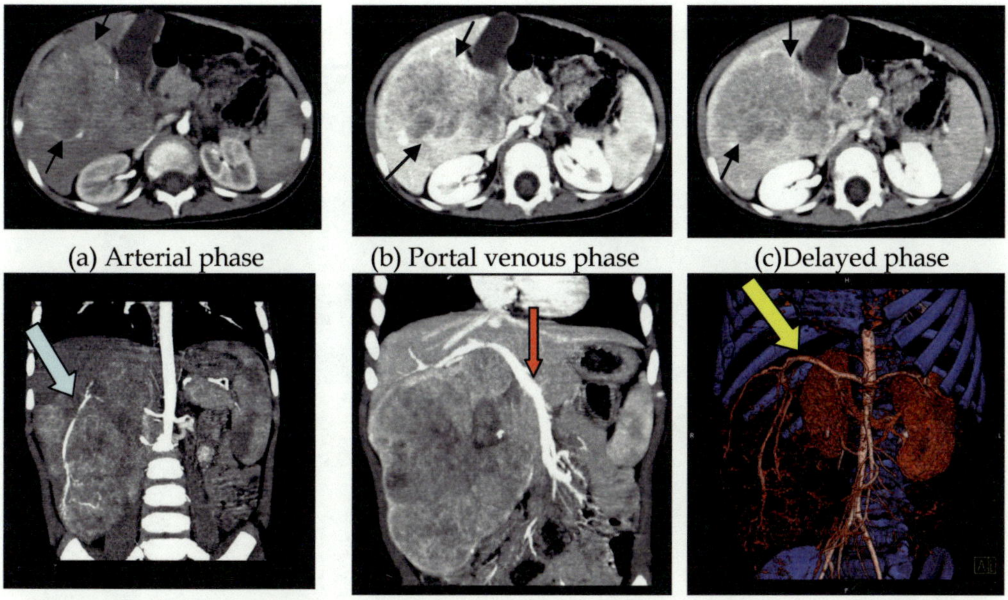

(a) Arterial phase (b) Portal venous phase (c)Delayed phase

(d) MIP of Arterial phase (e) MIP of Venous phase (f) Volume rendering(VR)

Fig. 4. A 2-year-old boy with HCC. Enhanced CT images of the abdomen shows an ill-defined heterogeneous mass (black arrowheads) with early arterial contrast enhancement and a rapid wash-out on portal venous phase and delayed phase(a、b、c);d. Maximum intensity projection reconstructed from the axial MDCT images obtained during the early arterial phase of contrast enhancement demonstrates artery in tumor (blue arrowheads);e. Maximum intensity projection obtained during the portal venous phase of contrast enhancement shows the relationship between tumor and portal veins (red arrowheads) ;f. Volume rendering(VR) shows the feeding arteries of the tumor (yellow arrowheads)

3.2 Benign tumors

3.2.1 Infantile hepatic hemangioma or hemangioendothelioma

Hepatic hemangiomas and hemangioendotheliomas are the most common vascular hepatic tumors in the first year of life (50% of the benign tumors) (Kuhn et al,2004, Helmberger et al,1999, Jha et al,2009). Most affected patients are young infants less than 6 months old

(85%), the male:female ratio being 1:2. The two lesions show distinct histopathological characteristics. Infantile hepatic hemangiomas are benign vascular lesions. Epitheliod hemangioendotheliomas are also primarily benign, endothelium lined vascular masses, but may show a malignant potential (Emre & McKenna, 2004). In the proliferative phase, there is characteristic hypercellularity, endothelial proliferation and dilatation of vascular spaces, leading to a characteristic 'cavernous appearance'. On unenhanced computed tomography (CT), hemangiomas and hemangioendotheliomas have a lower attenuation than the liver parenchyma with occasional hemorrhage(Fig. 5a). Calcifications may be seen in up to 40% of cases. On contrast-enhanced CT there is a characteristic intense, nodular peripheral rim enhancement with central progression (Fig. 5b,c,d). Central filling defects may occur in larger lesions due to central thrombosis or fibrosis. On delayed enhanced images, infantile hemangiomas and hemangioendotheliomas show a characteristic persistent enhancement, a distinct feature compared with other liver tumors.

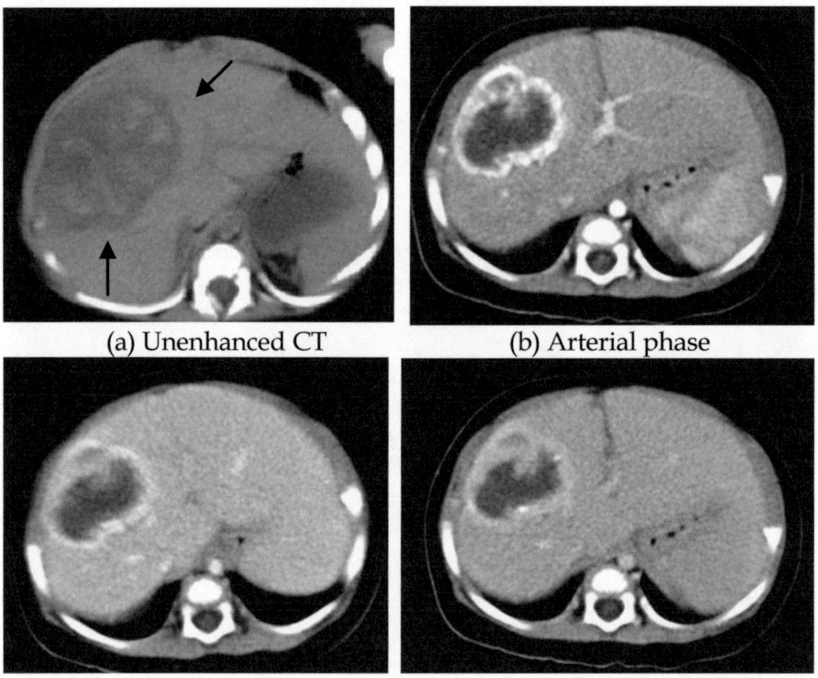

(a) Unenhanced CT (b) Arterial phase

(c) Portal venous phase (d) Delayed phase

Fig. 5. A 10-month-old girl with hemangioedothelioma . a Unenhanced axial CT slice with soft tissue window. The tumor (arrowheads) is seen as a well-defined, lobulated, low attenuation mass in the right lobe of the liver. Hyperintensity in the center of the lesion represents dystrophic calcification. b、c、d Contrast-enhanced CT showsr peripheral rim enhancement and persistent enhancement on delayed phase.

3.2.2 Mesenchymal hamartoma

It is the second most common benign hepatic lesion in the perinatal period. It is seen usually in children less than 2 years of age with a male:female ratio of 2:1. The tumor arises from mesenchymal tissue around the portal tract. Grossly, the lesion is not encapsulated and is typically composed of multiple cysts, filled with clear or mucoid fluid. (Stringer & Alizai, 2005; Chang et al,2006). CT images show a multilocular low-attenuation cystic mass with enhancing septae and stroma (Fig. 6). Calcification is generally not seen.

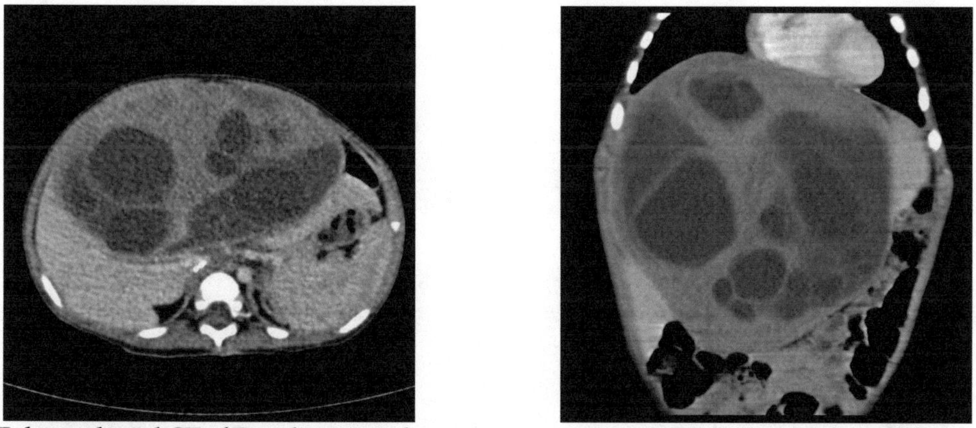

(a) Enhanced axial CT of Portal venous phase (b) Coronal reformats

Fig. 6. Huge mesenchymal hamartoma in a 12-month-old boy. a Enhanced axial CT shows multilocular low-attenuation cystic mass with enhancing septae and stroma. b On coronal reformats the mass was noted to occupy large areas in the abdomen

3.2.3 Hepatic adenomas

Adenomas are rare in the pediatric population. They are usually seen in teenagers with a female preponderance. They may be seen in patients with glycogenstorage diseases. Histologically, adenomas present as encapsulated, rounded masses, which consist of hepatocytes, Kupffer cells, rudimentary portal tracts and distorted biliary elements. The Kupffer cells in adenomas have a decreased or absent phagocytic activity, This is a distinctive feature compared with FNHs. CT demonstrates an isodense or slightly hypodense mass with a well-defined border due to the presence of a capsule. Hemorrhage may lead to a heterogeneous appearance. Adenomas typically show an early arterial enhancement followed by a rapid wash-out on enhanced CT.(Fig.7)

4. The value of CT scan in guiding the surgical treatment

For most hepatic malignancies, complete tumor resection or liver transplantation is essential for cure. Types of liver resection performed include left lobectomy; left lateral segmentectomy; right lobectomy; or trisegmentectomy (right lobe and medial segment of the left lobe). Therefore, a mass must be confined to the left or right lobe or the right lobe plus the medial segment of the left lobe to be considered resectable. If a lesion does not meet anatomic requirements for resectability at initial imaging, the child is often initially treated with chemotherapy, with or without radiation, and then re-imaged. Therefore, proper imaging of the liver is necessary and can shorten the surgical duration and increase the accuracy of the resection (Kinoshita et al.,2009; Dong et al.,2007)

The major role of liver imaging is to define accurately the extent of the lesion in relation to hepatic lobar anatomy and vascular and biliary structures for preoperative planning and to

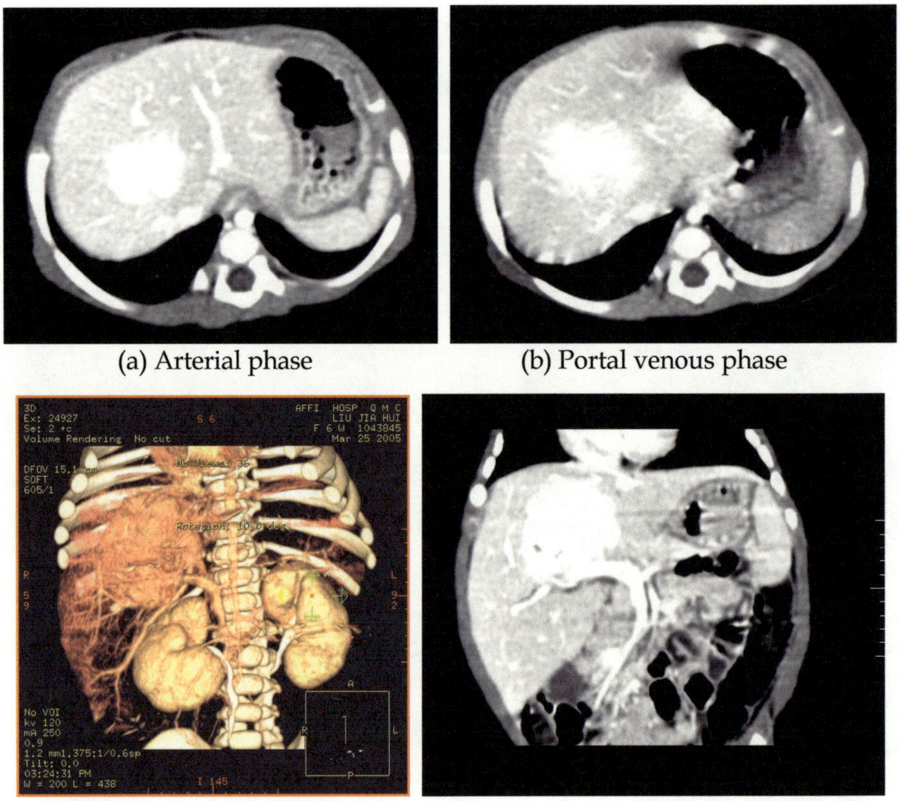

(a) Arterial phase (b) Portal venous phase

(c) Volume rendering(VR) (d)Coronal reformats

Fig. 7. A 3-year-old girl with hepatic adenomas Contrasted CT scans show an early arterial enhancement followed by a rapid wash-out on enhanced CT.

monitor tumor response to chemotherapy or radiation. Worldwide, computed tomography (CT) is undoubtedly the most frequently used diagnostic tool in the radiologist's armamentarium for studying the liver. The development and rapid clinical acceptance of single-detector helical (spiral) computed tomography (HCT) during the last decade and, more recently, the introduction of multidetector CT (MDCT) have resulted in significantly improvements of the ability to study the liver. In addition to technical advances, such as shorter scanning times, multiplanar imaging, and improved ability to perform multiphasic contrast-enhanced studies, newer and better intravenous contrast media and advances in postacquisition data processing techniques have renewed the enthusiasm for using hepatic CT scanning(Kinoshita et al.,2009;Frericks et al.,2004).(Fig.8)

Before the application of the three-dimensional imaging with spiral CT, angiography was the most common imaging approach to determine tumor location and relation to blood vessels. However, the invasiveness and the need for anesthesia limit the use of the approach. Although these scans may roughly determine the size and location of the tumor, the precise location of the tumor in relation to crucial blood vessels cannot always be accurately assessed. Therefore, the surgeon relies heavily upon surgical exploration; because one-stage resection cannot be guaranteed, some parents decline the treatment.

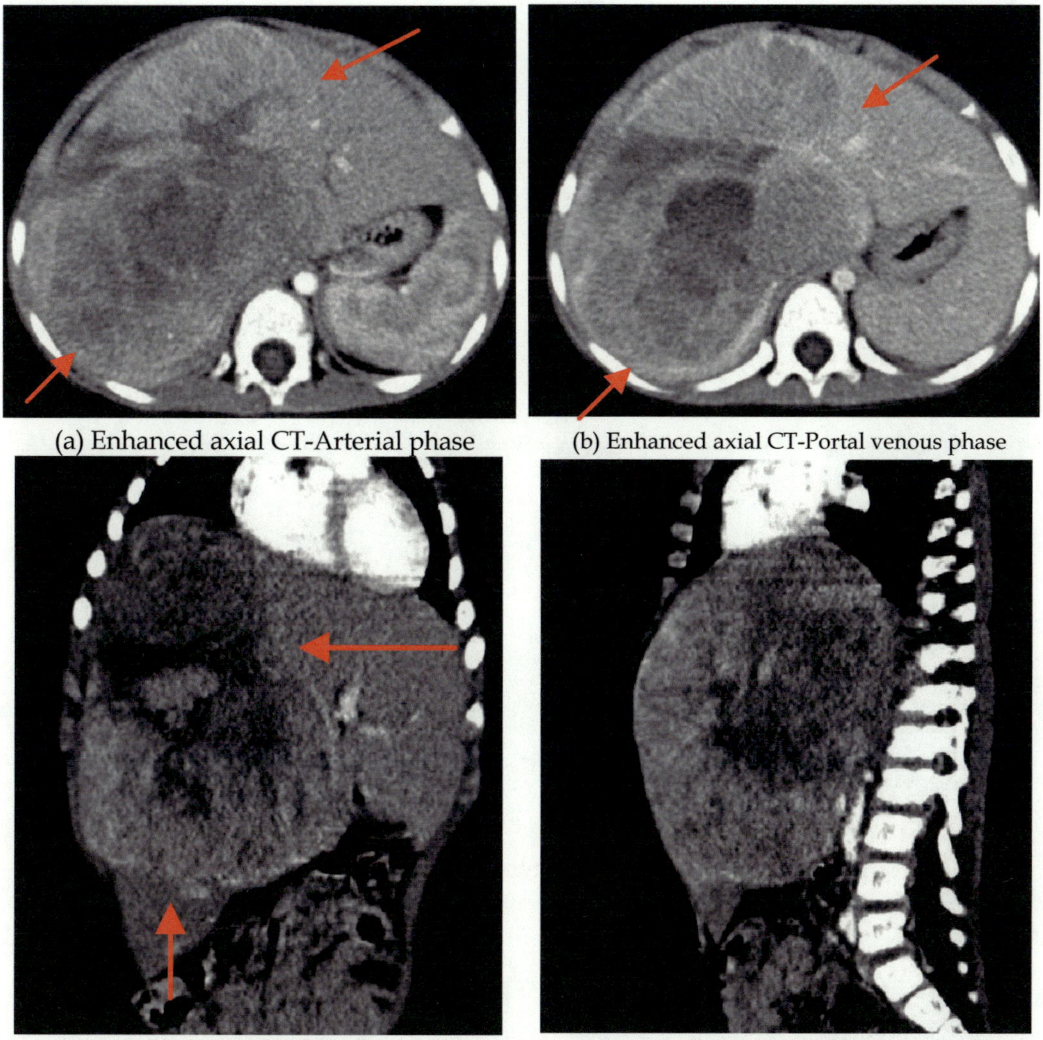

(a) Enhanced axial CT-Arterial phase

(b) Enhanced axial CT-Portal venous phase

(c) Coronal reformat

(d) Sagittal reformat

Fig. 8. Multiplanar imagings can show the extent of the lesion accurately(red arrowheads).

MDCT makes it possible to image the precise vascular anatomy including the anomalous branches, feeding arteries, or drainage veins (Kinoshita et al.,2009; Dong et al.,2007). the reconstructed images from MDCT were never inferior to those obtained by angiography. Therefore, when a chemoembolization by TACE is not necessary, this MDCT reconstruction is considered to provide a sufficient evaluation of the vessels. On the other hand, each image phase (arterial phase, equilibrium phase, portal phase) could be independently and simultaneously extracted or combined, respectively (Nievelstein RA et al.,2010). (Fig.9) (Fig.10) (Fig.11)

Furthermore, the software program for volumetry provides a proposed remnant liver volume and an optimal cut line of the liver. Various preoperative simulations can thus be considered. This volumetric analysis positively contributes to the safety of the procedure by assisting in the selection of the optimal operations.

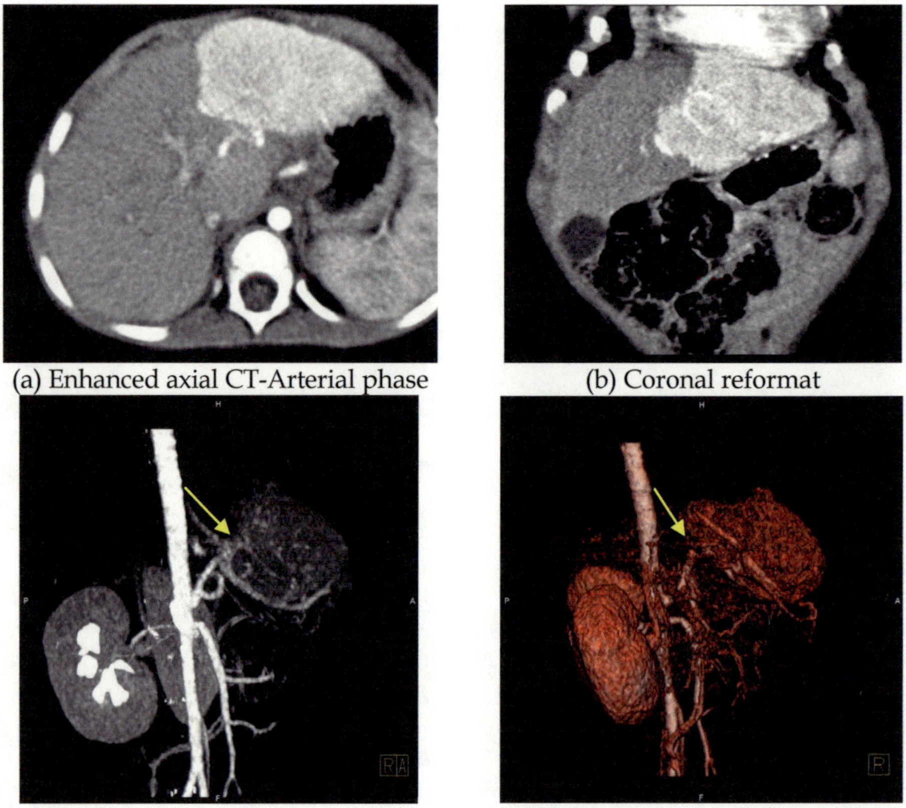

(a) Enhanced axial CT-Arterial phase (b) Coronal reformat

(c) Three-dimensional imaging (d) Three-dimensional imaging

Fig. 9. Multiplanar imagings can show the extent of the lesion accurately(a、b); The feeding artery of the tumor and its anomalous branches are detected by 3-D reconstruction images(yellow arrowheads). (c、d).

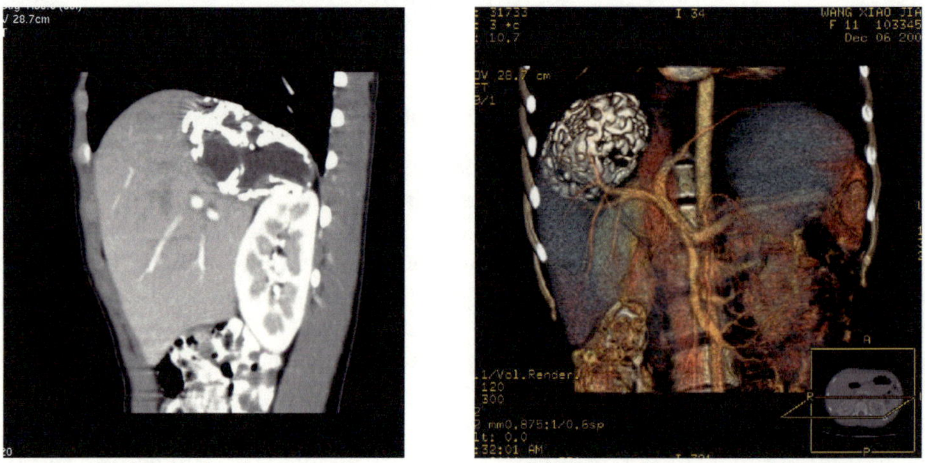

(a) Sagittal reformat (b) Three-dimensional imaging

Fig. 10. Multiplanar imaging and three-dimensional imagingshow the tumor very clear.

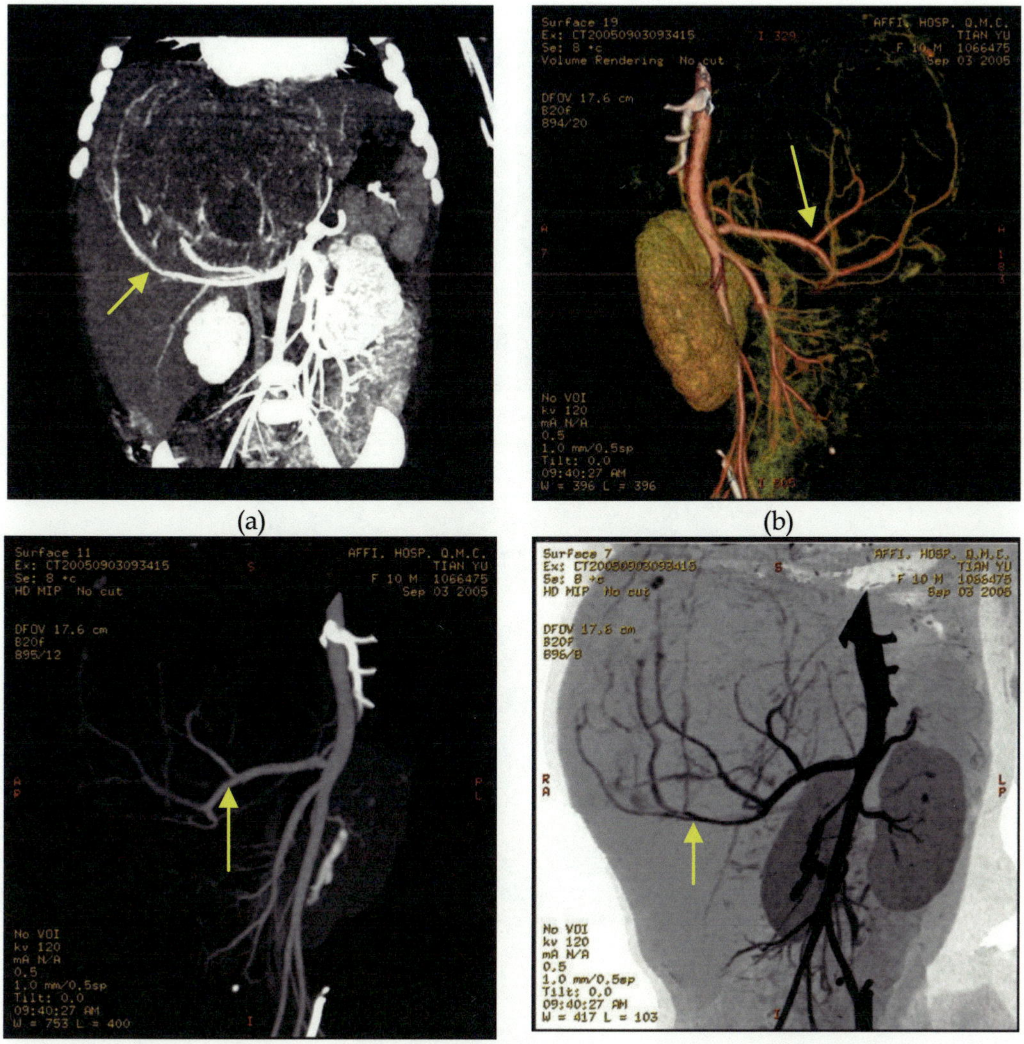

(a) (b)

(c) (d)

Fig. 11. CT angiography shows the feeding artery of the tumor and its anomalous branches(yellow arrowheads).

5. Clinical applications of CT 3-D reconstruction imaging for diagnosis and surgery in children with large liver tumors or tumors at the hepatic hilum

Multidetector CT (MDCT) scanners has opened new chapters in 3D imaging. These advances were made possible by the rapid acquisition of volumetric data in the lower case z-axis using thin slices and improved rendering algorithms, which facilitate exquisite 3D reformats, devoid of degradation by respiration and other physiological movements. The pace of progress is being hastened with the rapid developments in MDCT technology.

Curing the patients with liver tumor and prolong survival are current principles for surgeon, complete tumor resection without liver dysfunction is essential, especially for

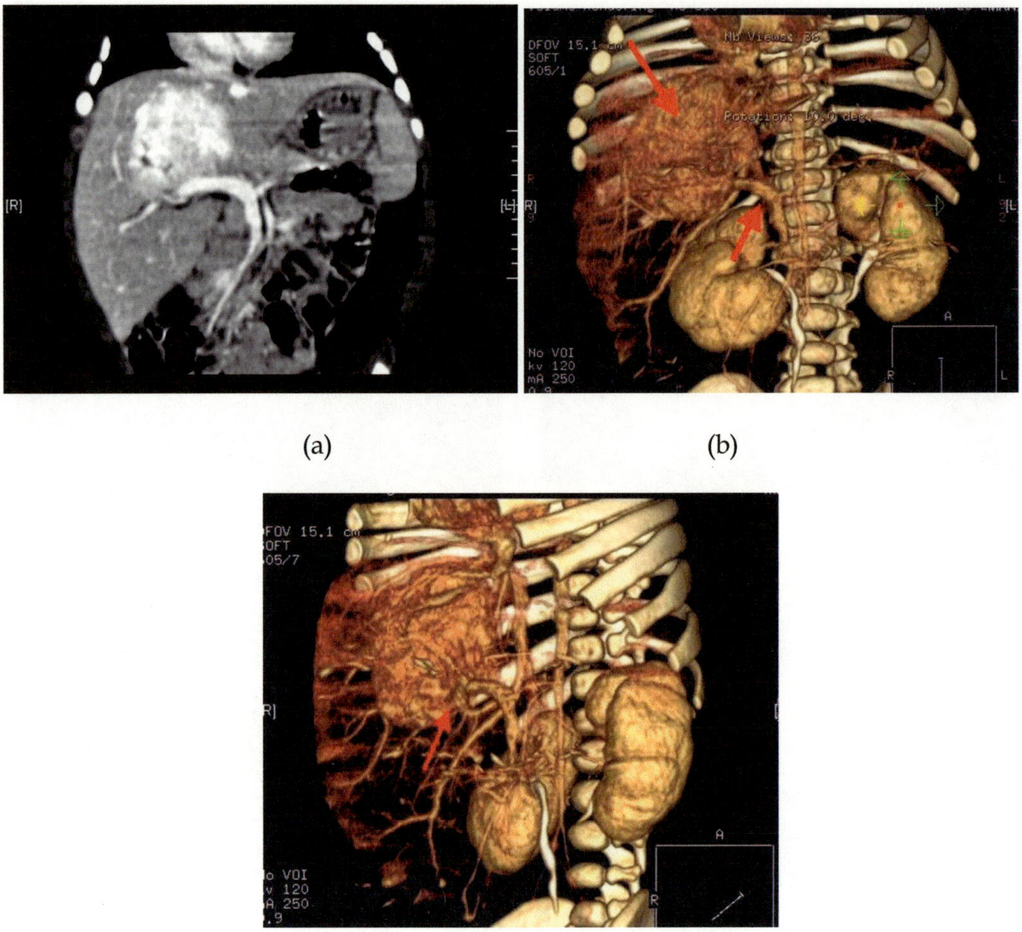

(a) (b) (c)

Fig. 12. a CT shows that the main portal vein is invaded by tumors at the hepatic hilum in the middle lobe. b CT 3-D imaging shows the margins of the tumors and their relationships with hepatic vessels. The arrows indicate tumors situated near the portal vein or in the middle lobe. The frontal (anteroposterior) image suggests that the main portal vein is completely embedded by the tumor. c After dynamically rotating the CT 3-D images, the branches arising from the main portal vein posterior to the tumor deviated from the tumor, indicating possible preservation of the main portal vein. This suggests that CT 3-D imaging could be used to guide the operation procedures

children with liver tumors. However, maintaining the integrity of hepatic blood vessels is a prerequisite for a successful resection, and this process is more difficult when the tumor is exceedingly large or located close to major hepatic vessels. Therefore, proper imaging of the liver is necessary and can shorten the surgical duration and increase the accuracy of the resection. Three-dimensional images can display the location of the tumor relative to blood vessels. In particular, rotatable dynamic images clearly illustrate the path and location of important blood vessels, thus facilitate surgical approach to the location of the tumor and determine the incision line. To some extent, three-dimensional imaging is superior to conventional enhanced CT imaging, particularly in helping the surgeon evaluate the feasibility of one-stage resection. For example, as shown in Fig.12, the tumor located at the hepatic hilum involving with the trunk of the portal vein, which may preclude a one-stage operation. Nevertheless, after dynamically rotating the three-dimensional CT images, we were able to see that a ramification originated from the trunk of the portal vein behind the tumor and leave away from the tumor; therefore, the trunk of portal vein could be reserved (Kinoshita et al..2009; Dong et al, 2007, Dong et al.,2009).

6. Conclusions

CT has always played a major role in the imaging of the liver. The development of multidetector row CT (MDCT) technology has helped CT to continue to excel in its already established indications (ie, hepatic lesion detection and characterization) and to add new clinical indications (ie, CT angiography, three-dimensional imaging). For children with liver tumors, proper imaging can shorten the surgical duration and increase the accuracy of the resection, especially using. three-dimensional images.

However, a major drawback of MDCT is the use of ionising radiation and, consequently, the risks of radiation-induced side effects. Therefore, reducing the radiation dose and its associated risks in children should be one of the major goals of the (paediatric) radiologist.

7. References

American Society of Anesthesiologists Task Force. (1996). Practice guidelines for sedation and analgesia by non-anesthesiologist: a report by the American Society of Anesthesiologists Task Force on sedation and analgesia by non-anesthesiologists. Anesthesiology,84:459–471.

Aytekin, Oto., Eric, P.& Tamm, Janio Szklaruk.(2005) Multidetector Row CT of the Liver,Radiol Clin N Am, 43 : 827 – 848.

Bae, KT.& Heiken, JP.(2005). Scan and contrast administration principles for MDCT, Eur Radiol,15 [suppl 5]:E46 –E59.

Bae, KT., Tao, C., Gurel, S., et al.(2007). Effect of patient weight and scanning duration on contrast enhancement during pulmonary multidetector CT angiography, Radiology,242 : 582–589.

Bae, KT., Shah, AJ., Shang, SS.et al.(2008). Aortic and hepatic contrast enhancement with abdominal 64-MDCT in pediatric patients: effect of body weight and iodine dose, AJR Am J Roentgenol, Nov;191(5):1589-94.

Bisset, GS III.& Ball, WS.(1991). Preparation, sedation and monitoring of the pediatric patient in the magnetic resonance suite, Semin Ultrasound CT MR,2:376–378.

Caoili, EM., Cohan, RH., Korobkin, M.; et al.(2002). Urinary tract abnormalities: initial experience with multi-detector row CT urography, Radiology,222:353–360.

Chang, HJ., Jin, SY., Park, C.; et al. (2006). Mesenchymal hamartomas of the liver: comparison of clinicopathologic features between cystic and solid forms, J Korean Med Sci ,21:63–68.

Cody, DD.(2002). AAPM/RSNA physics tutorial for residents: topics in CT. Image processing in CT, RadioGraphics,22:1255–1268.

Committee on Drugs, American Academy of Pediatrics. (1992).Guidelines for monitoring and management of pediatric patients during and after sedation for diagnostic and therapeutic procedures, Pediatrics,89:1110–1115.

Cote, CJ.(1994). Sedation for pediatric patient: a review, Pediatr Clin North Am,41:31–56.

Davey, MS.& Cohen, MD.(1996). Imaging of gastrointestinal malignancy in childhood, Radiol Clin North Am, 34:717-742.

Dong, Q., Xu, W., Jiang, B.; et al.(2007). Clinical application of computerized tomography 3-D reconstruction imaging for diagnosis and surgery in children with large liver tumors or tumors at the hepatic hilum, Pediatr Surg Int, 23: 1045-1050.

Dong ,Q., Jiang, B., Lu, Y.; et al.(2009). Surgical management of giant liver tumor involving the hepatic hilum of children, World J Surg, Jul;33(7):1520-1525.

Donnelly, LF.& Bisset GS III. (1998). Pediatric hepatic imaging. Radiol Clin North Am, 36:413–427.

Emre, S.& McKenna, GJ. (2004). Liver tumors in children, Pediatr Transplant,8:632–638.

Frericks, BB., Caldarone, FC., Nashan, B.; et al.(2004).3D CT modeling of hepatic vessel architecture and volume calculation in living donated liver transplantation,Eur Radiol, 14: 326-333.

Frush, DP., Bisset, GS III.& Hall, SC. (1996). Pediatric sedation in radiology: the practice of safe sleep, AJR,;167:1381–1387.

Frush, DP., Siegel, MJ.& Bisset, GS 3rd.(1997). From the RSNA refresher courses: challenges of pediatric spiral CT, RadioGraphics,17 : 939–959.

Frush, DP. (2008). MDCT in children: scan techniques and contrast issues. In: Kalra MK, Sanjay S, Rubin GD (eds) Multidetector CT: from protocols to practice, 1st edn. Springer Verlag, Heidelberg, pp 331–351.

Geleijns, J., Salvadó Artells, M., Veldkamp, WJH; et al. (2006). Quantitative assessment of selective in-plane shielding of tissues in computed tomography through evaluation of absorbed dose and image quality, Eur Radiol ,16:2334–2340.

Greenberg, M.& Filler, RM.(1997). Hepatic tumors. In: Pizzo PA, Poplack DG, eds. Principles and Practice of Pediatric Oncology, Philadelphia: Lippincott-Raven,717–732.

Helmberger, TK., Ros, PR., Mergo, PJ. et al. (1999). Pediatric liver neoplasms: a radiologic-pathologic correlation, Eur Radiol ,9:1339–1347.

Jha, P., Chawla, SC., Tavri, S.et al.(2009), Pediatric liver tumors--a pictorial review, Eur Radiol, Jan;19(1):209-219.

Kinoshita, Y., Souzaki, R., Tajiri, T.;et al..(2009). A preoperative evaluation for neo-infantile liver tumors using a three-dimensional reconstruction of multidetector row CT, Oncol Rep, Apr;21(4):881-886.

Krauss, B.& Green, SM. (2000). Sedation and analgesia for procedures in children, N Engl J Med, 342(13):938–945

Kuhn, JP., Slovis, TL., Haller, JO.et al. (2004). Caffey's pediatric diagnostic imaging, 10th edn. Mosby,Philadelphia.

Leswick, DA., Hunt, MM., Webster, ST; et al. (2008). Thyroid shields versus z-axis automatic tube current modulation for dose reduction at neck CT, Radiology, 249:572–580.

Maher, MM., Kalra, MK., Sahani, DV.et al,(2004).Techniques, clinical applications and limitations of 3D reconstruction in CT of the abdomen,. Korean J Radiol, Jan-Mar;5(1):55-67.

Nievelstein, RA., van Dam, IM.& van der Molen, AJ.(2010). Multidetector CT in children: current concepts and dose reduction strategies, Pediatr Radiol, Aug;40(8):1324-44.

Pereira, JK., Burrows, PE., Richards, HM.et al.(1993). Comparison of sedation regimens for pediatric outpatient CT, Pediatr Radiol,23:341–344.

Pobiel, RS.& Bisset, GS, 3rd.(1995).Pictorial essay: imaging of liver tumors in the infant and child, Pediatr Radiol,25(7):495-506.

Powers, C., Ros, PR., Stoupis, C.;et al. (1994). Primary liver neoplasm: MR imaging with pathologic correlation, Radiographics, 14: 459-482

Roche, KJ., Genieser, NB.& Ambrosino, MM. (1996).Pediatric hepatic CT: an injection rate, Radiology,26:502–507.

Roebuck, DJ.(2009). Assessment of malignant liver tumors in children,Cancer Imaging, Oct 2;9 Spec No A:S98-S103.

Sahani, D,, Saini, S., Pena, C., et al. (2002).Using multidetector CT for preoperative vascular evaluation of liver neoplasms: technique and results,AJR Am J Roentgenol Am J Roentgenol,179:53–59.

Scuza, RA.& Narla, LD.(1992). Primary endodermal sinus tumor of the liver detected by CT, Pediatr Radiol , 22:449–450.

Shankar, VR. (2008).Sedating children for radiological procedures: an intensivist's perspective, Pediatr Radiol, May;38 Suppl 2:S213-217.

Siegel, MJ. (1998).Protocols for helical CT in pediatrics. In: Silverman PM, ed. Helical (Spiral) Computed Tomography. Philadelphia: Lippincott-Raven:179–224.

Siegel, MJ.(1999). Liver and biliary tract. In: Siegel MJ, ed. Pediatric Body CT. Philadelphia: Lippincott Williams & Wilkins;:141–174(a).

Siegel, MJ.(1999). Practical CT techniques In: Siegel MJ, ed. Pediatric Body CT. Philadelphia: Lippincott Williams & Wilkins:1–41(b).

Siegel, MJ.(2001). Pediatric liver imaging,Semin Liver Dis,May;21(2):251-269.

Siegel, MJ., Chung, EM.& Conran, RM.(2008). Pediatric liver: focal masses,Magn Reson Imaging Clin N Am, Aug;16(3):437-452.

Siegel ,MJ. (2008).Practical CT techniques. In: Siegel MJ (ed) Pediatric body CT, 2nd edn. Lippincott Williams & Wilkins, Philadelphia, pp 1–32.

Strain, JD., Campbell, JB., Harvey, LA.et al.(1988). IV Nembutal: safe sedation for children undergoing CT, AJR, 151:955–959.

Stringer, MD.& Alizai, NK. (2005). Mesenchymal hamartoma of the liver: a systematic review, J Pediatr Surg ,40:1681–1690.

Taghon, TA., Bryan, YF.& Kurth, CD. (2006). Pediatric radiology sedation and anesthesia, Int Anesthesiol Clin, 44:64–79.

Vollmar, SV.& Kalender, WA. (2008).Reduction of dose to the female breast in thoracic CT: a comparison of standard-protocol, bismuthshielded, partial and tube-current-modulated CT examinations, Eur Radiol,18:1674–1682

5

Cone-Beam Volumetric Imaging in Craniofacial Medicine

Corega Claudia, Avram Adrian,
Nocini Pier Francesco and Bertossi Dario
*Eberhardt-Karls University, Iuliu Hatieganu University,
University of Verona Germany, Romania,
Italy*

1. Introduction

Few new technological developments have revolutionized medical diagnostics as extensively as has x-ray technology. Even before Wilhelm Conrad Rontgen officially announced his discovery on December 28, 1895, it was used among others by the Austrian physician Guido Holzknecht.

With the development of x-ray computered tomography (CT) in the 1960s and its first use for clinical studies in 1972 by Sir Godfrey Hounsfield, radiological tomography attained widespread use and today is one of the essential imaging techniques in medical radiology. It is a technically mature and clinically widely accepted method and complements classical x-ray panoramic radiography in many areas.

The development of spiral CT and the introduction of multislice detector systems in 1998 further accelerated CT techniques and led to the ability to acquire volume data.

A subsequent development of CT technology, digital volume tomography, as we will refer to it in this bookchapter has been established in recent years. The technology is frequently used in craniofacial radiology because of its characteristic low radiation dose (1-2), high spatial resolution and lower cost compared with CT. Its technology and a lot of possible applications in craniofacial medicine are discussed in this chapter.

Currently voxel-based craniofacial medicine and surgery are becoming increasingly popular. Furthermore they are a popular tool for diagnosing, planning, monitoring and evaluation of craniofacial morphology, growth and various treatment procedures.

The aim of this work is:

a. to describe the principles of Cone-Beam Tomography
b. to make a brief description of the existing CBCT devices.
c. to highlight the use of 3D diagnosis in craniofacial medicine.

2. Principles of cone-beam tomography

Image reconstruction in modern computed-assisted imaging techniques such as magnetic resonance imaging (MRI), single-photon emission CT (SPECT) and positron emission tomography (PET) is based on mathematical algorithms that permit axial tomographic imaging of the human body without superimpositioning. The progressive development of

detector technology and reconstruction mathematics and the reduction of radiation exposure have allowed the generation of increasing numbers of single-slice images, particularly in CT.
In contrast to the classical process of radiology, where a single slice is sharply imaged but all other layers in the beam path overlay the desired image, the digital imaging process of CT permits the use of computer-supported reconstruction algorithms to generate image slices of the human body without superimpositions. (El-Mohri,Y et al.,2011)
This is always based on the superimposition-free measurement of the distribution of a tissue layer in a transverse slice. Integrals are measured over this distribution along curves. The separation of the individual slices is performed by the measurement process itself: that is, focus and detector are always in the plane of the slice to be examined, and the electromagnetic beam scans only this slice. Consequently, image reconstruction in the CT process is a two-dimensional issue.
This 2 D issue generates a 3D image and this reconstruction algorithm is based on the one developed by Feldkamp in 1984. The radiation doses are also measured in Sievert or microSievert. Koyama et al.,2010 demonstrated that a conventional CT multislice acquisition is 1,5 to 12,3 times the dose of a CBCT, which equals to 3 -5 panoramic x-rays. (Table 1).

Panoramic x-ray	2,9-9,6
Maxillary CBCT	17,6-656,9
Mandibular CBCT	124,9-250,3
TOTAL	145,4-916,8
CT	50,3

Table 1. Radiation doses in microsievert for various conventional X-ray versus CBCT

These doses are extremely lower if compared to a conventional CT. Expecially in orthodontics and maxillo-facial and plastic surgery there is always a need for a combination of CT scans, panoramic and cephalograms, and this can be nowadays achieved in a single step with the CBCT machine. (Kaeppler, 2010)

3. CBCT devices

The first CBCT machine was a fixed unit and its introduction opened new horizons in the craniofacial medicine. In the operating theaters the use of a CBCT has been restricted to a few cases due to the lack of space for such a machine or due to the efforts required by patient transportation for the image acquisition, not always possible in various pathology.
Once this fixed CT unit has been developed for the craniofacial medicine, the work has been proceeding on a mobile 3D imaging system for use in the operating room. Such a system coupled to a navigation system would be helpful in shortening procedures and preventing complications in complex surgical procedures of the visceral and osseous cranium. This problem was solved by the introduction of CBVI (cone-beam volumetric imaging) into mobile C-arms and permits the integration of the most current Newtom 5G (QR Verona Systems, Italy), Galileos (Sirona, Germany), BrainLAB (USA), Medtronic (USA), Praxim and Stryker (USA) navigation systems. This digital volume tomography with mobile C-arms requires less space, effort and provides better patient access than conventional intraoperatory CT scans.

4. 3D Diagnosis in craniofacial medicine

In pre- and postnatal development, malformations can affect any part of the head and neck. These malformations can have a genetic or environmental etiology and their diagnosis is of great importance for the dental practitioners. An extensive study of the anatomical features of malformations, possible due to the reduced amount of radiontions produced by CBCT, can be useful both for therapeutical and research purpose, providing the basis for a successful treatment plan and setting the anatomical landmarks that may recur in syndromes. (Bamgbose et al.,2008)

4.1 Abnomalies in tooth number and morphology

These abnormalities justify the use of radiological images in the dental and jaw region but results must be always compared with the clinical findings.

The dental practitioners' task is to correctly assess the information that is obtained in the images in order to set up the necessary therapeutic procedures. The 3D CBCT images supply the additional information and allow a more accurate treatment planning so that the dentist can define the appropriate therapeutic procedures; very often, in fact, radiological findings may significantly differ from the clinical findings, resulting in remarkable changes in clinical treatment planning. (Song et al., 2010)

4.2 Various manifestations of eruption disturbances

Eruption disturbances require an accurate determination of tooth position relative to the adjacent anatomical structures. 3D Diagnosis facilitates this task and also allows a prognosis regarding the course of continuing therapy. In orthodontic treatment planning, the assessment of the position and degree of teeth impaction and ankylosis, bone quality and the spatial relationships with the adjacent dental structures permits a prognosis for the successful orthodontic adjustments. The extent of the surgery required in some cases in order to facilitate the eruption or for extraction purposes can be determined given the characteristics of the malformation (e.g. ankylosis), thus assessing the operative risk. By means of accurate CBCT metric diagnosis, surgery can be optimally prepared and the surgical access can be planned to protect tissue. Depending on the degree of displacement, navigation-guided surgery can be used for a minimally invasive surgical approach. The resulting spatial orientation shortens the surgical time and reduces the degree of postoperative symptoms. In Figure 1 and 2 one might notice the third molar impaction in panoramic digital imaging extracted from CBCT and detail (slice). (Becker et al., 2010)

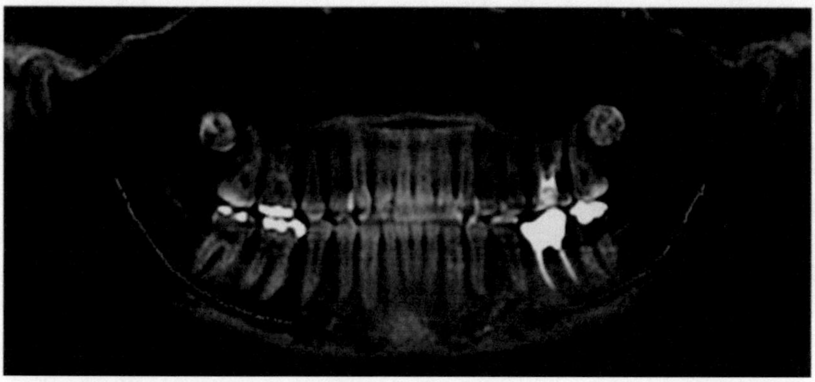

Fig. 1. Third molar impaction in the maxilla

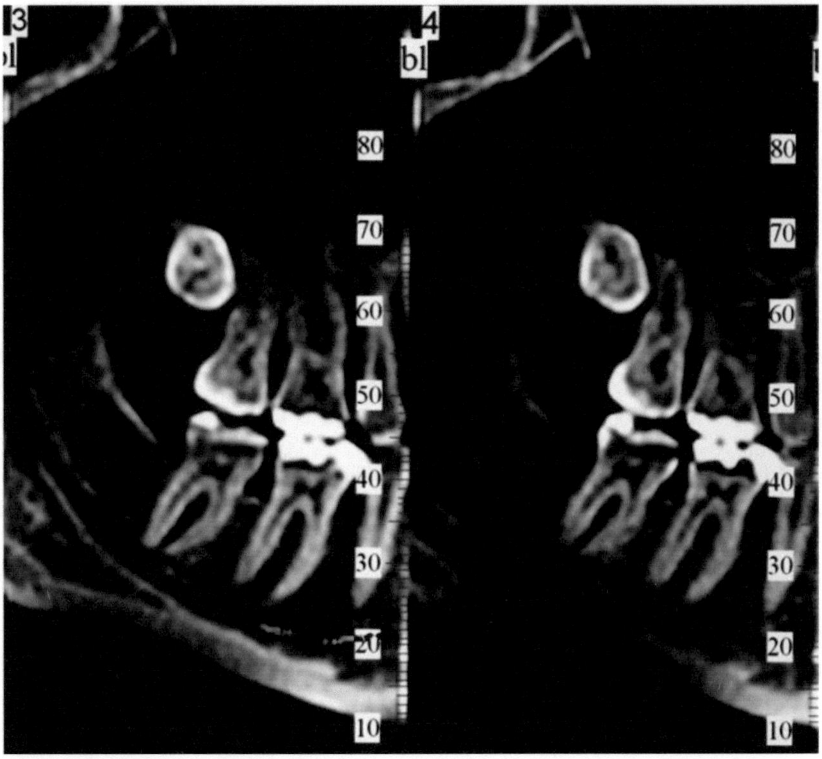

Fig. 2. Third molar impaction (slice detail)

4.3 Cystic changes in the maxilla and the mandible, non-neoplastic lesions, diseases of the maxillary sinus, diseases of the salivary glands, malignant and non-malignant tumors of the maxilla and the mandible

The broad spectrum of these lesions require precise radiodiagnostic assessment. CBCT permits the individual selection of the planes, meeting the demand for dynamic multiplanar imaging without distortions. In particular, the channel of the inferior alveolar nerve relative to a cyst or a tumor can be visualized with sufficient accuracy for planning mandibular surgery. Given the high contrast of the pathological proceses of the maxilla, CBCT is highly suitable for maxillary sinus diagnosis. Although MRI may be more effective in analyzing the bony and soft tissues involvement in this cathegory of pathologies, the details that CBCT can provide concerning the peculiarities of the inferior alvolar nerve are hardly matched by other methods of investigation, regardless of the possible artifacts that may occur due to the interference of dental materials (Rosenberg et al., 2010). Fig 3 and 4 highlight the distance from a cystic lesion in a Gorlin-Goltz syndrome to the inferior alveolar nerve , thus facilitating the surgical approach.

4.4 Periodontal diseases and preprosthetic surgery

CBCT assists in evaluating and analyzing tridimensionally a periodontal disease as well as the preprosthetic surgery situation. Intraosseous defects with one, two, three walls can be distinguished and furcation involvement can be classified. CBCT images are more likely to correspond with the clinical situation for horizontal and vertical bone loss. Unusual features

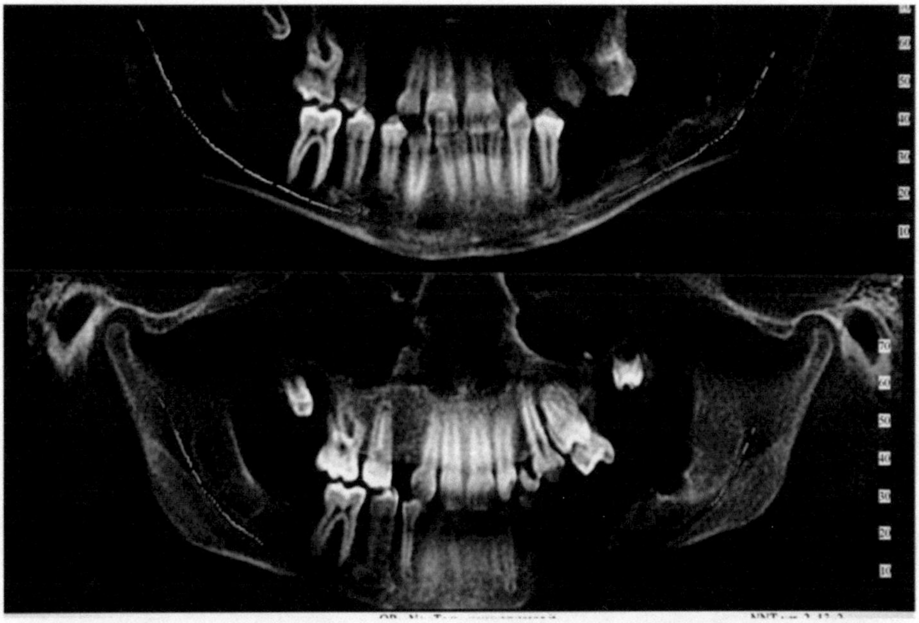

Fig. 3. Distance between the cyst and alveolar nerve in a Gorlin Gotz syndrome

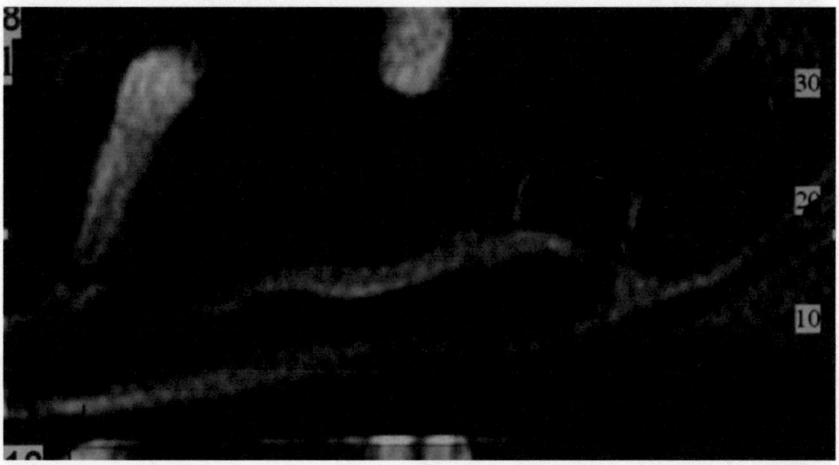

Fig. 4. The distance between the cyst and alveolar nerve in a Gorlin Gotz syndrome (detail)

are more readily identified and localized by radiology and it is more likely to estimate the real dimensions of the defect precisely prior to the surgical procedures, thus conferring to the surgeon a considerable advantage in terms of treatment planning and prevention of complications. The same is for wider bone defects, in which we can observe exactly the mandibular nerve and the maxillary sinuses as welll as transverse defects which have to be treated with expansion or grafts without any distortion (Danfort et al., 2010, Heiland et al., 2008, Boeddinghaus et al., 2008).

Maxillary and mandibular bone atrophy is accurately visualised on a 3D reconstruction or in CBCT slices (Fig.5 and 6). The clinical situation after bone grafting is revealed in the same

projection postoperatively (Fig. 7 and 8). Also CBCT slices reveal details about the extent of mandibular atrophy and the position of the inferior alveolar nerve.
CBCT is used more and more in implant surgery in order to acquire detailed anatomical informations, to produce a 3D stereolitographic model and finally to generate the surgical guide.

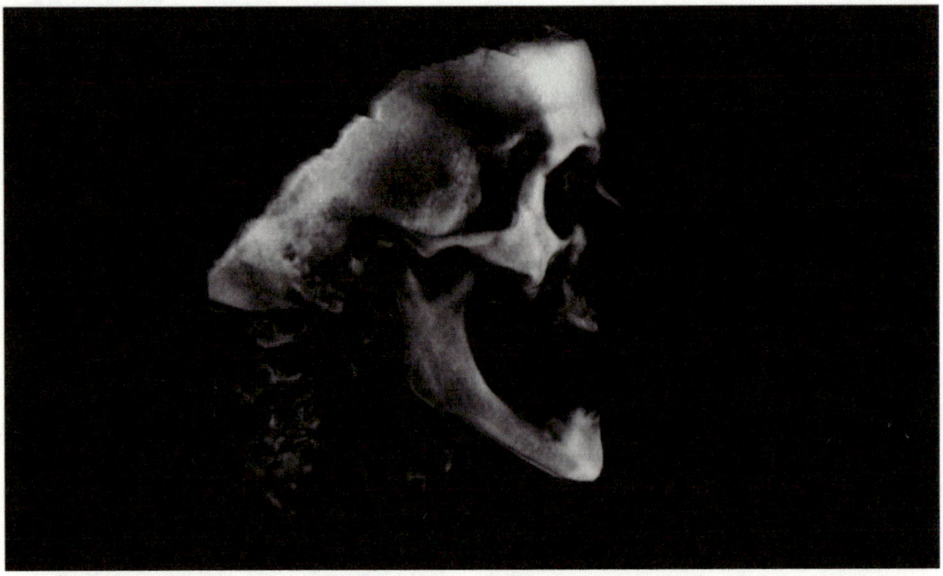

Fig. 5. Maxillary and mandibulary bone atrophy- 3D reconstruction

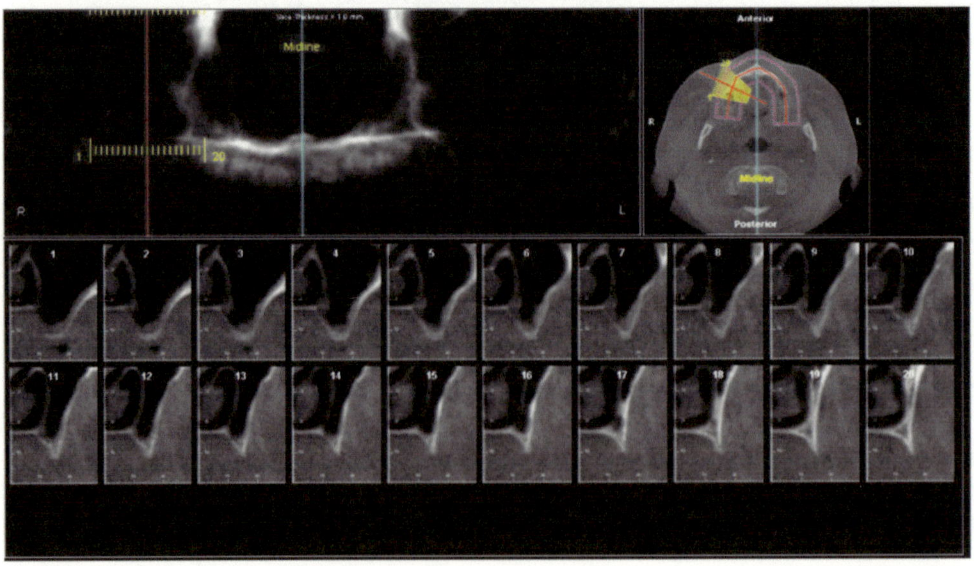

Fig. 6. Bone atrophy of the maxilla (detail)

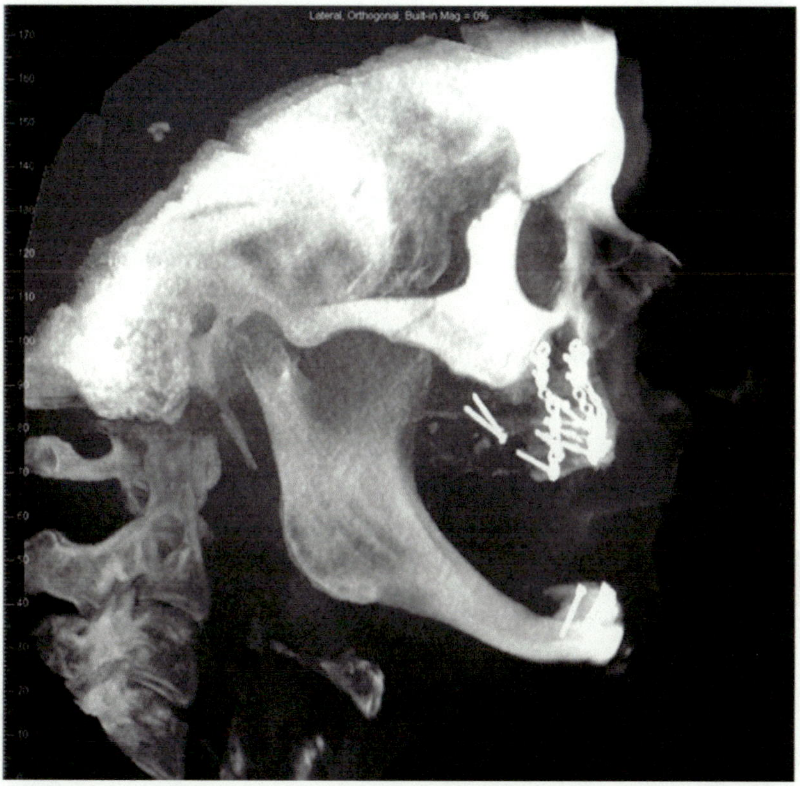

Fig. 7. 3D Reconstruction of the clinical situation after bimaxillary bone grafting

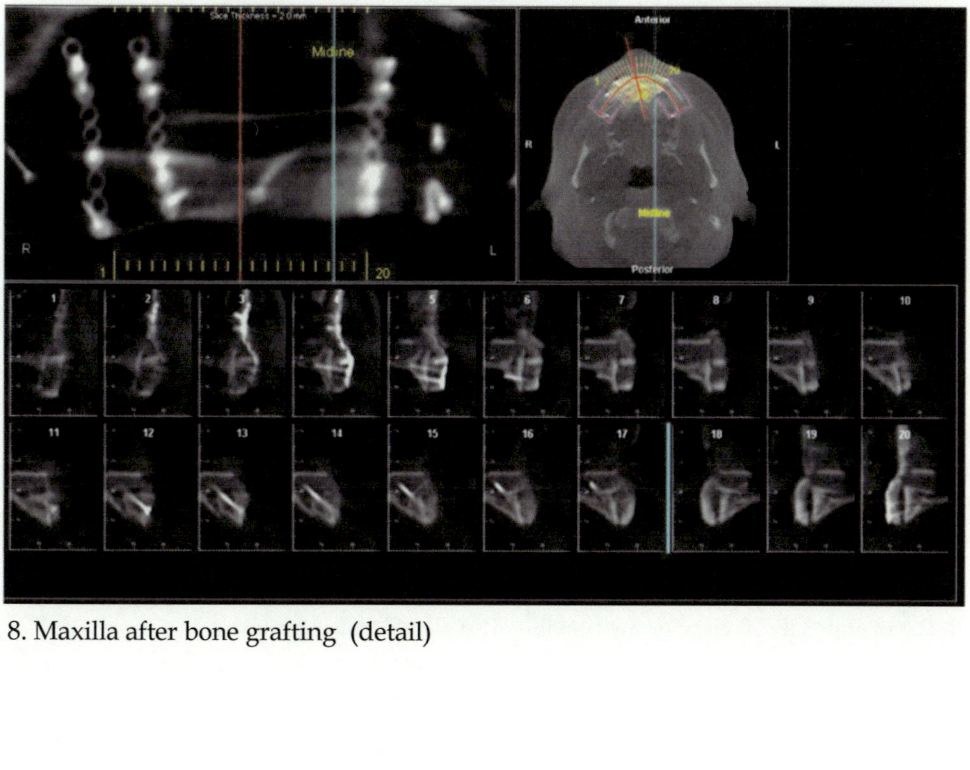

Fig. 8. Maxilla after bone grafting (detail)

4.5 Orthodontic diagnosis and treatment planning

Malocclusions can involve a deviation in tooth position as well as sagittal, vertical and transverse changes in the positional relationship between maxilla and mandible. Each malocclusion can derive from functional, dentoalveolar and skeletal changes. The individual findings obtained in orthodontics permit the establishment of a differential diagnosis and the combination of the individual findings into an overall orthodontic summary, which can be addressed in orthodontic therapy.

Radiographic 3D diagnosis provides the orthodontist with information that might greatly influence the treatment plan. Dentoalveolar malpositions in mesiodistal or buccolingual directions can be precisely evaluated and taken into account in therapeutic planning. Furthermore, the cause of malpositions of groups of teeth can be identified with 3D diagnostics. Both 3D reconstructions of the skull and bidimensional projections can be achieved from a single radiographic exam, with a lower x-ray dose and a more natural shape of soft-tissue facial mask. When examinating skeletal deviations, 3D visualization offers new possibilities for evaluating craniofacial structures and will allow a more precise differential diagnosis in the future. Given all the previous considerations and the great values of the achievable data, it is possible to substain that the use of CBCT as gold-standard for the analysis of the cranio-maxillo-facial region in orthognathic surgery is desirable, since it will permit to merge the advantages of traditional cephalometric studies and new databases that can be developed from the volumetric data collectable (Lyoid et al., 2011, Tucker et al., 2010, Swennen et al., 2009).

A 3D shot of the postsurgical position of the upper maxilla after a Le Fort I osteotomy is possible due to the panoramic view and through a 3D reconstruction based on the CBCT acquisition.

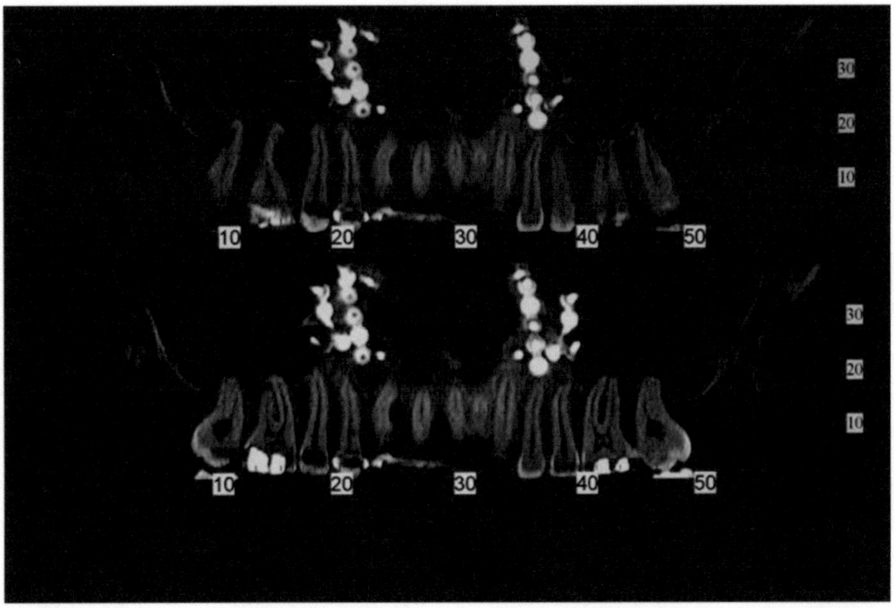

Fig. 9. Panoramic CBCT view of the maxilla after a Le Fort I osteotomy

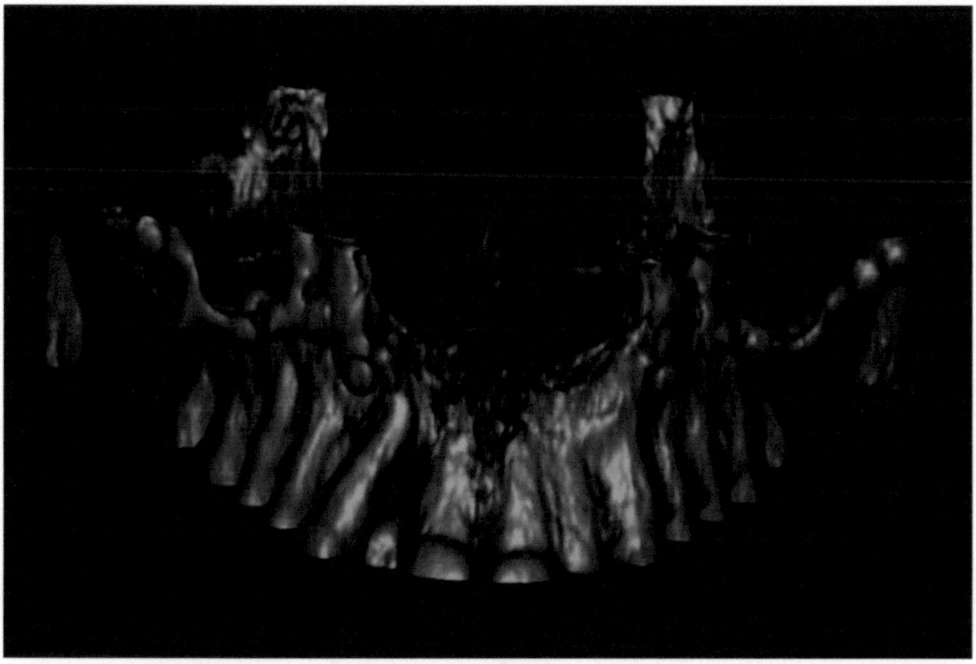

Fig. 10. 3 D view of the maxilla after a Le Fort I osteotomy

4.6 Traumatology

Traumatology is an important part of the craniofacial pathology. Dentoalveolar injuries include tooth fractures and luxations as well as alveolar process fractures and are among the most frequent injuries in the oro-maxillofacial region. In addition to the clinical diagnosis, a 3D radiological diagnosis is also necessary. CBCT combines the three dimensions necessary for diagnostics with the information-rich OPG, displacing classic dental radiological techniques.

Midfacial fractures and mandible fractures require always a 3D radiological diagnosis, since even a combination of various conventional radiological procedures cannot display all fracture lines. CBCT is always preferred to CT, as the radiation exposure is lower. Although the CBCT is characterized by a low-contraxt resolution and MRI is still considered the gold standard for the study of soft tissues, the minor amount of radiation exposition and the lesser amount of artifacts due to foreign bodies make CBCT more and more preferred in this kind of pathologies (Melo et al., 2010).

4.7 Diseases of the TMJ

This type of pathology can affect different anatomical structures and hence different tisues. In contrast to most of the other disease of the maxillofacial region, a wide variety of imaging procedures can be used to visualize the affected structures. (Fig.11, Fig.12)

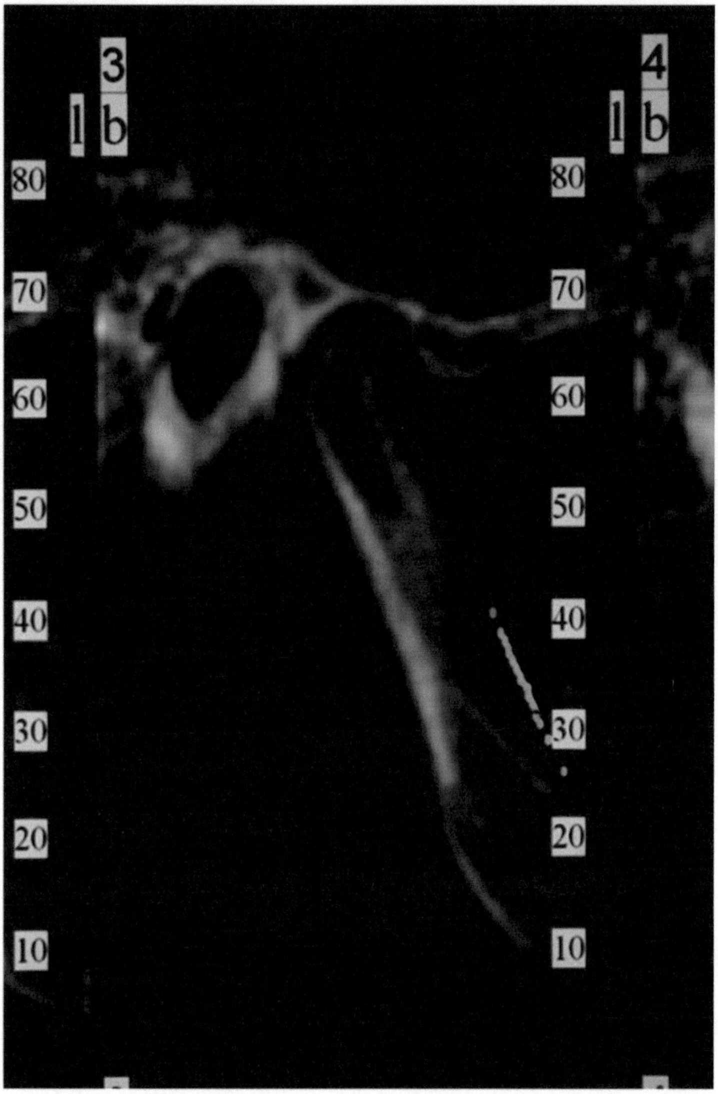

Fig. 11. TMJ arthritis

The use of CBCT allows osseous changes in the temporomandibular joint (TMJ) to be portrayed at a much higher sensitivity than the conventional radiological techniques. The advantages are a high resolution and the 3D nature of the image. The advent of the CBCT has substantially expanded the options for diagnosing TMJ joint disease, giving the maxillofacial and plastic surgeons access to 3D information of the region without requiring a radiologist in developmental, primary and secondary acquired diseases of the joint. Moreover, a joint study with CBCT and MRI technique may result in greater accuracy and better timing in diagnosis and treatment, resulting in greater recovery rate for the patient and a higher success rate for the clinician (Miloglu et al., 2011, Tecco et al., 2010). The position of the TMJ joint before and after orthognathic surgery can be visualized and measured on the CBCT scan.

4.8 Craniofacial malformations and syndromes (cleft lip and palate, genetic syndromes)

CBCT allows anatomically precise informations in 3D to be obtained regarding the type of cleft, the extent of defect and the residual defects after secondary osteoplasty. It also makes treatment planning more effective as the anatomical relations of the cleft are clearly apparent and easier to evaluate than 2D images.

Craniofacial asymmetries, the quality of the bone and the affected structures can be easily detected in CBCT images in various syndromes, thus enabling the orthodontist and the maxillofacial surgeons to establish the timing and the sequences for the specific treatment goals. Anatomical features and landmarks of rare syndromes can be studied and determined with greater precision, conferring on the clinician and on the researcher a valuable tool in terms of early diagnosis and prognosis of the functional recovery of the patient (Oberoi et al., 2010)

4.9 Maxillofacial and plastic computer-assisted surgery

In recent years, computer assisted surgical methods in the head and neck area have been continuously advanced. Initially optical navigation methods were the main focus. Clinical applications pertain nowadays to reconstructive and craniomaxillofacial surgery (CMF surgery).CMF planning modules facilitate a virtual 3D representation using CBVI and CBCT data sets. The diagnosis and examination of the facial asymmetries has been significantly simplified using the 3D imaging, moreover all surgical steps- maxillofacial and plastic procedures can be planned in a virtual environment. With the aid of bone- and tooth-supported cutting and drilling templates drafted on the computer, the so-called "surgi-guides" the results of the planning can be transferred exactly to the in vivo procedure. Surgical splints cand be produces using rapid prototyping. Plastic surgery procedures such as rhinoplasty can be also designed using the computer-assisted surgery and the CBCT images. The precision of CBCT and the development of more sophisticated software allowed the rehabilitation of extreme atrophies of the jaws, that would have had otherwise no surgical indication. In effect, only the joint work of the clinician, the radiologist and the technician can merge the surgical skills with the finest definition of the image and the mastery of an intraoperatory surgical guide, resulting in the minimization of the clinical failure and in the achievement of clinical success and patient satisfaction even in the most complicated cases. This model is applicable not only in oral surgery, but also in greater surgical reconstruction following oncological or traumatic injury, leaving the room for further technological improvement and for the development of new forms of interdisciplinary cooperation (Mischkowski et al., 2007).

The improvement in the airway diameter can be measured after rhinoplasty and also after soft palate surgical procedures in clefts surgical procedures in clefts.(Fig 12)

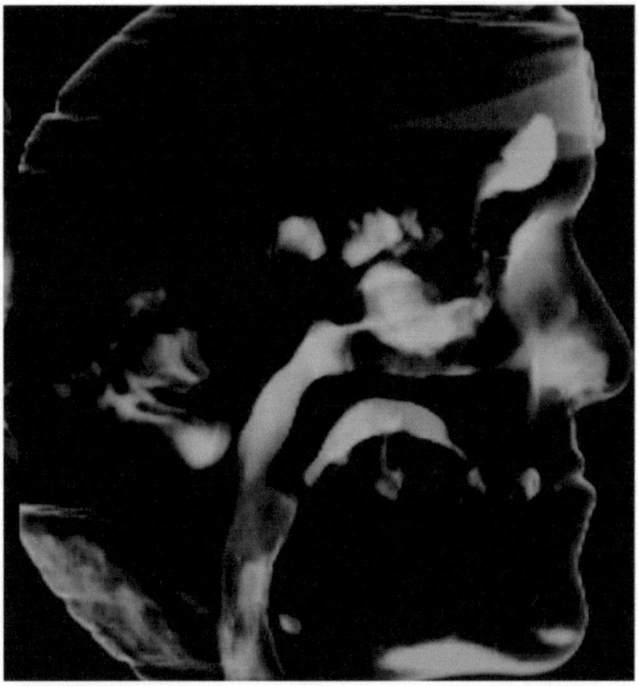

Fig. 12. Airway assesment on CBCT

A detailed surgical approach for functional nasal defects is easy to establish after a CBCT scan. Meanwhile the availability of nasal septal cartilage for grafting the secondary nose defects is extremely precise. (Fig 13, Fig 14).

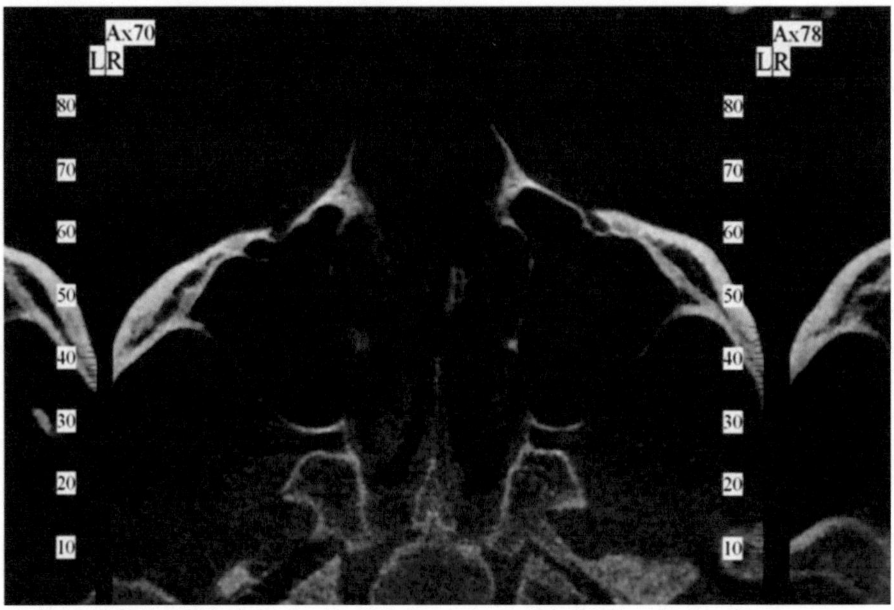

Fig. 13. Nasal septum analysis

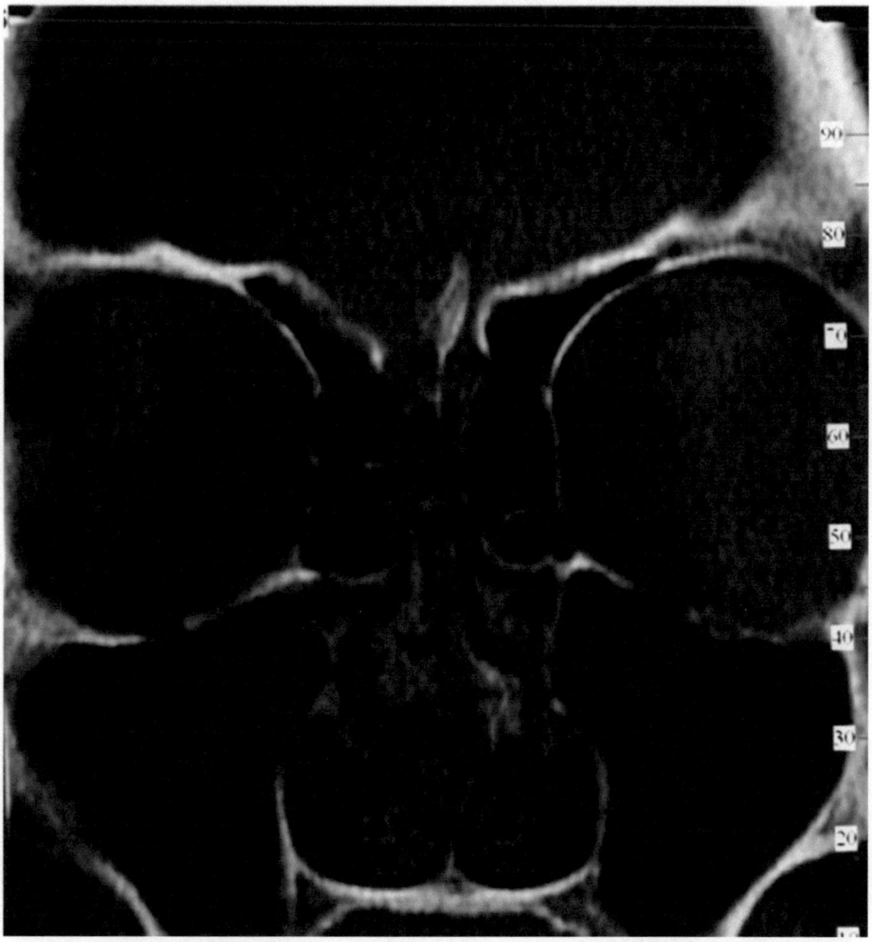

Fig. 14. Nasal septum deviation

The bone contours for cosmetic remodelling can be detected acurately on the CBCT slices. (Fig 15)

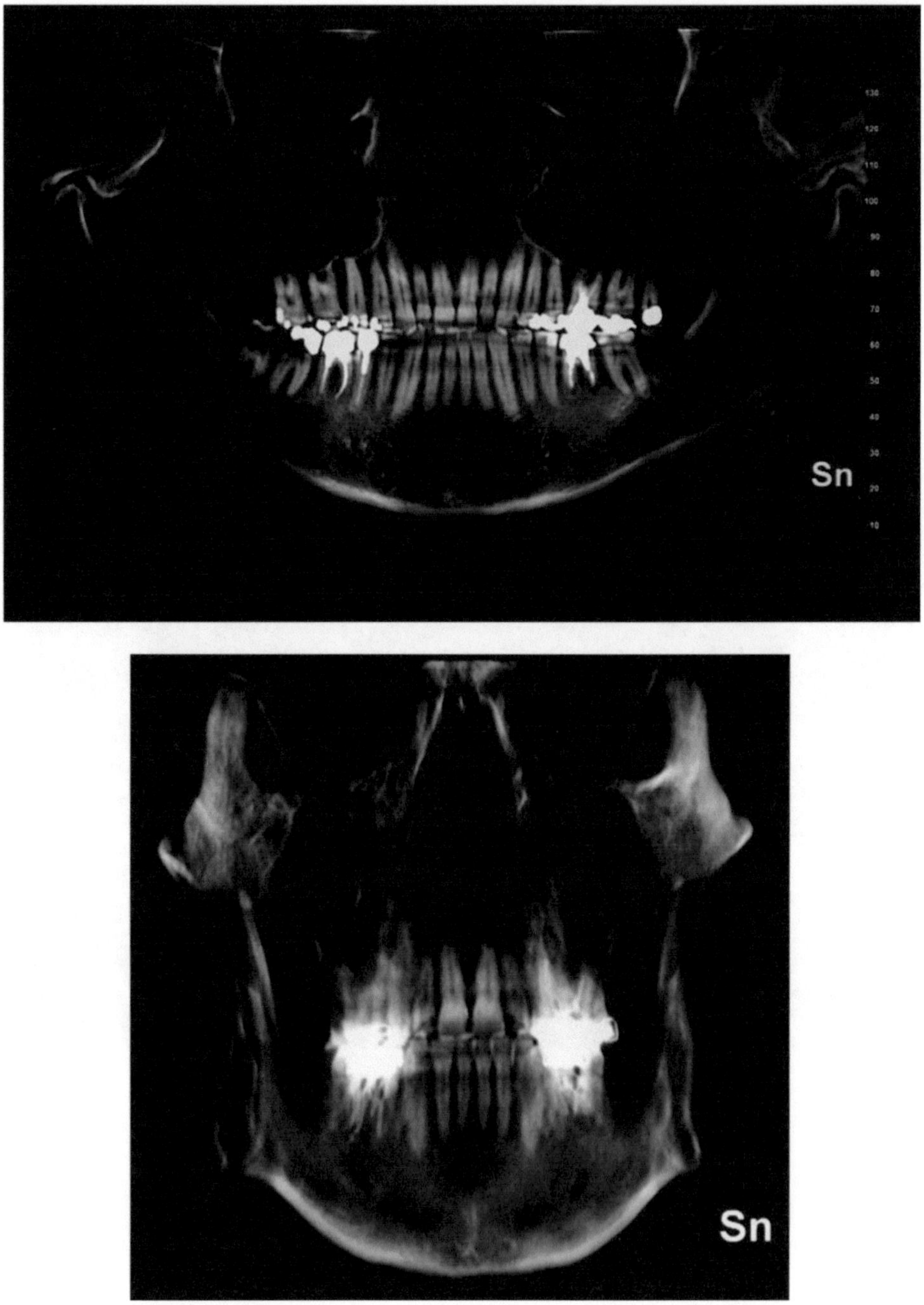

Fig. 15. Bone contours analysis for cosmetic remodelling

5. Conclusions

Modern 3D imaging with CBCT facilitates an exact diagnosis and evaluation of all craniofacial pathology and provides a precise tool for diagnosis, treatment planning, monitoring and evaluation of the underlying morphology, of the growth and various modern treatment procedures in dentistry, orthodontics, maxillofacial and plastic surgery. The huge margins of development for the technique and its possible applications in these fields are undoubtedly the forewords for further research and will result in greater advantages and tools for the clinician, with the ultimate increase in patient benefit.

6. References

Bamgbose, BO.; Adeyemo, WL.; Ladeinde, AL.; Ogunlewe, MO.(2008). Conebeam computed tomography (CBCT): the new vista in oral and maxillofacial imaging. *Nig Q J Hosp Med*. 2008 Jan-Mar;18(1):32-5

Becker, A.; Chaushu, S.; Casap-Caspi, N. (2010) .Cone-beam computed tomography and the orthosurgical management of impacted teeth. *J Am Dent Assoc*. 2010 Oct;141 Suppl 3:14S-8S

Boeddinghaus, R.; Whyte, A. (2011). Current concepts in maxillofacial imaging. J *Craniofac Surg*. 2011 Mar;22(2):669-73

Danforth, RA et al. (2003). Cone beam tomography: an imaging option for diagnosis of complex mandibular thord molar anatomical relationships. *J Calif Dent Ass* .2003;31:847-52.

El-Mohri, Y.; Anthonuk,LE.; Zhao,O.; Jiang, H.; Liu, L. (2011). Low-dose megavoltage cone-beam CT imaging using thick, segmented scintillators. *Phys Med Biol*, Vol 21, 56(6):1509-27

Heiland, M.; Pohlenz, P.; Blessmann, M.; Werle, H.; Fraederich, M.; Schmelzle, R.; Blake, FA. (2008). Navigated implantation after microsurgical bone transfer using intraoperatively acquired cone-beam computed tomography data sets. *Int J Oral Maxillofac Surg*. 2008 Jan;37(1):70-5

Kaeppler, G. (2010). Applications of cone beam computed tomography in dental and oral medicine.*Int J Comput Dent*. 2010;13(3):203-19

Koyama, S.; Aoyama, T.; Oda,N.; Yamauchi-Kawaura, C. (2010) .Radiation dose evaluation in tomosynthesis and C-arm cone-beam CT examinations with an anthropomorphic phantom. *Med Phys*. 2010 Aug;37(8):4298-306.

Lloyd, TE,; Drage, NA.; Cronin, AJ. (2011). The role of cone beam computed tomography in the management of unfavourable fractures following sagittal split mandibular osteotomy. *J Orthod*. 2011 Mar;38(1):48-54

Melo, SL.; Bortoluzzi, EA.; Abreu, M Jr.; Corrêa, LR.; Corrêa, M.(2010). Diagnostic ability of a cone-beam computed tomography scan to asess longitudinal root fractures in prosthetically treated teeth. *J Endod* . 2010 Nov;36(11):1879-82

Miloglu, O.; Yilmaz, AB.; Yildirim,E.; Akgul, HM.(2011). Pneumatization of the articular eminence on cone beam computed tomography: prevalence, characteristics and a review of the literature. *Dentomaxillofac Radiol*. 2011 Feb;40(2):110-4

Mischkowski, RA.; Pulsfort, R.; Ritter, L.; Neugebauer, J.; Brochhagen, HG.; Keeve, E.; Zöller, JE. (2007). Geometric accuracy of a newly developed cone-beam device for maxillofacial imaging. *Oral Surg Oral Med Oral Pathol Oral Radiol Endod*. 2007 Oct;104(4):551-9

Oberoi, S.; Gill, P.; Chigurupati, R.; Hoffman, WY.; Hatcher, DC.; Vargervik K. (2010). Three-dimensional assesment of the eruption path of the canine in individuals with bone-grafted alveolar clefts using cone-beam computed tomography. *Cleft Palate Craniofac J*. 2010 Sep;47(5):507-12

Rosenberg, PA.; Frisbie, J.; Lee, J.; Lee, K.; Frommer, H.; Kottal, S.; Phelan, J .; Lin, L.; Fisch, G.(2010). Evaluation of pathologists (histopathology) and radiologists (cone beam computed tomography) differentiating radicular cysts from granulomas. *J Endod*. 2010 Mar;36(3):423-8

Song, CK.; Chang, HS.; Min, KS.(2010). Endodontic management of supernumerary tooth fused with maxillary first molar by using cone-beam computed tomography. *J Endod* 2010;13(3):203-19.

Swennen, GR.; Mollemans, W.; De Clercq, C.; Abeloos, J.; Lamoral, P.; Lippens, F,.; Neyt N.; Casselman, J.; Schutyser, F.(2009). A cone-beam computed tomography triple scan procedure to obtain a three-dimensional augmented virtual skull model appropriate for orthognathic surgery planning. J Craniofac Surg. 2009 Mar;20(2):297-307.

Tecco, S; Saccucci, M.; Nucera, R.; Polimeni, A.; Pagnoni, M.; Cordasco, G.; Festa, F.; Iannetti, G.(2010). Condylar volume and surface in Caucasian young adults subjects. *BMC Med Imaging*. 2010 Dec 31;10:28

Tucker, S.; Cevidanes, LH.; Styner, M.; Kim, H.; Reyes, M.; Proffit, W.; Turvey, T. (2010). Comparison of actual surgical outcomes and 3-dimensional surgical simulations. *J Oral Maxillofac Surg*. 2010 Oct;68(10):2412-21

6

Medical CT Image Classification

Hongmei Xie
Northwestern Polytechnical University
China

1. Introduction

With the rapid development of CT imaging technology, CT images that include various human body part like stomach, head, face, back,chest and pelvis are obtained in order to help doctors diagnose some illness like brain tumor, lung cancer, and so on. However, the efficient usage of these large amounts of image data is limited by the current image processng level and also by doctor's experience, knowledge and some other subjective factors like whether the doctor is tired or not. Thus proper imaging, segmenting, transferring, classificaton and processing of the image by computer software is necessary.

How to process all the available image data and make computer aided diagonosis system(CAD) be a reality is one of the hotspots in recent research. Recently there are some researches that focus on this specific field. **Yoshida** et al.(2004), proposed a lung disease detection method based on Generic Algorithms(GA) and template matching. **El-bazl** et al.**(2003)**, proposed a novel CAD system based on the symmetrical feature of lung and also based on that tumors appear to be round . These methods are effective for some specific patients. However, sometimes the oversimplified algorithm can not get ideal results becasue of the heterogeneity of human body.

This chapter introduces a scheme that uses NCut(Normalized Cut) image segmenter, novel edge features and SVM(Support Vector Machine) classifier to implement CT image classfication and brain tumor detection. Using real data, the propsoed algorithm was tested and some basic conclusions were given out.

2. Integration of NCut segmentation and SVM classifier

Shi J,Malik J(2000) proposed Normalized Cut(Ncut) as a good image segmentation method and soon NCut drew great attention in recent years because it maximizes the similarity of the same group and the dissimilarity of different groups simutaneously. Support vector machine(SVM) is proposed by V. Vapnik in 1963. And it is a promising statistical learning technique for machine learning. Therefore the problem of regression or time series analysis and pattern recognition like classification and decision can be solved by SVM. The medical diagnosis problem is a problem of pattern recognization and then in essence it is a classification problem. Of course, Ncut can not be followed by SVM classifiier directly since the output of Ncut is seveval subimages obtained from NCut segmenting while the input of SVM classifier is a high-dimensional feature vector. So to match the above 2 tools we need find an effective and efficient way to extract and then select the features.

For feature extraction, we get the multi-resolution edge by wavelet transformation and then compute the mean and variance of the edge matrix as a novel feature component besides traditional grey and texture features.

Here some more detail information should be given out to make our newly proposed algorithm more clearly and implementable. As shown in Figure 1 and Figure 2, the training and classification system shared one common interface, i.e. the same interface can be used as either training or classifying aims. The main difference lies in that for training procedure, Ncut segmentation is performed based on some prior information about the medical structure of the human body part (e.g. For brain tumor CAD system, we set the number of partition be about 10). Then for a given sample image, we get the best number by try some very close partition number. Since for the training sample images, the tumor's relatively precise information is known. So then we can extract the corresponding subimages and exact the features and then train the SVM classfier using different kernal functions or some kind of combination of the different kernals(see also Figure2 for intuitive description).

For the diagonosis system, we use scheme shown in Figure1. Here we load the trained classifier implicitly. Because the well-trained classifier can be used as a reference and it is very helpful for the CAD system to work well.

The main interface of the proposed computer aided diagnosis (CAD) is as shown in Fig.1.

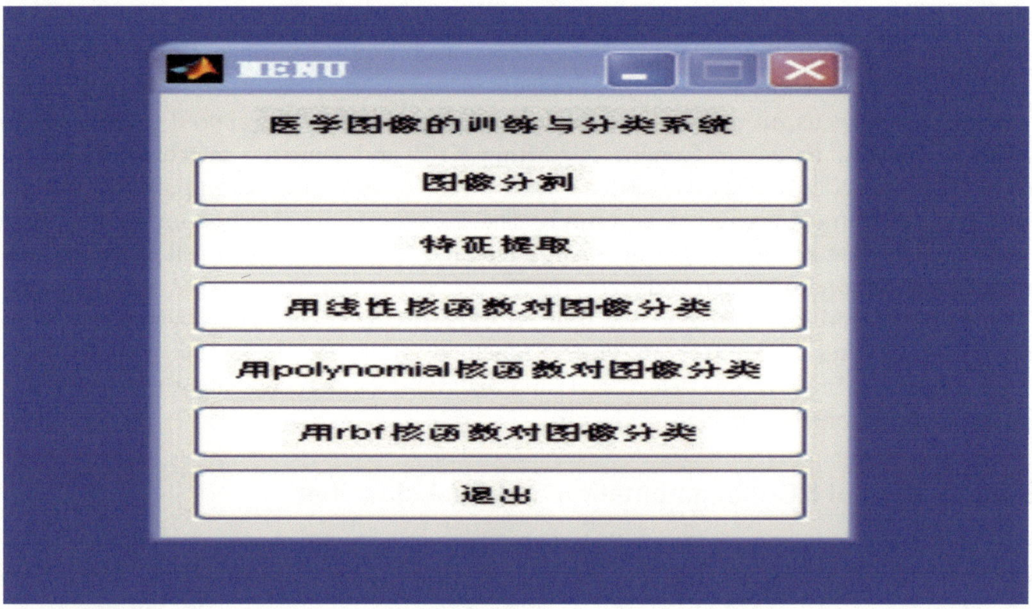

Fig. 1. Main interface of the software

The novel scheme can be briefly described as following: First,we perform image segmentation using NCut in order to get the ROI(Region of Interest). Meanwhile, this step is also helpful to reduce the data amount to be processed later. Then feature extraction using various selected math analysis tools was done for the ROI and the corresponding symmetric region and the feature spaces are constructed based on the extracted features. After that we trained the SVM classifier using selected samples and features. Finally,Computer Aided Diagnose (CAD) results can be get using the trained SVM classifier and real CT images.

Experiments with brain CT images shows that the new algorithm can make correct diagnose and thus help doctor to perform their work more efficiently.
Note that prior to the diagnosis phase, we need get some well-trained data for SVM classfier using some classical trainng dataset which is obtained from hospital and was well agreed by medical experts. Then we have some well-trained SVM classifier using linear, polynomial, radial basis function(RBF) various kernal function.
The expression of the polynomial, Gauss and Sigmoid kernal functions are as follows:

1. polynomial: $k(x,x_i)=[(x_i,x)+1]^q$
2. Gauss: $K(x,x_i)=exp[-\sigma|x-x_i|^2]$
3. Sigmoid: $K(x,x_i)=tanh(\sigma(x\cdot x_i)+c)$

Here, for each kind of the kernal function, there is one or two key parameter. For polynomial, the order q, for
Gauss kernnal it's the variance-related parameter σ and for Sigmod kernal σ and c.

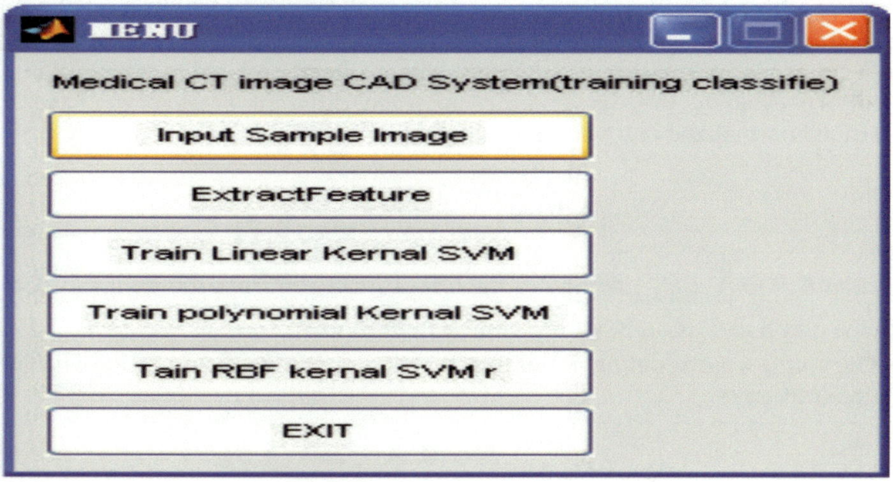

Fig. 2. Main interface of the training process

2.1 NCut-based image segmentation

Till now, researchers have proposed a lot of methods for image segmentation. These methods can be broadly classified into the following catergories: 1)Local filtering method ; 2) Active contour or snake; 3) Region growth ,split and merge algorithm like K-means, JSEG(J-value segmentation) and EM(Expectation Maximum); 4) Level set method that is based on the global minumum of energy function; 5) Mean shift method that is based on statistical iteration. The major drawback of the mentioned methods is that they fail to find global optima for the high-dimensional, nonliear problem and some of them can not guarantee the continuity since they use only the local information so they can not guarantee the continuity of the edge. NCut is proposed by J.Shi and J.Malik in 1997 to perform the task of image segmentation and image clustering. NCut has three major features: 1) It converts the problem of image segmentation into the one of graph partition; 2) It uses a global optimum criteria; 3) It maximizes the similarity of the same group and the dissimilarity of different group at the same time.

2.1.1 Math basis for NCut image segmentation

For a given input image or feature set, a weighted unidirectional graph is constructed first. In the graph, each pixel or feature point stands for one node in the graph. Then a global minimum normalized cut in the graph is searched for so as to divide the nodes in the graph. After all the nodes is partitioned, the image segmentation or feature set clustering is done.

The set of points in a feature space are represented as an arbitrary unidirectional graph $\mathbf{G} = (\mathbf{V}, \mathbf{E})$. Assume we divide the given graph $\mathbf{G} = (\mathbf{V}, \mathbf{E})$ into two independent disjoint parts $\mathbf{A}$ and $\mathbf{B}$, i.e. $\mathbf{A} \cap \mathbf{B} = \Phi$ and $\mathbf{A} \cup \mathbf{B} = \mathbf{V}$.

The partition can be done by simply removing the edges connecting the two parts. The dissimilarity of these two parts can be defined as the summation of all the weights that have been removed. It is called cut:

$$cut(\mathbf{A}, \mathbf{B}) = \sum_{i \in A, j \in B} w(i, j) \tag{1}$$

Where $w(i, j)$, the weight on each edge, is a function of similarity between node i and j.

The optimal bipartitioning of a graph is the one that minimize the cut value. However, minimum cut is not optimal cut because cut value is directly related to the number of edges in the cut. To evaluate the dis-similarity between different groups, we have the new measure called normalized cut(Ncut) as following:

$$Ncut(\mathbf{A}, \mathbf{B}) = \frac{cut(\mathbf{A}, \mathbf{B})}{assoc(\mathbf{A}, \mathbf{V})} + \frac{cut(\mathbf{A}, \mathbf{B})}{assoc(\mathbf{B}, \mathbf{V})} \tag{2}$$

Where $assoc(\mathbf{A}, \mathbf{V}) = \sum_{u \in A, v \in V} w(u, v)$ is the total conncetion from the nodes in A to all the nodes in the graph and $assoc(\mathbf{B}, \mathbf{V})$ has similar definition.

In the same spirit, we can define a measure for total normalized association within groups for a given partition as:

$$Nassoc(\mathbf{A}, \mathbf{B}) = \frac{assoc(\mathbf{A}, \mathbf{A})}{assoc(\mathbf{A}, \mathbf{V})} + \frac{assoc(\mathbf{B}, \mathbf{B})}{assoc(\mathbf{B}, \mathbf{V})} \tag{3}$$

Where $assoc(\mathbf{A}, \mathbf{A})$ and $assoc(\mathbf{B}, \mathbf{B})$ represent total weights of edges connecting nodes within $\mathbf{A}$ and $\mathbf{B}$ respectively.

Another important property is that $Ncut(\mathbf{A}, \mathbf{B})$ and $Nassoc(\mathbf{A}, B)$ is related by the following equation:

$$Ncut(\mathbf{A}, \mathbf{B}) = 2 - Nassoc(\mathbf{A}, \mathbf{B}) \tag{4}$$

Hence, the partition criteria minimize the disassociation between different groups and maximize the association between different groups are in fact identical and thus can be met simutaneously.

Although NCut is computational complex since it is actually an NP complete problem. An approximate discrete solution can be found using the algorithm desribed in the next part.

2.1.2 Implementation of image segmentation

Given a partition of nodes of a graph V into two sets A and B, let $\mathbf{x}$ be an indicator vector of size N ($N = |\mathbf{V}|$) and $x_i = 1$ stands for node i belongs to set A while $x_i = -1$ indicates that node i is in set B. Let $d_i = \sum_j w(i,j)$ be the total connection from node i to all the other nodes. With these definitions for $\mathbf{x}$ and d, we can rewrite $Ncut$ as:

$$Ncut(\mathbf{A},\mathbf{B}) = \frac{cut(\mathbf{A},\mathbf{B})}{assoc(\mathbf{A},\mathbf{V})} + \frac{cut(\mathbf{A},\mathbf{B})}{assoc(\mathbf{B},\mathbf{V})}$$
$$= \frac{\sum_{x_i>0,x_j<0} -w_{ij}x_i x_j}{\sum_{x_i>0} d_i} + \frac{\sum_{x_i<0,x_j>0} -w_{ij}x_i x_j}{\sum_{x_i<0} d_i} \qquad (5)$$

Let $\mathbf{W}$ be an $n \times n$ symetric matrix and with $\mathbf{W}(i,j) = w_{ij}$, and let $\mathbf{D}$ be a diagonal matrix with d_i on its diagnoal, i.e. $\mathbf{D} = diag(d_1, d_2, \cdots, d_N)$.

Denote $b = \frac{\sum_{x_i>0} d_i}{\sum_{x_i>0} d_i}$ and $y = (1+x) - b(1-x)$, where 1 be an Nx1 vector of all ones. Thus the global optimum problem can be simplified as(for detail derivation see ref[2]):

$$min_{\mathbf{x}} Ncut(\mathbf{x}) = min_{\mathbf{y}} \frac{\mathbf{y}^T(\mathbf{D}-\mathbf{W})\mathbf{y}}{\mathbf{y}^T\mathbf{D}\mathbf{y}} \qquad (6)$$

Subject to

$$y_i \in \left\{ 1, \frac{-\sum_{x_i>0} d_i}{\sum_{x_i<0} d_i} \right\}, \text{ and } \mathbf{y}^T D \cdot 1 = 0 .$$

If y is relaxed to take on only real value, we can minimize Eq.(6) by solving the generalzed eigenvalue

$$(\mathbf{D}-\mathbf{W})\mathbf{y} = \lambda \mathbf{D}\mathbf{y} \qquad (7)$$

Eq.(7) can be rewrite as a standard eigenvalue system as below:

$$\mathbf{D}^{-\frac{1}{2}}(\mathbf{D}-\mathbf{W})\mathbf{D}^{-\frac{1}{2}}\mathbf{z} = \lambda \mathbf{z} \qquad (8)$$

where $\mathbf{z} = \mathbf{D}^{\frac{1}{2}}\mathbf{y}$.

The important result that we used here is that the second smallest eigenvector of the generalized eigensystem (7) is the real value solution to the normalized cut problem. Using the vector that corresponding to the second smallest eigenvalue, we can segment each image into two parts. Then an iterative method is used to segment every part of the image.

2.1.3 Segmentation results

Before NCut Image Segmentation and Support Vector Machine Classifier for Computer Aided Diagnosis, sometimes a brief pre-processing procedure should be done in order to classify one given CT image into its corresponding coarse class so that one can put the images under their proper folders. The software we developed using VC platform and the initial software interface is given out as in the following figure (Fig.3).

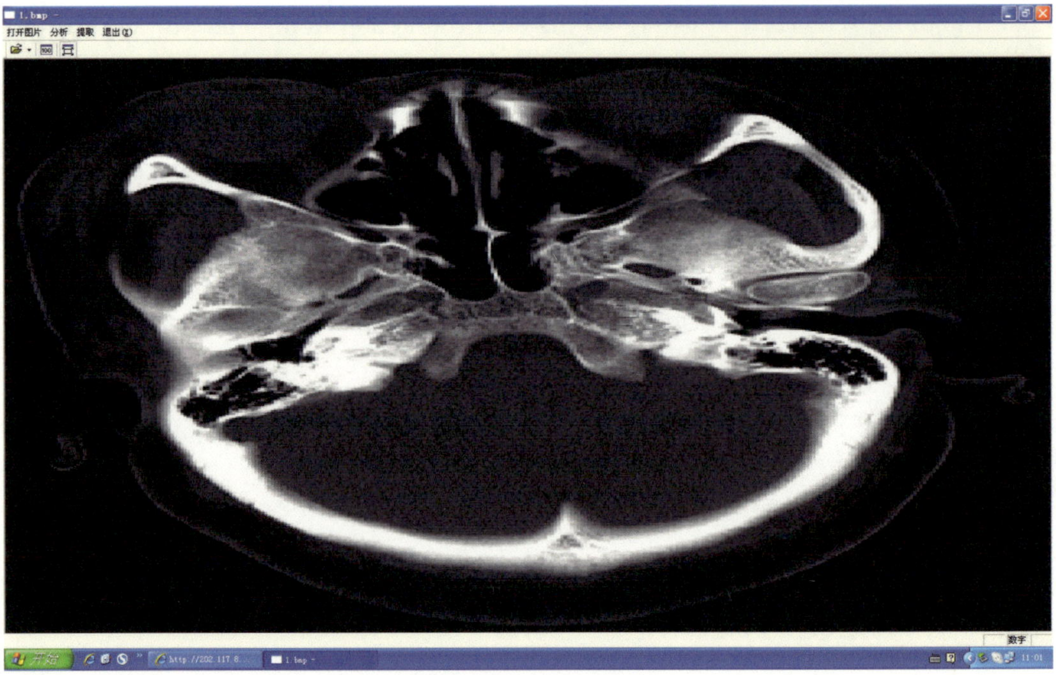

Fig. 3. Initial interface for coarse classification

Then, using the implementation procedure discussed above, we simulated the performance of image segmentation on the platform of Matlab7.0 software.

For a given CT brain image that is known to have a tumor somewhere, we perform the image segmentation task and annotate different regions using different colors. And the original and resultant images are shown in shown in Fig4 and Fig5 respectively. From Fig5, it can be seen that the image has been segmented into 10 parts and the edge of different parts is obvious. From Fig5, the possible tumor part has been annotated as blue part, and the shape and size of the corresponding part can be get by its coordinates and the distance between the edge points.

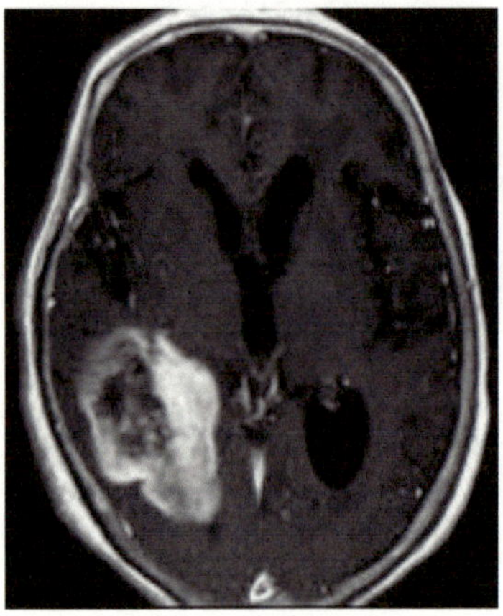

Fig. 4. Original brain CT image

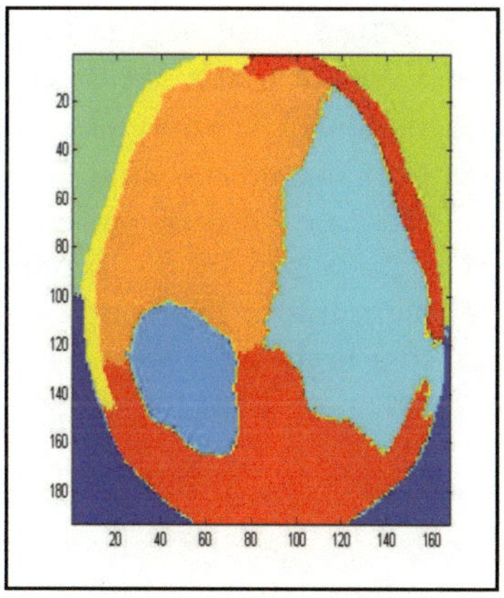

Fig. 5. Image segmented

2.1.4 Feature components for SVM classifier

After the processing described in the former part,the region of brain tumor has been extracted. Next, we need distinguish tumor and normal tissue by machine learning method. To do this, it is significant to describe different tissues with proper features. Many useful image features like grey descriptors, geometry feature and texture characteristics has been proposed to do these. Athough this features has solid mathmetical foudation, they can not fully describe the featurs of medical CT image. Here we proposed to use multi-resolution edge feature as an additional feature and compute the mean and variance of the matrix of edge pixels as basic features. The motivation of our novel feature component is that the tumor image has high space resolution and it has rich edge, grey and texture information.To get the new edge feature components, we get the multi-resolution edge by wavelet transformation and searching maximum modulos first, and then compute the mean and variance of the edge matrix.

Combining traditional feature and the novel featurs proposed here, the features used in this part is summed up in Table1. altogether we use 22 dimensional features to train and test our SVM classifier.

Feature Class and dimension	Description of the feature component
Edge (2-D)	Mean of the edge matrix Variance of the edge matrix
Grey（4-D)	Mean of the grey value Variance of the grey value Bias of the grey value Peak value of the grey value
texture（16-D)	Energy Contrast Correlation Entropy

Table 1. Features used in the CAD system

2.1.5 Classification using the integrated NCut segmenting and SVM classifier

We focuse on how to label different part of images with different names and describe their corresponding size and location using lots of unknown brain CT images.

This part we proposed to use support vector machine (SVM) to classify the image under test. Support vector machine(SVM) is one kind of pattern recognition which is based on statistical learning theory and it is proposed by V. Vapnik in 1963[3].Its basic idea is to tranform a nonlinear dividing problem into a linear one by some kind of kernal function. The sample space will be mapped to a high dimensional or even infinite dimension feature space (also called Hibert space). Then an optimal hyperplane for classification or regression is found.

SVM has the following advantages:

1. It's designed to use limited samples to get optimum solution for practical problem;
2. It can ensure to find the global rather than local optimum solution.
3. The generalization ability of SVM is very good with relatively less computation complexity.

Therefore SVM has drawn increasing adoption in many fields. However, one major problem is that the computation is complex, the idea of kernal funciton sovles this difficluty. By proper selected kernal function, we can greatly reduce the time of training without lost of any precision.

The problem is a nonlinear classification one, therefore we use nonlinear SVM that uses kernel function $K(x_i,x)$. The kernel function can be polynomial, Gauss and Sigmoid functions.

First, we describe the dataset used and the illustration is given out in Table 3. Specifically, our test in mainly focusing on brain CT images to detect brain tumour.

For other body part's images, using coarse-to-fine classification for large amounts of the incoming CT images we can classify the input CT images to its corresponding class based on the imaging part. The algorithm can be described as following:

Step 1. Extract and select features like grey, edge and texture features. Note the features used here may be different from the ones that used in the CAD system presented in this chapter. Because for efficiency, the features used here is global instead of local. So we can use more statistical feature to represent one kind feature. E.g. we propose to use 5-D edge features (the length of the region, the area of the region, etc) to quantify the edge feature.

Step 2. Use Euclidean distance as the measurement for classification. The definition of Euclidean is d=sqrt(∑(xi1-xi2)^ 2) i=1,2, ...n

The hardware platform for the simulation is as following: CPU is Intel Core Duo (1.6GHZ) and momery is 1024MB. The software platform is Windows XP as OS and Matlab7.0 code for Ncut-based image segmentation and LibSVM-2.86[5] for SVM training and testing. Some VC++6.0 codes are also developed for interoperating and interface.

For training procedure, the image used here is 512×512. First we selected 100 brain CT images as training samples and extracted 124 possible tumour images. And among the 124 sub-images, 68 images are positive samples and 56 images are negative images. And then the 22-D features for each sub-image are extracted according to Table1. After that, the extracted features are sent to SVM to train the SVM classifier.

In table 2, detail information about the data used is given out.

Image Type & features	Brian CT	Head CT
Data size	402MB	92.1MB
Data source	Provided by a hospital in Xi'an, , China	Provided by a hospital in Xianyang, Xi'an, China
Number of patients	37	10
Sex portion	20 males and 17 females	6 males and 4 females

Table 2. Descripton of the used data

Next, for testing procedure, we selected 50 brain CT images. Among which we detected 60 possible tumour regions. And 30 sub-images are positive samples while 30 are negative samples. And we set penalty parameter as 100,150 and 200 respectively. And the optimum parameter value can be get by comparing the value of classification precision. Note here the classification precision (P) is calculated as:

$$P=Nc/Nt \tag{9}$$

Where Nc and Nt stands for the number of correct classified samples and the number of total samples respectively.

Tumour identification and quantization is important for the future cure. So CAD brain tumor diagnosis has potential applications. The method presented in this paper gives a useful implementation of this CAD system. Furthermore the proposed Ncut-based image segmentation is also useful for other application like CBIR(Content-based Image Retrieval) system.

And from pririo knowledge, the region of tumor image can be get by simply click that region and then we can show it in Fig.5 or save it in a file so that the region can be used later as training sample in the following steps.

Penalty factor	P for Polynomial kernal	P for RBF kernal	P for Sigmoid kernal
C=100	93.3%	96.7%	93.3%
C=150	90%	93.3%	90%
C=200	83.3%	86.7%	86.7%

Table 3. Influence of different SVM parameters

In our experiments, the optimum parameter values are get by comparing different kernal function and penalty factors.

To sum up in this part, brain CT Computer Aided classification & Diagnosis software system was discussed.

Based on the mainly 2 references discussion and analysis, we solved the main steps of CT image process, like image reading, image segmentation, feature extraction and feature-based classification steps. This chapter's first contribution is that a coarse-to-fine classification is proposed. And the main part (NCut-based segmentation and SVM classifier) are illustrated. For the CAD system, firstly by extracting features like colour histogram, edge and texture features and then using SVM classifier.

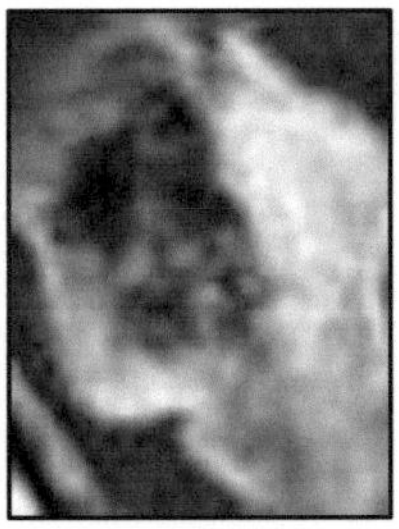

Fig. 6. Brain tumor

The specific method used in this chapter is NCut segmentation, multi-feature exaction and SVM classification. And the software tools used is Matlab7.0 and VC6.0 programming, compiling and debugging environment.
The software works well in Matlab7.0 for current data. What's New and good: Combined NCut segmentation and SVM classification.

3. Selective higher level classification

In the case that we get a CT image and the higher level class like the imaging part and the specific patient of the input image is unknown, a coarse CT image classification is proposed. And the basic idea is shown as Fig. 7.

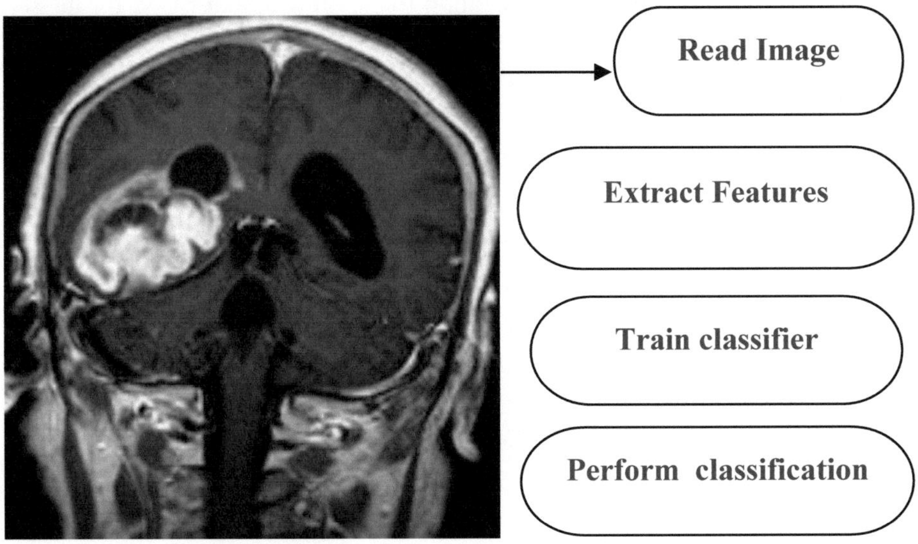

Fig. 7. Flowchart of coarse classification

For the coarse classification of the input image, grey features are used. First, the CT image is input and some normalizing work is done so as to make the size or resolution of the CT image to be uniform.
Then histogram of the input CT image is calculated and plotted. Based on histogram data and its statistical features like mean, variance, etc, the classification information is given out. Then based on the following equations (i.e. the Euclide-distance-based classification).

$$X_{train} = \{x_{tn1,}x_{tn2,}\cdots,x_{tnm,}\}$$

$$X_{test} = \{x_{tm1,}x_{tm2,}\cdots,x_{tmm,}\}$$

Where m is the dimension of the feature vector.
And the euclide-distance based classifying procedure can be described as:

For k=1 to numofclass

$$\text{Compute } d_{euk} = \sqrt{\sum_{i=1}^{m}(x_{tni} - x_{tmi})^2}$$

And find the minimum d_{euk} and classify the input image as kth class.
For a given input CT image, it is used either as training samples or test sample. In the latter case, then the resultant class label is given out the image is saved in the proper folders. (Note in some cases this pre-processing can be skipped if the exact information of imaging part is known.)

Imaging body part	Back	head	face	stomach	pelvis	chest
Data size	1402MB	403MB	89.2MB	52.9MB	39.6MB	477MB
Number of patients and sex portion	18 10 males and 8 females	37 20 males & 17 females	18	10 6 males and 4 females	3 (all females)	13(7 males and 6 females)
Total image size	1.16GB					

Table. 4. Descripton of the dataset used for coarse classification

Last the coarse classification results is given out in table 5.
Using histogram features as the main discriminitive base and te Euclide distance as the classifying criteria, we get the resultant resuts shown in table 5. One can see the precision rate is relatively high and acceptable. Thus we draw the conclusion that the propsoed coarse classificaton is simple and effective. This coarse classification may be very useful for the the following CT image-based disease detection and diagnosis.

4. Discussions of the novel algorithm for CAD system

The CAD system consists of two separate components. The first one is a coarse classification subsystem which is implemented by global feature extraction and Euclide-distance based classifier.
The second subsystem is the part that is composed of image segmentation, feature extraction, classifier training and classifier test. NCut is one of the novel proposed segmentation algorithms. Actually, some newly occurred algorithm can be used to

	stomach	head	pelvis	Back	face	chest
Total sample number	52.9MB	1346	131	450	320	1526
# of training samples	34	270	27	90	64	306
# of training samples	134	1076	104	360	256	1220
# of correct classified images	121	1035	100	353	213	1218
Precision rate	90.30%	90.19%	96.15%	98.08%	83.20%	99.84%
Total time cost	Approximately 355 seconds					

Table 5. Coarse classification results

substitute the NCut image segmentation according to the system needs. U. von Luxburg proposed using sparse representation to implement the image segmentation task. J. Mairal used Sparse signal models for local image discrimination tasks, proposing an energy formulation with both sparse reconstruction and class discrimination components, jointly optimized during dictionary learning. The approach improves over the state of the art in texture segmentation experiments using the Brodatz database, and it paves the way for a novel scene analysis and recognition framework based on simultaneously learning discriminative and reconstructive dictionaries. Our future work can be to use the sparse representation substitute our Ncut based segmentation provided that the newly proposed algorithm is proved to be better than our method.

For the classifier part, the SVM classifier has been proven to be good enough for the task. And future work can be done to improve the processing speed and also to improve the data amount that the system can handle. Therefore, parallel SVM classifier design and implementation is our future work field.

5. Conclusion

From the simulation results, we draw the conclusion that the NCut-based segmentation is correct and the parameter setting is reasonable. And this system can help doctors to make a reasonable and correct decision.

Diagnosis software was designed. For about 500MB image dataset we tested the software. The time cost is about 350 seconds and the average correct rate is about 90%. Actually 1.17GB image data was provided to be tested. This much detail work should be done.

There is a predefined parameter (the number of segmentation) for NCut segmentation, currently we set the number of segmentation to be 10 parts for brain CT image. In future work, much more detail work should be done to make the parameter more adaptive for other parts' CT image.

Although the software work well for the current software environment and dataset but for newly matlab version we met some portable problem since the NCut part only works on Matlab7.0 version and what's more important is that more modification should be done to make the software more flexible in order to make it work without matlab platform.

On the one side, future work should be focus on the multi-kernel learning so as to improve the performance of the SVM classification.

On the other side, coarse-to-fine classification for medical CT image need be done for large amount of raw data. The coming medical CT image retrieval based on imaging body part and also Computer Aided classification is undergoing developing. We propose to parallel the traditional Euclidean distance-based coarse classification and implement it in the parallel platform or even the internet-based cloud environment in order to put the image into their corresponding imaging part fast and cost-effectively. Then fine segmentation based on NCut and the specific part's biological information, and lastly SVM classifier should be used to detect and analyze the ill tissue.

Moreover, much more data should be analyzed and the software development can be developed using merely C or Java platform in order to make the software product more portable and can be used in the newly occurred cloud computation environment.

6. Acknowledgment

The work is supported by Chinese Educational Department's returned Oversea Scholar's fund NAYX0001. The author would also like to give her sincere thanks for Dr. Baoping Wang for the abundant CT data obtained from the hospital that his wife is currently working with.

7. References

Yoshida Hiroyuki (2004). Local contra lateral subtraction based on bilateral symmetry of lung for reduction of false positives in computerized detection of pulmonary nodules. ieee transactions on biomedical engineering, volume: 51, issue: 5, may 2004 pages: 778-789

El-Bazl A, Farag, AA, Falk R, et al(2003). Automatic Identification of Lung Abnormalities in Chest Spiral CT Scans. 2003 IEEE International Conference on Acoustics, Speech, and Signal Processing, 2003. Proceedings. (ICASSP '03). Volume: 2, 6-10 april 2003, pages: ii - 261- 4 vol.2

Shi J,Malik J(2000). Normalized Cuts and Image Segmentation. IEEE Transections on Pattern Analgsis and Machine Intelligence, 2000,22(8):888-905

Nello Cristianini,John Shawe-Taylor(2005). An Introduction to Support Vector Machines and Other Kernel-based Learning Methods[M], Beijing: Press of machenical industry, 2005

Chih-Jen Lin(2008).A simple and easy-to-use support vector machines tool for classification〔EB/OL〕. http://www.csie.ntu.edu.tw/~cjlin/

Bach F R, Lanckriet R G, Jordan M I(2004). Multiple Kernel Learning, Conic Duality, and the SMO Algorithm[J]. Proc of the 21st International Conference on Machine Learning. 2004

U. von Luxburg "A Tutorial on Spectral clustering", available at www.springer.com

J. Mairal, et al., "Discriminative Learned Dictionaries for Local Image Analysis", IEEE conf. on CVPR, Anchorage, Alaska, (2008) 1--8

Part 2

Diagnosis

7

Distraction Osteogenesis of the Maxillofacial Skeleton: Clinical and Radiological Evaluation

Mehmet Cemal Akay
Ege University, Faculty of Dentistry, Department of Oral and Maxillofacial Surgery, Turkey

1. Introduction

Bimaxillary deficiencies (BMD) are frequently observed in adult patients and an increasingly recognized major orthodontic problem. Transverse skeletal deficiency (TSD) is a common clinical problem associated with narrow basal and dentoalveolar bone. An adequate transversal dimension is an important factor of stable occlusion and it positively effects facial esthetics and mastication. Narrow and V-shaped dental arch, dental crowding, posterior cross-bite, unesthetic black buccal corridors upon smiling and BMD are generally interrelated (Matteini & Mommaerts, 2001; Mommaerts, 1999; Mommaerts et al., 2004a; Proffit et al., 1996; Ramieri et al., 2005; Vanarsdall, 1999). Additionally, mouth breathing results in many clinical problems such as, xerostomia, an increased caries incidence and recurrent upper air way infections in these cases. Ideal functional reconstruction should achieve sufficient alveolar height and thickness, allowing for permanent restoration of dentition, maxillo-mandibular occlusion, mastication, deglutition, mandibular continuity, sensibility of the mucosa, lip competence and speech. The general aim of oral reconstruction is to restore both normal physiology and facial esthetics. Attention to the transverse deficiencies is vital in planning treatment for a patient who requires an increase in the lateral dimension of the mandible or maxilla.

2. Traditional treatment modalities for BMD

Traditional treatment options include compensating orthodontics, functional appliances, and orthopedic devices. Arch wire expansion, Schwarz plates, and proclination can all produce alveolar expansion. When these patients are treated using classical orthodontic appliances, the duration of the treatments increase and risks such as root resorption, undesired movements of anchorage teeth, and relapse occur. These therapies show relatively stable results for younger patients, particularly those who presented with lingually tipped teeth that need to be decompensated (Mommaerts, 1999; Neyt et al., 2002).
Orthognathic surgery techniques for the treatment of BMD are used for many years. However, in these methods, mucosa can not adopt to rapid movement of bone fragmants after the osteotomies. Therefore, in the postoperative period, relapse, functional and esthetic

problems ocur (Guerrero et al., 1997; Little & Riedel, 1989; Mommaerts & Vande Vannet, 2004). Distraction osteogenesis technique (DO) offers a solution for these problems.

3. Distraction osteogenesis

Distraction osteogenesis, also called callus distraction, callotasis, osteodistraction and distraction histogenesis is a surgical process used to reconstruct skeletal deformities and lengthen the long bones of the body (Ilizarov, 1989a, 1989b). The human body possesses an enormous regenerative capacity. DO takes advantage of this regenerative potential to induce the regeneration and remodeling of bone, cartilage, nerve, muscle, blood vessels, and skin. DO is defined as the creation of neoformed bone and adjacent soft tissue after the gradual and controlled displacement of a bone fragment obtained by surgical osteotomy. With this procedure, bone volume can be increased by gradual traction of a fracture callus formed between osteotomized bony segments. When the desired or possible length is reached, a consolidation phase follows in which the bone is allowed to keep healing. DO has the benefit of simultaneously increasing bone length and the volume of surrounding soft tissues. Clinically, this offers a distinct advantage because several craniofacial anomalies have soft tissue hypoplasia in addition to deficient bony structures. Neurovascular elements contained within distracted bony segments are also stimulated to regenerate. Experimental studies in dogs demonstrate regeneration of the mandibular canal containing both neural and vascular elements. However, the functional level of the regenerated neurovascular structures is less than normal (Imola et al., 2002; Imola et al., 2008).

3.1 History of DO technique

However, bone distraction is not a new concept, DO of the craniofacial skeleton has become increasingly popular as an alternative to many conventional orthognathic surgical procedures. For patients with mild to severe abnormalities of the craniofacial skeleton, distraction techniques have increased the number of treatment alternatives. DO initially used in orthopedic surgery by Codivilla in 1905. Abbott (1927) contributed in the improvement of Codivilla method by incorporating pins instead of casts used by Codivilla. Allan (1948) was the first to incorporate a screw device to control the rate of distraction. Research into osteogenic distraction originated in the fields of orthopedics and traumatology. However, the complication rate remained high and the technique was not understood until Gavriel Ilizarov, a Russian orthopedic surgeon, performed detailed studies in 1952. Ilizarov found that succesful distraction depends of the stability of fixation, the rate of daily distraction, and the preservation of the local soft tissue envelope and vascular supply. Mandibular lengthening by gradual distraction was reported in 1973 by Synder et al. who used an extraoral device in a canine study; new bone formation at the elongated site was demonstrated later by Karp et al. (1990). The first clinical results of craniofacial DO were reported in 1992 by McCarthy et al. in a small series of patients with congenital mandible deformities. Authors successfully elongated the mandible by up to 24 mm. Interest in craniofacial distraction was slow to grow initially, with sporadic experimental reports appearing throughout the ensuing 2 decades. However, in the early 1990s, experimental investigation intensified following reports that examined lengthening canine mandibles and the use of DO to successfully close canine segmental lower jaw defects. Thereafter, several studies demonstrated the ability to apply DO at several different sites, including the mandible, lower maxilla, midface, and cranial vault, within a variety of animal models. Since then, several larger series with longer follow-up periods have appeared. More recently, the technique has been successfully used for midface and upper craniofacial skeletal defects. DO is particularly useful for treating cases of severe bony hypoplasia where the surgical movement required to correct the malocclusion is outside the range predictably achievable with routine orthognathic surgery techniques.

Orthognathic surgery and DO have three steps in common. Both techniques require osteotomies, mobilization of segments, and a period of stabilization. The only difference between these two techniques is that, in distraction, the bone segments are slowly moved over time to their final position, whereas in conventional orthognathic surgery, this movement is immediate and it is accomplished intraoperatively. In DO, many tissues besides bone have been observed to form under tension stress, including mucosa, skin, muscle, tendon, cartilage, blood vessels, and peripheral nerves.

3.2 Types of DO technique

DO has been categorized into monofocal, bifocal, and trifocal types, depending on the number of foci at which osteogenesis occurs (Figure 1A-C). Monofocal elongation DO currently represents most of the clinical applications in the craniofacial skeleton.

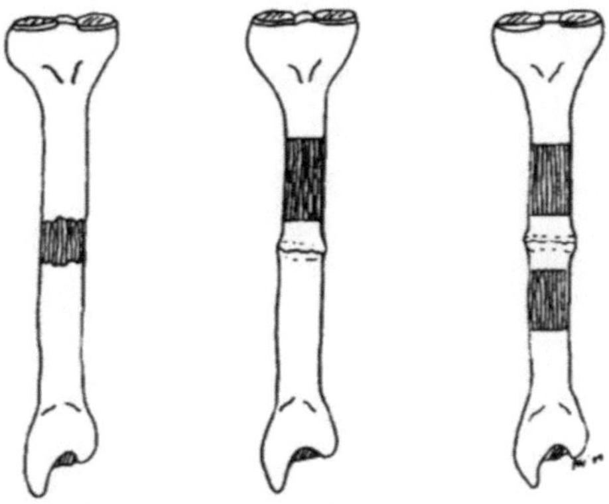

A: Monofocal distraction is used to lengthen abnormally shortened bones and involves separation of 2 bone segments across a single osteotomy.
B: Bifocal distraction is used to repair a segmental defect and requires creation of a transport disk, which is then distracted across the defect until it docks with the opposing bony segment.
C: Trifocal distraction is similar to bifocal distraction attempts to halve the distraction time by transporting 2 disks from opposite ends of a defect to dock in the middle. Arrows indicate distraction vectors; large arrow heads, distraction regenerate; and small arrow heads, docking site.

Fig. 1. Three types of distraction osteogenesis have been described: Monofocal, bifocal, and trifocal. (Reprinted from Costantino et al. (p543)

3.3 Types of distractors: internal and external

One of the primary planning considerations in maxillofacial distraction osteogenesis is the use of either an external distraction framework or an internal device. Critical to this decision is an evaluation of the goals of the distraction process (McCarthy et al. 1996, 1998). The external devices have the powerful advantages of allowing bone distraction in three planes and allowing the surgeon to alter the direction, or vector, of the distraction process while the distraction is proceeding. The external distractors allow for easier adjustment of the direction of the distraction. However, the longer the distance from the axial screw of the distractor to the callus, the less effective the distraction. Pensler et al. (1995) first reported this principle of "molding the regenerate" in 1995. The "molding" takes advantage of the ability to manipulate the semisolid state of the nonmineralized, and hence nonrigid, bone in the distraction gap. This allows for "fine-tuning" of the distraction process while the distraction is proceeding, and thus permits dental relationships to be adjusted before the patient enters the consolidation phase of bone healing (Luchs et al. 2002). The external framework also allows greater amounts of ultimate expansion length. Expansions of 40 mm or greater have been reliably obtained. The disadvantages of an external frame distractor are the creation of a facial scar and the increased distance from the body of the distractor to the bone surface, leading to a longer "moment arm" at the pin-bone interface and an increased possibility of pin loosening. In addition, there is the need for "pin care" by the patient at the percutaneous pin sites (Gosain et al. 2002). The goal of distraction with internal devices is generally more modest, in the range of 25 mm or less. This is a consequence of the constraints placed on the physical size of the device and the ability to fit it within the mouth. In addition, the direction of the distraction cannot be altered after the device is placed. Development of miniature, internal distraction devices have made this clinically feasible and practical.

3.4 Physiologic process of DO

Several factors influence the physiologic process of DO, and these can be separated into 2 basic groups: bone healing factors and distraction factors as Table 1:

Local Bone-Healing Factors	**Systemic Bone-Healing Factors**	**Distraction Factors**
Osteoprogenitor supply	Age	Rate of distraction
Blood supply	Metabolic disorders	Frequency of distraction
Infection	Vitamin D deficiency	Latency period
Soft tissue scarring	Connective tissue disease	Rigidity of fixation
Bone stock	Steroid therapy	Adequate consolidation period
Prior radiation therapy	Calcium deficiency	Length of regenerate

Table 1. Factors that affect physiologic process of DO (Imola et al. 2002, 2008)

Factors that affect bone healing can be local or systemic in nature. Viability of osteocytes and osteoblasts is essential to provide an adequate source of osteogenic activity at the distraction site. Hence, careful surgical technique should be used to minimize thermal or mechanical injury to the periosteum and endosteum, which are the main sources of osteoblast precursors. Similarly, an adequate blood supply to the distraction site is critical to osteogenesis. Arterial insufficiency may lead to ischemic fibrogenesis within the regenerate, yielding a loose, irregular collagen network instead of the desirable dense, regular collagen pattern. Venous outflow obstruction has been associated with cystic degeneration of the regenerate. The clinician, therefore, needs to ensure that the soft tissues that surround the site of the proposed distraction are well vascularized. Early studies in long bones concluded that both an intact periosteum and endosteum were critical to successful osteogenesis; therefore, many advocated that a corticotomy be performed only through a minimal periosteal opening. More recently, however, investigators have demonstrated that the periosteum alone can provide sufficient osteogenic capacity for a healthy regenerate, and this is especially true in the well-vascularized membranous bone of the craniofacial skeleton. Prior radiation therapy to the distraction site has been shown to not adversely influence the results of distraction in the canine model, and when using DO to repair segmental defects, the status of the surrounding soft tissues will likely be the key factor that influences outcome (Gantous et al. 1994).

3.5 Distraction phases

DO is divided into 3 distinct phases, namely the latency phase, the distraction (activation) phase, and the consolidation phase. Of these, the 2 early phases are of relatively short duration and are not associated with substantial morbidity or complications. The consolidation phase, however, entails a prolonged period of immobilization, which may result in serious complications.

Latency is that period immediately following the osteotomy and application of distractor; it ranges from 1 to 7 days. In most cases, the osteotomy creates an initial defect of approximately 1.0 mm. The basic principles of using new fresh burrs, using constant irrigation during the drilling process, and minimizing thermal injury to the bone must be strictly followed in this technique. Furthermore, the actual placement of the pins and/or screws should be meticulous. If a pin or screw needs to be backed out, it is often better to drill a new hole and place the pin/screw with a fresh placement than to risk unstable and inadequate fixation that will loosen and lead to failure of the distraction process. After the latency phase is the activation phase. To achieve targeted bone growth, a rigid stretching device delivers tensile force to the developing callus at the site of the bone cut. During this phase, the distraction device is activated by turning some type of axial screw, usually at 1 mm/day in four equal increments of 0.25 mm each. Once activation is complete, the third and final phase is the consolidation phase (Fig. 2). Typically, the consolidation phase is twice as long as the time required for activation (Ilizarov, 1988). Today, many different devices are being used clinically, with many different distraction protocols.

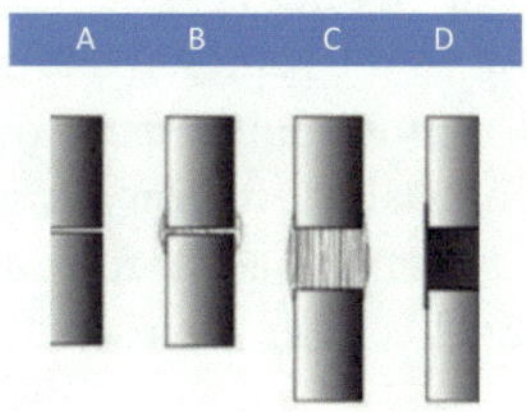

Fig. 2. Distraction phases: A) Osteotomy, B) Latency period, C) Distraction period, D) Consolidation period

In younger patients, distraction using the corticotomy of the external cortex is possible because the bone is very soft and pliable. However, in adults it is possible that the distraction device could deviate or distraction could fail due to resistance because the internal cortex does not fracture. Latency, rate, and rhythm of distraction are variables that influence the quality of the regenerate. Of these factors, the effect of latency is the most controversial (Aronson, 1994; Chin, 1999; Chin & Toth, 1996). Most craniofacial surgeons have empirically applied the conclusions from long bone studies and recommend waiting periods of 4 to 7 days following osteotomy and before initiating the distraction process. In younger children, the high rate of bone metabolism favors a shorter waiting period. Some clinicians, however, use a zero latency period and begin distracting right at the time of appliance insertion. They claim no adverse effects on outcome while substantially shortening the treatment period (Chin & Toth, 1996; Toth et al. 1998). Waiting too long before distraction (beyond 10 to 14 days) substantially increases the risk of premature bone union. In contrast to latency, the rate and rhythm (frequency) of distraction are believed to be important factors (Aronson, 1994). If widening of the osteotomy site occurs too rapidly (>2 mm per day), then a fibrous nonunion will result, whereas if the rate is too slow (<0.5 mm per day), premature bony union prevents lengthening to the desired dimension. These findings in long bones have been empirically applied to the craniofacial skeleton, and most studies have described a rate of 1.0 mm per day. According to Ilizarov's work in long bones, the ideal rhythm of DO is a continuous steady-state separation of the bone fragments (Ilizarov, 1971, 1988, 1989a, 1989b). However, this is impractical from a clinical standpoint, and therefore, most reports recommend distraction frequencies of 1 or 2 times daily. A 1-mm/day rate of distraction (2 x 0.5 mm) and a 5- to 7-day latency seem to be generally accepted as the gold standards in the field of craniofacial distraction osteogenesis (Guerrero et al. 1997; Bell et al. 1999; Mommaerts, 1999; Braun et al. 2002; El-Hakim et al. 2004; Iseri & Malkoc, 2005; Gunbay et al. 2008a; Gunbay et al. 2008b; Gunbay et al. 2009). In the craniofacial skeleton, most authors advocate 4 to 8 weeks, with the general rule that the consolidation period should be at least twice the duration of the distraction phase (Aronson, 1994; Chin & Toth, 1996; Polley & Figueroa, 1998; Shetye et al. 2010). Distraction in load-bearing bones, such as the mandible, is an indication for a longer consolidation time. Appliance rigidity during distraction and consolidation is a critical element to ensure that bending or shearing forces do not result in microfractures of the immature columns of new bone within the regenerate, which lead to focal hemorrhage and cartilage interposition (Aronson, 1994).

The histophysiolgy of DO is based on the slow steady traction of tissues, which causes them to become metabolically activated, resulting in an increase in the proliferative and biosynthetic functions. The premise then is that the newly generated bone between distracted bony ends will result in a stable lengthening and behave as "new" bone, appropriately responding and adapting to the regional environmental loads placed on it.

DO takes place primarily through intramembranous ossification. Histological studies identified 4 stages that result in the eventual formation of mature bone.

Stage I: The intervening gap initially is composed of fibrous tissue (longitudinally oriented collagen with spindle-shaped fibroblasts within a mesenchymal matrix of undifferentiated cells).

Stage II: Slender trabeculae of bone are observed extending from the bony edges. Early bone formation advances along collagen fibers with osteoblasts on the surface of these early bony spicules laying down bone matrix. Histochemically, significantly increased levels of alkaline phosphatase, pyruvic acid, and lactic acid are noted.

Stage III: Remodeling begins with advancing zones of bone apposition and resorption and an increase in the number of osteoclasts.

Stage IV: Early compact cortical bone is formed adjacent to the mature bone of the sectioned bone ends, with increasingly less longitudinally oriented bony spicules; this resembles the normal architecture.

As the bone undergoes lengthening, each of these stages are observed to overlap from the central zone of primarily fibrous tissue to the zone of increasingly mature bone adjacent to the bony edges. By 8 months, the intervening bone within the distraction zone achieves 90% of the normal bony architecture. It is believed that the architecture is maintained and that the bone responds to normally applied functional loads (Imola et al. 2008).

3.6 Indications of DO

Current usage falls into 3 broad groups as follows:

a. **Lower face (mandible)**

- Unilateral distraction of the ramus, angle, or posterior body for hemifacial microsomia
- Bilateral advancement of the body for severe micrognathia, particularly in infants and children with airway obstruction as observed in the Pierre Robin syndrome
- Vertical distraction of alveolar segments to correct an uneven occlusal plane or to facilitate implantation into edentulous zones
- Horizontal distraction across the midline to correct crossbite deformities or to improve arch form

b. **Mid face (maxilla, orbits)**

- Advance the lower maxilla at the LeFort I level
- Complete midfacial advancement at the LeFort III level
- Closure of alveolar bony gaps associated with cleft lip and palate deformities
- Upper face (fronto-orbital, cranial vault)
- Advancement of the fronto-orbital bandeau, alone or in combination with the mid face as a monobloc or facial bipartition
- New use of distraction as a means of cranial vault remodeling by gradual separation across resected stenotic sutures

Established indications for craniofacial DO include the following:

a. **Congenital indications**

- Nonsyndromic Craniofacial Syndrome - Coronal (bilateral or unilateral) or sagittal
- Syndromic Craniofacial Syndrome (Apert, Crouzon, and Pfeiffer syndromes)
- Facial clefts, cleft lip and palate
- Patients with severe severe sleep apnea
- Hemifacial microsomia
- Severe retrognathia associated with a syndrome (eg, Pierre Robin syndrome, Treacher Collins syndrome, Goldenhar syndrome, Brodie Syndrome), especially in infants and children who are not candidates for traditional osteotomies
- Bimaxillary crowding with anterior-posterior deformity
- Bimaxillary deficiencies (Lengthening and widening)
- Asymmetry
- Mandibular hypoplasia due to trauma and/or ankylosis of the temporomandibular joint

b. **Acquired indications**

- Reconstruction of posttraumatic deformities (midfacial retrusion or mandibular collapse)
- Insufficient alveolar height and/or width (Maxillary or mandibular alveolar distraction)
- Reconstruction of oncologic and/or aggressive cystic jaws defects

- Previously failed bone graft sites
- Insufficient soft tissue coverage
- Patient is not a candidate for a bone graft

3.7 Advantages and disadvantages of DO

Generally, facial deformities have been corrected by conventional osteotomy of the jaws and bone grafting. Conventional osteotomy has some advantages, such as the possibility of shorter hospital stays and obtaining precise preferable occlusion. However, despite these advantages the amount of mobilization may be limited and is determined by the preoperative orthodontic treatment obtaining a stable occlusal relationship between the maxilla and mandible. In addition, operative blood loss may be massive, occasionally requiring blood transfusion, with an autogenous bone graft being mandatory when rigid fixation materials are used. Intermaxillary fixation is required for 2 to 4 weeks after the operation. Relapse by absorption of the grafted bone is unclear. The advantages of distraction osteogenesis compared with conventional osteotomy are that it reduces operative times and blood loss, bone grafts are naturally unnecessary, and bone is distracted in conjunction with the surrounding soft tissues and nerves. These adaptive changes in the soft tissues decrease the relapse risk and allow the treatment of severe facial deformities. In addition, the length of distraction can be set freely and regulated within the limits of the device. Comparatively small relapses are another major advantage of distraction. Distraction also offers enormous advantages in jaw bones because they are covered with special fixed mucosa gingiva. Distraction in the maxillofacial area also has several merits because intermaxillary fixation is not necessary, no temporomandibular dysfunction is left, and fine adjustment of occlusion is possible. However, distraction osteogenesis has some disadvantages such as technique sensitive surgery, equipment sensitive surgery, possible need of second surgery to remove distraction devices and patient compliance. From a surgical standpoint, an adequate bone stock is necessary to accept the distraction appliances and to provide suitable opposing surfaces capable of generating a healing callus. Therefore, in patients who have undergone several craniofacial procedures in the past, the facial skeleton may exist in several small discontinuous fragments unsuitable for distraction. In these cases, bone grafting the gaps first may be possible, followed by distraction on a delayed basis.

3.8 Complications of DO

Complications can be divided into 3 groups: A) Intraoperative, B)Intradistraction, and C) Postdistraction complications.

a. The intraoperative complications concern the surgical procedure (eg, malfracturing, incomplete fracture, nerve damage, and excessive bleeding) and device- related problems (eg, fracture and unstable placement).
b. Intradistraction complications concern those arising during distraction (eg, infection, device problems, pain, malnutrition, and premature consolidation).
c. Postdistraction complications concern the late problems arising during the period of splinting and after removal of the distraction devices (eg, malunion, relapse, and persistent nerve damage (Samchukov et al. 2001).

The infection rate associated with distraction osteogenesis in general is reported as varying between 5% and 30% (Samchukov et al. 2001). However, these complications are mainly related to the application of external distraction devices. Infection is nevertheless mentioned as the most common complication during distraction. Notwithstanding that bacterial contamination is possible during the weeks of distraction and consolidation, the preventive administration of antibiotics during both the placement and the removal of the devices, along with good oral hygiene, appear to be sufficient to reduce the infection rate to an acceptable level.

4. Distraction osteogenesis for maxillofacial application

4.1 Alveolar Distraction Osteogenesis (ADO)

Insufficient bone height leads to overloading of osseointegrated implants and jeopardizes the longevity of the prosthetic restoration. A common pattern for vertical bone deficiency in this location is the loss of bone due to periodontitis or to trauma or subsequent to dental extraction. If socket preservation is not done, the alveolus narrows and alveolar vertical dimension is often reduced.(Froum et al. 2002; Vance et al. 2004) Vertical regeneration of resorbed alveolar ridges is still a challenging surgical procedure, especially in case of extensive bone atrophy. Several augmentation techniques have been proposed, even in cases with limited bone support and inadequate nourishment. These procedures often involve the use of bone substitutes or the harvesting of autogenous bone from a donor site. Autogenous bone is believed to be the most effective bone graft material and is still regarded as the "gold standard" for augmentation procedures because of its osteogenic potential. However, this graft has a limited availability; furthermore, the surgical harvesting procedures might cause additional morbidity. (Cricchio & Lundgren, 2003; Nkenke et al. 2002; Sasso et al. 2005)
Difficulties have been encountered to simultaneously augment the width and height of the deficient ridge. Crestal split technique is efficient in lateral widening but not vertical augmentation (Palti, 2003). Onlay bone graft or guided bone regeneration technique is especially useful for augmenting the ridge width but, to some extent, has limited advantages in increasing the ridge height (Nkenke et al. 2002; Simion et al. 1994). The interpositional bone graft procedure also has technical difficulty in a limited edentulous ridge. Additionally autogenous bone graft this graft has a limited availability; furthermore, the surgical harvesting procedures might cause additional morbidity. (Cricchio & Lundgren, 2003; Sasso et al. 2005). The various bone graft techniques can lead to wound dehiscence, infection, and possibly total failure of bone graft because of lack of appropriate soft tissue coverage in those traumatized areas. In addition, early membrane exposure may cause infection that may compromise the final outcome of the rehabilitation. This technique has been mainly applied to limited defects with vertical bone gains ranging from 2 to 7 mm, on average (Jovanovic et al. 1995; Simion et al. 1994).
ADO is a process used for vertical and horizontal distraction of the atrophic mandibular and maxillary alveolar ridges. This technique provides a very good quality of the neogenerated bone, with adequate characteristics for implant osseointegration. Alveolar distractors may be classified as intraosseous (endosseous) or extraosseous (subperiosteal) according to their insertion techniques (Fig.3-Fig.9). Extraosseous distractors are placed over the buccal surface of the alveolus subperiosteally, whereas intraosseous ones are placed through the transport segment and fixed to the basal segment by microplates toward the vector of distraction. The first devices used for distraction surgery of the upper & lower jaws were large and

protruded through the patient's skin. The results were often satisfactory, but the facial scars and esthetic compromise of such devices made the process an option for only the more extreme cases. In the last few years the technology of distraction devices has progressed to the point where the distraction devices are all intraoral; thus avoiding the unsightly facial scars. Recently, new distraction devices have been developed to permit this nascent technique to be employed in the growth of bone for dental implants. In such cases a small section of the jaw bone is surgically cut and then gently distracted to grow both height or width of bone. After a short healing period dental implants can be placed. In alveolar distraction, the vertical bone gain may reach more than 15 mm, it is obtained in amore 'physiologic'way, with no need of bone transplantation, thus reducing morbidity. Another main advantage may include a progressive elongation of the surrounding soft tissues with very limited risk of wound dehiscence and bone exposure. In most distraction cases the need for extensive bone grafting is eliminated. The final result, be it advancement of the jaws or the growing of bone for implants, is often reached in less time than with grafting, with superior results, and less patient discomfort (Gunbay et al. 2008b; Uckan et al. 2002).
ADO is not an uncomplicated procedure, and the occurrence of relapse of the distracted segment seems to necessitate an overcorrection of 15–20%. Survival of dental implants inserted into distracted areas has been shown to be satisfactory.

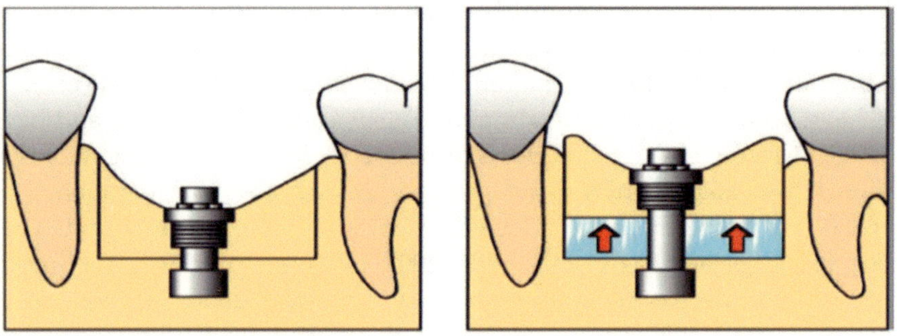

Fig. 3. OsteoGenic Distractor System

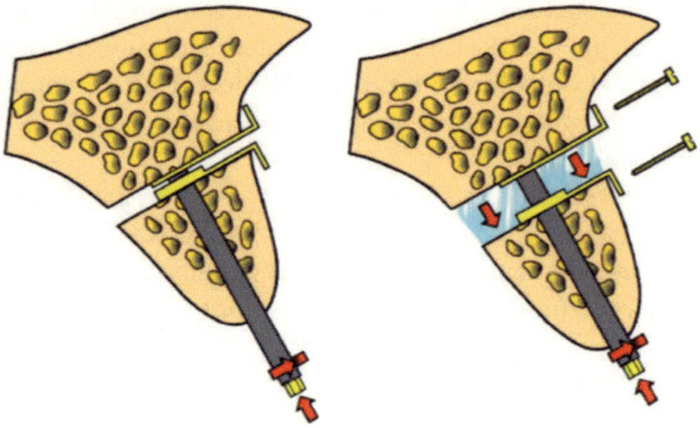

Fig. 4. LEAD Distractor System

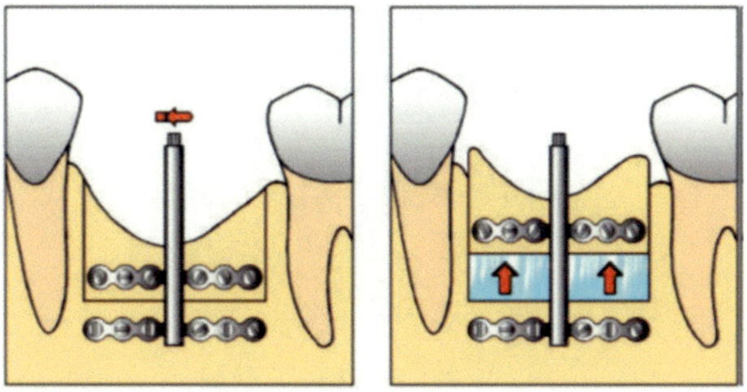

Fig. 5. TRACK 1.0 Distractor

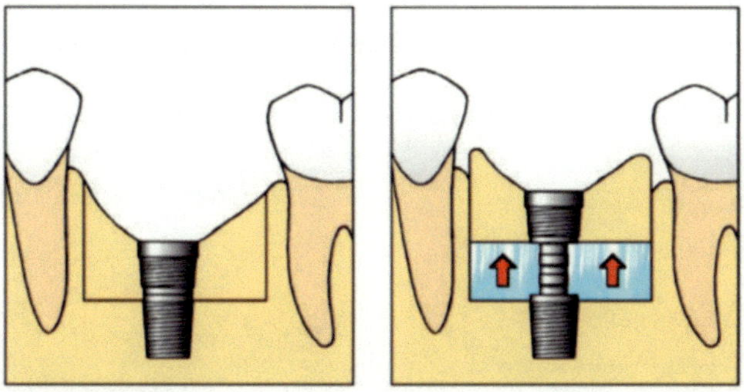

Fig. 6. DISSIS Distractor-Implant.

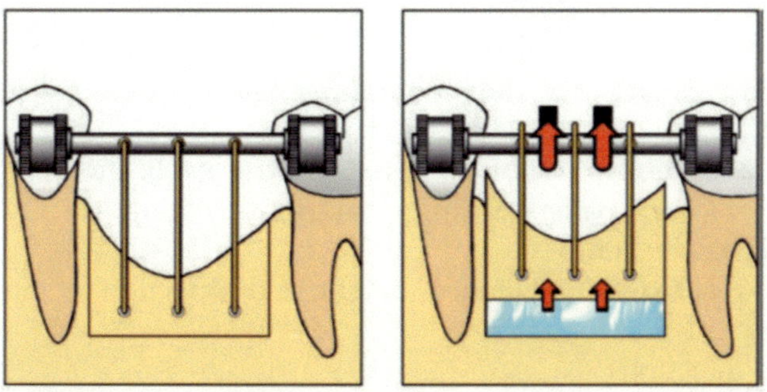

Fig. 7. ROD5 Distractor.

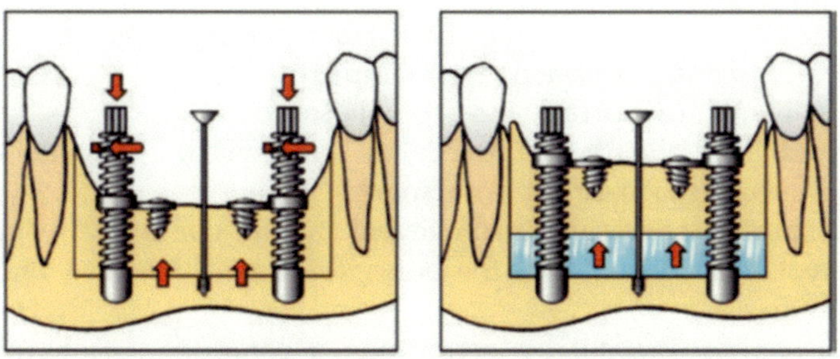

Fig. 8. GDD Distractor. (Fig.3-Fig.8 Reprinted from Cano et al. 2006)

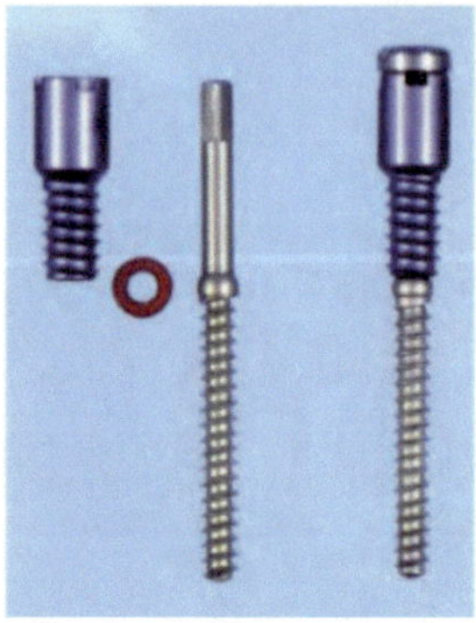

Fig. 9. The Endodistraction Implant System: The cortical screw is placed inside a hollow Implant, which rests on top of the shoulder of the threaded rod. A silicon seal inside the hollow implant prevents contact of saliva to bone (Krenkel and Grunert, 2007)

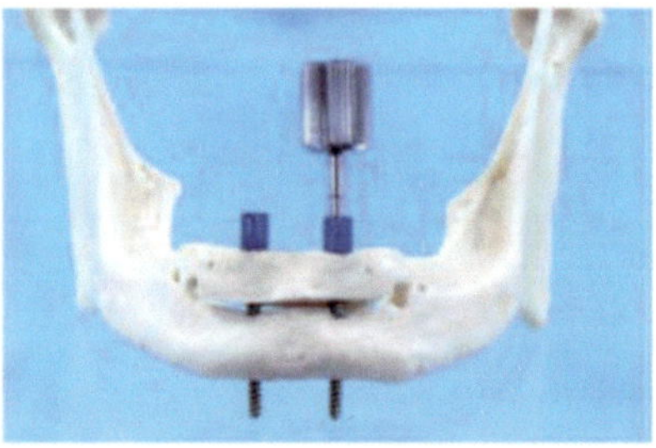

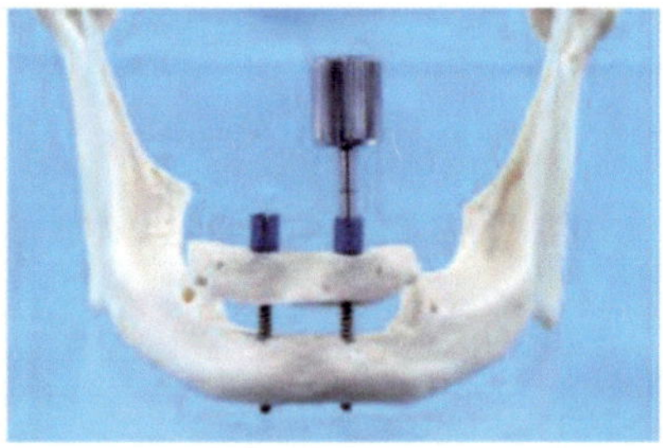

Fig. 9.a.b. Endodistraction Implant before (a) and after (b) distraction (Krenkel & Grunert, 2007).

An ideal distraction device for the edentulous jaws should include the following characteristics:

1. Minimal trauma for tissues and blood vessels during application
2. Maximal comfort for the patient during speaking and eating
3. Not compromising aesthetics
4. Guarantee for reaching the planned height and direction of augmentation of the alveolar ridge
5. Minimal risk of infection
6. Chance for continuing distraction in case of problems or pitfalls during the primary distraction period
7. Minimal invasive removal
8. Perfect stabilization of the new formed bone when placing implants
9. No limitations for using any type of dental implants

Complications of alveolar distraction and possible solutions

Infection of distraction chamber. Prevent by prophylactic antibiotic treatment and adequate mucosal covering. Treatment: Antibiotics.

Fractures of transported or basal bone. Prevent by the use of very fine blades in the osteotomy and avoiding expansion of the bone. Treatment: Suspend the distraction and treat with osteosynthesis.

Premature consolidation. Prevent by performing a complete osteotomy and using the appropriate distraction rate and distraction vector. Treatment: Repeat osteotomy.

Consolidation delay and absence of fibrous union. Prevent with a correct stabilization of the distractor. Treatment: Delay distractor withdrawal until consolidation; in absence of fibrous union, carry out debridement of the area and reconstruct using other regeneration techniques.
Slight resorption of the transported fragment. Prevent with an overcorrection of the defect of around 2 mm.
Wound dehiscence. Prevent by smoothing the sharp edges of the transported fragment. Treatment: Resuture soft tissues to prevent infection of the distraction chamber.
Distractor instability. Prevent by prior evaluation of the bone density and distractor model used. Treatment: Specific, depending on the distractor design.
Deviations from the correct distraction vector. Prevent with prior evaluation of the thickness of the mucosa and vestibular and lingual muscle insertions. Treatment: Early correction with acrylic plates or orthodontic corrective devices.
Neurological alterations. Prevent with correct localization of osteotomy and placement of retention screws. Treatment: Immediate withdrawal of screws; microsurgery.
Distractor fractures. Prevent with evaluation of the occlusion and avoidance of interferences. Treatment: Immediate withdrawal of fractured fragments and their repositioning according to the phase of the process.
High cost of distractors.
Need for the collaboration of the patient or family member for activation of the distractor.
(Cano et al. 2006)

4.2 Transpalatal Distraction Osteogenesis (TPDO)

Transverse maxillary deficiency is frequently observed in adult patients and may be responsible for unilateral or bilateral posterior cross-bite and anterior teeth crowding. This defect may be associated with a sagittal or vertical jaw discrepancy. In some cases, the transverse deficiency is apparent (relative) and resolves with jaw repositioning, but in all other cases it is essential to include transverse augmentation in the treatment plan, in order to achieve stable, satisfactory occlusion. Different approaches can be considered for correction. Orthodontic devices may move the teeth buccally, but do not augment bone transversally. Consequently, they can only be applied to small discrepancies. Since the comprehensive fundamental clinical investigations carried out by Derichsweiler in 1956, rapid expansion of the midpalatal suture has become an established, proven method for treating children and adolescents with severe transverse maxillary deficiencies combined with crossbite. Generally, non-surgical expansion is indicated in patients under the age of 12 years and is associated with complications when used in skeletally mature patients (Mommaerts, 1999). In adults, this technique has frequently led to complications such as buccal tipping, extrusions, root resorption and fenestrations of the alveolar process at the supporting teeth absorbing the force (Mommaerts, 1999; Moss, 1968; Neyt et al. 2002).
For many years, maxillary width discrepancies have been corrected in pediatric patients solely by orthodontic therapies, such as slow orthodontic expansion (SOE) and rapid palatal expansion (RPE), and in adult patients by surgical treatments such as surgically assisted rapid palatal expansion (SARPE) and 2-segment Le Fort I-type osteotomy with expansion (LFI-E). Although commonly performed, these therapies present some problems related to the tooth-borne appliances (ie, SOE, RPE, SARPE), including alveolar bone bending, periodontal membrane compression, root reabsorption and lateral tooth displacement and extrusion (Glassman et al., 1984). Longterm stability remains problematic as well (Haas

1980). Relapse is the main problem after a LFI-E maxillary osteotomy combined with a midpalatal osteotomy (Koudstaal et al. 2005), probably due to the lack of a palatal retention appliance, fibrous scar retraction, and palatal fibromucosal traction (Matteini & Mommaerts, 2001). An increment in the transverse diameter obtained entirely via bone formation, with no dental compensation, the absence of dental or osseous relapse, and no dental or periodontal damage, represents the ideal goal in treating the narrow maxilla. DO has been proven to ensure new bone formation at the osteotomy site without fibrous scarring in the maxillofacial skeleton (Nocini et al. 2002). TPDO is a new method for treating transversal maxillary deficienciy using the DO procedure, which has proven very valuable in other surgical fields (Mommaerts, 1999). Transpalatal distraction device is a bone-borne appliance that directs the forces mainly to the palatal helves close to the center of resistance of the maxillary bone without tooth movement; it also leaves all of the crowns clear for orthodontic access (Mommaerts et al., 1999). Additionally, most of the maxillary expansion is orthopaedic (Aras et al. 2011; Koudstaal et al. 2006). TPDO is an effective and largely painless technique for maxillary expansion free of complications and relapses. Since no teeth are used for distractor fixation but the alveolar processes undergo bodily lateral distraction below the osteotomy lines, all problems induced by forces acting upon anchorage teeth are eliminated (Fig.10-11). Moreover, the use of these appliances is not dependent on the number of anchorage teeth available. TPDO has been used extensively in the expansion of maxillary collapse in non-congenital defects (Gunbay et al. 2008a; Koudstaal et al. 2006; Mommaerts, 1999). Recurrence of the collapse and alveolar bone effects are among the reported complications (Gunbay et al. 2008a; Mommaerts, 1999; Suri & Taneja, 2008). Transverse maxillary expansion with a bone-borne transpalatal distractor has been used with favourable results in congenital and acquired transverse maxillary deficiency (Gunbay et al. 2008a; Koudstaal et al., 2006; Mommaerts, 1999; Suri & Taneja, 2008; Vyas et al. 2009).

In many studies, effects of transversal expansion have been examined by posteroanterior cephalometric measurements in dentoalveolar, maxillary base and nasal regions. Innovation of computed tomography (CT) technology, now makes it possible to acquire radiographic images with high resolution and diagnostic reliability that allow investigators to evaluate the changes at different levels of maxilla and nasal cavity (Aras et al. 2011; Garrett et al. 2008; Gunbay et al. 2008a; Phatouros & Goonewardene, 2008; Podesser et al. 2007).

Considering the problems encountered, no major surgical complications are expected from transpalatal distraction, except for the potential damage to the periodontal tissues adjacent to the midline osteotomy. In TPDO technique, especially vertical osteotomy is very important because this can damage dental structures. Close root proximity between the maxillary central incisors presents a problem in the surgical management of a maxillary palatal expansion. If the roots of the teeth are too close together in the area of the planned interdental osteotomy, the roots must be diverged to create adequate room for the bone cut. Vertical osteotomy must be done carefully. Any incorrect placement of a TPD may also damage the surrounding blood vessels and premolar or molar roots. Bony anchorage can bring about a number of complications, which have not been studied so far. In the searched TPD literature, wound infection, epistaxis, haematoma in cheek, maxillary sinusitis, infraorbital hypoaesthesia, palatal ulceration, displacement or loosening of transpalatal modules and abutment plates, extrusion of osteosynthesis screws, segmental tilting and dental complications due to vertical osteotomy were mentioned (Aras et al. 2011; Gunbay et al. 2008a). Minor difficulties that result from mechanical failure of TPD device might be eliminated with refinement of the instrumentation.

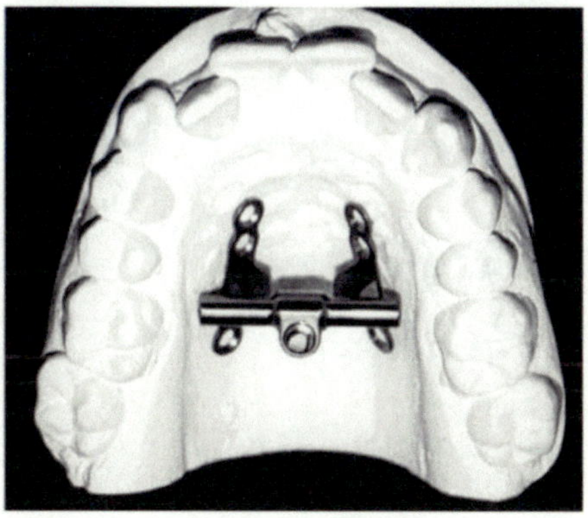

Fig. 10. Palatal distractor on a dental cast (Reprinted from Gerlach & Zahl 2003).

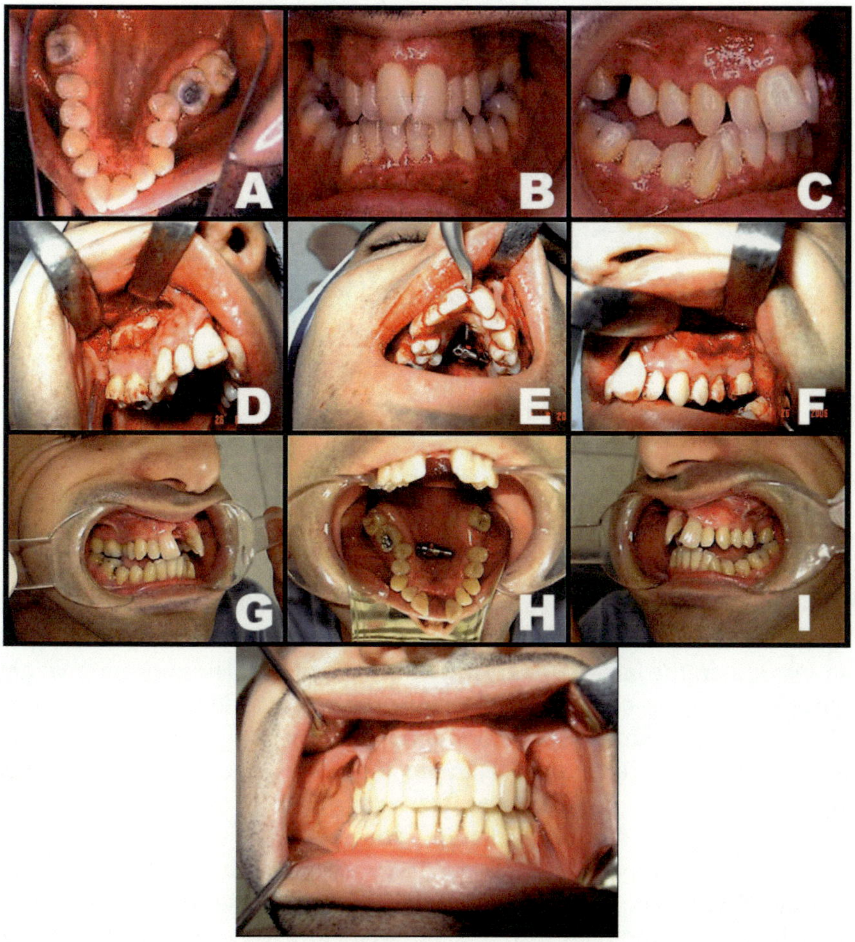

Fig. 11. Clinical appearence of our 1.case with severe maxillary deficiency, before treatment (A-C), of osteotomies (D-F), and in postdistraction period (G-I). Clinical appearence of the patient - 7 years after orthodontic treatment)

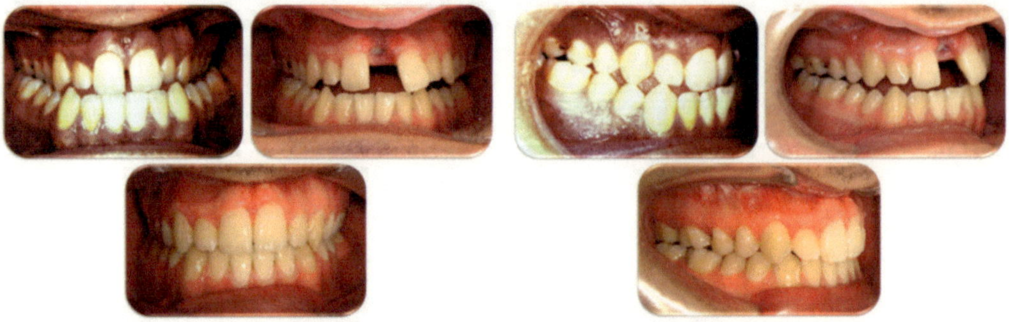

Fig. 12. A. Clinical appearence of our 2. case, the pretreatment, postdistraction period and after orthodontic treatment

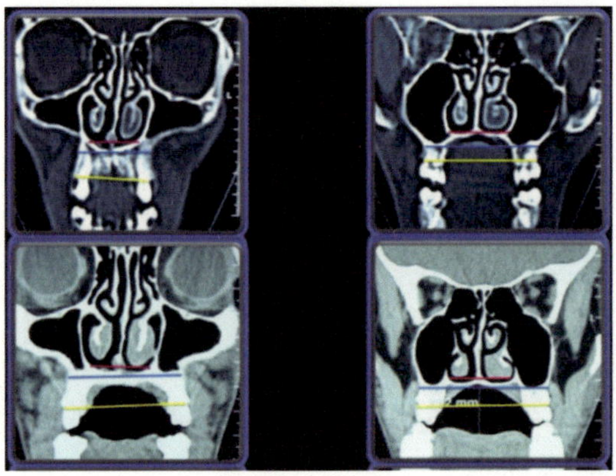

Fig. 12. B. CT measurements at the maxillary canine and first molar region-Pre and postdistraction period.

4.3 Transmandibular Distraction Osteogenesis (TMDO)

Mandibular transverse deficiency (MTD) and crowding of the anterior teeth are problems shared by most orthodontic patients. MTD is a common clinical problem associated with narrow basal and dentoalveolar bone (Del Santo et al. 2000, 2002; Guerrero et al. 1990). Attention to the transverse deficiencies is vital in planning treatment for a patient who requires an increase in the lateral dimension of the mandible. The conventional approaches for correcting mandibular crowding are extraction of teeth, dentoalveolar expansion or interproximal enamel reduction. Orthodontic treatment options include functional appliances, and orthopedic devices. MTD in mix dentition stage are commonly treated with orthodontic expansion using lip bumpers, Schwarz's device, or functional devices. These therapies Show relatively stable results for younger patients, particularly those who presented with lingually tipped teeth that need to be decompensated (McNamara & Brudon, 1993). But mandibular expansion or incisor protrusion in the anterior area is generally unstable and tends to relapse toward the original dimension and with a compromised periodontium created by moving teeth out of their supporting alveolar bone in the long term (Blake & Bibby, 1998; Guerrero et al. 1997; Herberger, 1981). Previously in adult patients, the sole correction technique of symphyseal osteotomy has been proposed as a solution for treatment of MTD. However, this surgical procedure has not been well accepted because of lack of rigid fixation, need to use bone grafts, risk of periodontal problems that may occur when the bone segments are rapidly and excessively separated and increased risk of relapse (Conley & Legan, 2003). The mandible was the initial site of application of distraction osteogenesis in the face. The mandible's structure is similar to the tubular structure of the long bones of the skeleton. Principles learned by orthopedic surgeons over the previous 80 years from distraction of the long bones of the lower extremity were rapidly adapted to this new location (Synder et al. 1973; Michieli & Miotti, 1977). Since first described by McCarthy et al. in 1992, DO of craniofacial bones has increasingly become a mainstay in bone regeneration. DO has provided a powerful tool for treatment of many mandibular deformities that previously could not be successfully treated by the conventional methods of orthognathic surgery, free tissue transfer, or nonvascularized bone grafts (Havlik & Bartlett, 1994; McCarthy et al. 1996, 1998).

Transmandibular symphyseal distraction (TMSD) technique solve rapidly MTD problems. TMSD can be performed to increase the transverse dimension of the mandibular basal bone if the aim is to correct arch length deficiency by expanding the basal bone (Guerrero et al. 1997; Gunbay et al., 2009; Mommaerts et al. 2005, 2008; Uckan et al. 2005, 2006). With this clinical procedure, the mandibular geometry is definitively changed. Theoretically, greater stability could be expected if the expansion is performed slowly, allowing better adaptation of the soft tissues, and allowing bone to grow in the osteotomy site. Guerrero et al. (1990) pioneered the use of rapid surgical mandibular expansion for correcting MTD. Although vertical midsymphyseal osteotomy technique for treatment of MTD is used for many years, many investigators reported that in this method, mucosa and periodontal ligaments can not adopt to rapid movement of bone fragmants after osteotomy. Compared with distraction osteogenesis, vertical midsymphyseal osteotomy is a more extensive surgical procedure involving a higher risk of relapse, a longer operative time, the requirement of bone grafts and internal fixation (Guerrero et al. 1997; Martin, 1998).

TMSD is a successful surgical alternative to orthodontic dental compensation, removal of tooth mass by interproximal stripping, or extractions in cases of transverse anterior mandibular discrepancy (Guerrero et al. 1990, 1997; Gunbay et al., 2009; Mommaerts, 2001; Mommaerts et al., 2004a, 2004b; Mommaerts & Vande Vannet, 2004; Mommaerts et al., 2005). Several authors have proven the efficacy of this technique in animal experiments (Bell et al. 1999; El-Hakim et al. 2004) and in small clinical series (Kewitt & Van Sickels, 1999; Weil et al. 1997). The distraction device itself can be tooth-borne (Alkan et al. 2006; Braun et al. 2002; Del Santo et al. 2000, 2002; Guerrero et al. 1997; Iseri & Malkoc, 2005; Orhan et al. 2003; Tae et al. 2006), bone-borne (Bell et al. 1999; Braun et al. 2002; El-Hakim et al. 2004; Gunbay et al. 2009; Iseri & Malkoc, 2005, Mommaerts, 2001), or a combination of both (Duran et al., 2006; Uckan et al. 2005, 2006). There are some conflicts on the use of different types of symphyseal distractor. Toothborne distractors have some serious disadvantages such as periodontal problems, buccal root resorption and cortical fenestration, segmental tipping and anchorage-tooth tipping, loss of anchorage. In TMSD technique, the forces act directly on symphyseal bone region. Therefore no tooth tipping and other unwellcome dental effects are expected and most of the mandibular expansion is orthopaedic. Many authors state that the bone-borne devices applied directly to the symphysis lead to greater skeletel effect than dental effects.

One of the most important potential side effects of TMSD is alteration of temporomandibular joint function. Harper et al. (1997) studied the impact of a tooth-borne appliance for mandibular symphyseal DO in monkey's mandibular condyle. They found that the histologic changes in the condyles were minor, limited to atypical morphology. Using computer modeling, Samchukov et al. (1998) showed lateral rotational movement of the condyles subsequent to mandibular widening, and reported 0.34-degree condylar rotation for every 1 mm of widening at the mandibular midline. Fortunately, the human temporomandibular condyle is known to have some degree of physiologic adaptability (Gunbay et al. 2009; Uckan et al. 2006)

The location of the TMD device are another important issue. This is critical because this may affect the ratio of skeletal/dental expansion. An obliquely positioned distractor may result in asymmetric expansion (Basciftci et al. 2004; Orhan et al. 2003).

Complications at the level of the periodontal and endodontal status of the incisors and at the Temporomandibular Joints (TMJ) have been reported in another study (Mommaerts et al. 2005). Gunbay et al. (2009) reported that, the follow-up cephalograms and CT scans showed the transverse skeletal stability of the distraction procedure and no permanent temporomandibular dysfunction. The effect of the procedure on the condyle was 2.5 degrees to 3 degrees of distolateral rotation as calculated using the CT scans. The authors think that moderate symphyseal expansion will not cause clinical problems in the TMJ area. On the other hand, bony anchorage can bring about a number of complications, which have not been studied so far. In the TMSD literature some complications such as seriously hemorrhage and infection, damage to the inferior alveolar nerve and dental structures, pseudoarthrosis, jaw fractures and breakage of distractor device were reported (Bayram et al. 2007; Del Santo et al 2002; Gunbay et al., 2009; Kewitt & Van Sickels 1999; Uckan et al, 2006). Alkan et al. (2007) reported some complications of bone-borne distractors such as high cost, long operation time, and need for removal distracton in a second operation. The main problem during symphyseal transverse DO with the bone-borne Transmandibular Distractor device appears to be high local infection rates and patient discomfort due to delayed union. (Mommaerts et al. 2008; Gunbay et al. 2009) Mommarets et al. (2008) suggested that in order to prevent late local infections, the device could be removed at the end of the distraction period and replaced by titanium or resorbable osteosynthesis plates. Because of the design of the TMSD, food remnants are easily stuck on activation rods and leads to chronic hyperplastic gingival infections. Therefore patients must be instructed to clean the device thoroughly on a daily bases and a regular visit to an oral hygienist should be arranges. The main advantage of the TMSD is that the device is located intraorally and preferred by the patients. Due to the design the TMSD is easily placed and activated. The use of this appliance is not dependent on the number of anchorage teeth available. Moreover, orthodontic appliances can be installed at an earlier date than when tooth-borne expanders are used. There is no need for dental anchorage that might cause damage to the dentition or dental tipping.

Although TMSD has become an extremely alternative technique for the maxillofacial surgeons, there is no consensus in literature regarding osteotomy techniques used in distraction osteogenesis procedure, type of distractor used, effects of the distraction loads on TMJ, dental and skeletal structures, cause and amount of relapse and whether or not overcorrection is necessary. In TMSD technique, especially vertical osteotomy is very important because this can damage dental structures. Close root proximity between the mandibular central incisors presents a problem in the surgical management of a TMSD. If the roots of the teeth are too close together in the area of the planned interdental osteotomy, the roots must be diverged to create adequate room for the bone cut. Vertical osteotomy must be done carefully and accurately. From the surgical point of view, treatment planning should include analysis of a recent periapical radiograph of the incisor roots to determine the need for orthodontic root separation before surgery. 3–5 mm space between the apices of the central teeth is necessary to safely perform an interdental vertical osteotomy, without compromising periodontal health or tooth vitality. Removing bone and damaging the periodontal ligament along the root surfaces of adjacent teeth can result in periodontal defects or ankylosis of the involved lower central teeth during the following years. In cases of severe dental crowding on the midline, Mommaerts at al. (2008) currently prefer to place the interdental osteotomy at a site where there is a natural diastema at the apical level, which is frequently between the canine and lateral incisor. To prevent deviation of the chin, a vertical osteotomy is performed in the midline to 5 mm below the apices of the incisors. The two vertical osteotomy lines are then connected with an oblique subapical osteotomy. Mussa & Smith (2003) suggested creating a diastema pre-operatively using orthodontics. However, since severe crowding is the primary indication for symphyseal widening, nonextraction orthodontic widening is very difficult.

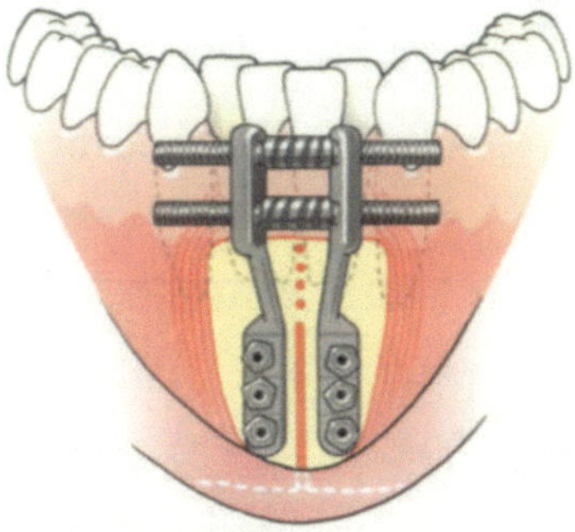

Fig. 13. Symphyseal vertical midline osteotomy, avoiding the mentalis muscles but endangering the apices of the central incisors when these are juxtaposed (Mommaerts et al. 2008).

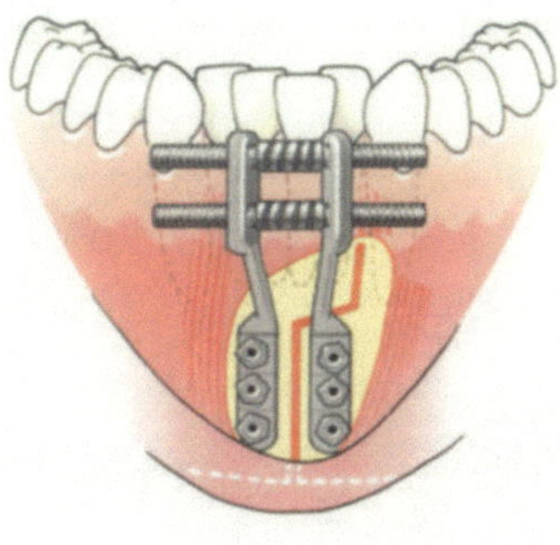

Fig. 14. Step osteotomy in the symphysis. The alveolus between the canine and lateral incisor is often much wider than between the central incisors (Mommaerts at al. 2008).

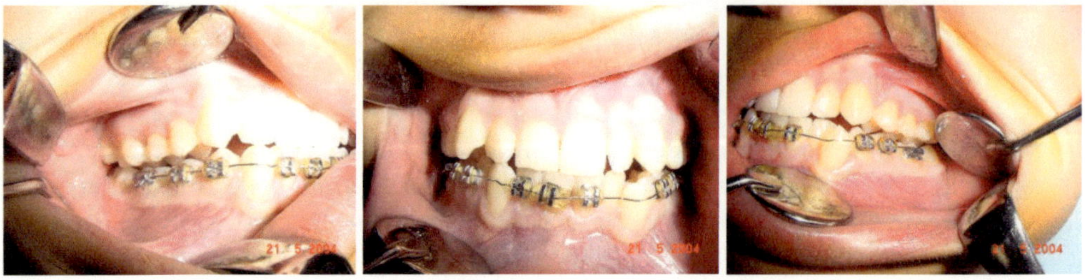

Fig. 15. A. Our case 3. Clinical appearence before TMSD treatment

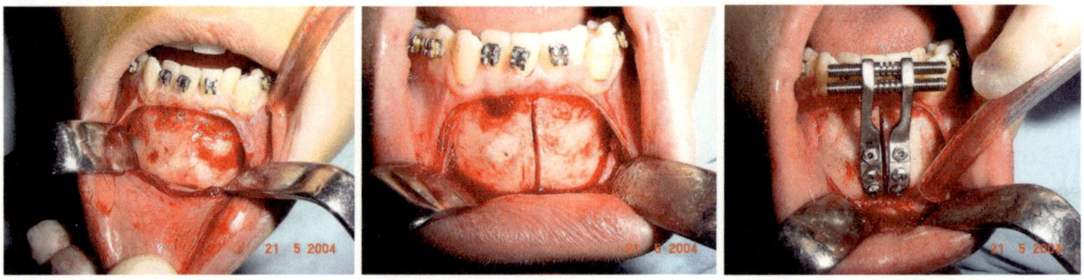

Fig. 15. B. Our case 3. Clinical appearence of osteotomies and predistraction period

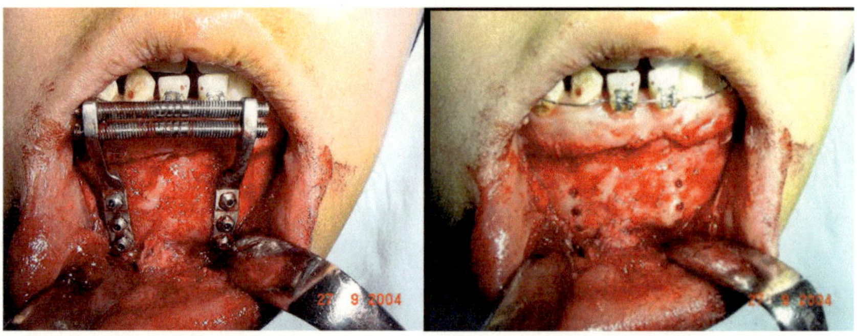

Fig. 15. C. linical appearence of new regenerated bone in postconsolidation period

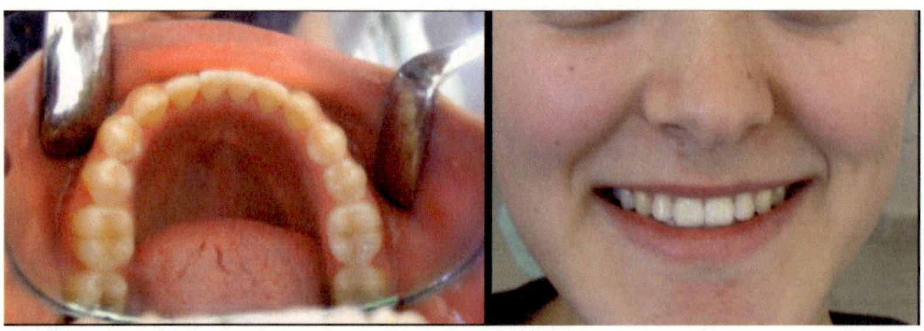

Fig. 15. D. Clinical appearence of postorthodontic treatment period

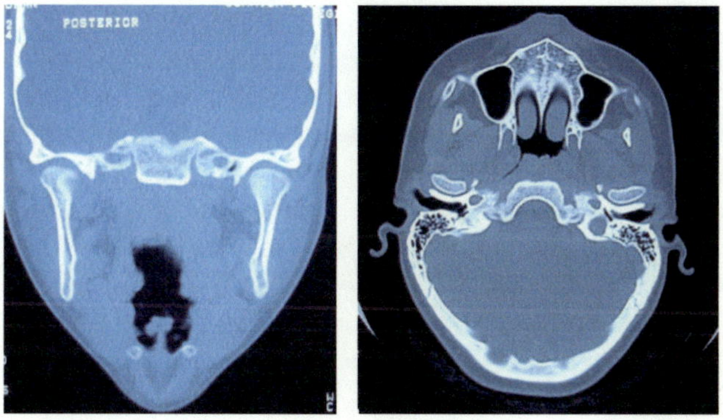

Fig. 15. E. CT imaging. In predistraction and postorthodontic treatment period

5. Conclusion

There are different treatment modalities for bimaxillary deficiencies in the recent literatures. Many surgeons find it difficult to decide which technique offers better results, and are also uncertain about the factors which might influence their techniques of choice. Distraction osteogenesis of the craniofacial skeleton has become increasingly popular as an alternative to many conventional orthognathic surgical procedures. For patients with mild to severe abnormalities of the craniofacial skeleton, distraction techniques have increased the number of treatment alternatives. Many of the adult distraction cases are significantly compromised, requiring a multidisciplinary approach to treatment. It is very important to consider surgical and dental concerns during distraction osteogenesis treatment planning. These concerns include predistraction orthodontics, osteotomy design and location, selection of the distraction device, distraction vector orientation, duration of the latency period, the rate and rhythm of distraction, duration of the consolidation period, postdistraction orthodontics and functional loading of the regenerate bone. DO represents an exciting new development in craniofacial surgery with several potential benefits, including less invasive surgery, the ability for earlier intervention, and the potential for correction of more severe deformities with improved posttreatment stability. The exact role of distraction osteogenesis relative to conventional techniques requires ongoing assessment. Improvement of the technique and of the devices used, with an adjusted protocol, could lead to a reduction in the number of complications. In the presented chapter, advantages and disadvantages of DO techniques are discussed under the light of the current literatures.

6. References

Abbott, J.S., (1927) Letters to the Editor. *Am J Public Health* (NY), Vol. 17, No.12, pp: 1256- 1257

Alkan, A., Arici S. & Sato S., (2006) Bite force and occlusal contact area changes following mandibular widening using distraction osteogenesis. *Oral Surg Oral Med Oral Pathol Oral Radiol Endod,* Vol.101, pp: 432-436

Alkan, A., Ozer M. & Bas B. Et al., (2007) Mandibular symphyseal distraction osteogenesis: review of three techniques. *Int J Oral Maxillofac Surg* Vol.36, pp: 111–117

Allan, F.G., (1948) Bone lengthening. *J Bone Joint Surg Br,* Vol.30B, No.3,: 490-505

Aras, A., Akay M.C. & Cukurova I., et al., (2010) Dimensional changes of the nasal cavity after transpalatal distraction using bone-borne distractor: An acoustic rhinometry and computed tomography evaluation. *J Oral Maxillofac Surg,* Vol.68, No. 7, pp: 1487-1497

Aronson, J., (1994) Experimental and clinical experience with distraction osteogenesis. *Cleft Palate Craniofac J* Vol. 31, pp: 473-482.

Basciftci, F.A., Korkmaz H.H. & Iseri H., et al., (2004) Biomechanical evaluation of mandibular midline distraction osteogenesis by using the finite element method. *Am J Orthod Dentofacial Orthop,* Vol.125, pp: 706-715

Bayram, M., Ozer M. & Alkan. A., (2006) Mandibular symphyseal distraction osteogenesis using a bone-supported distractor. *Anle Orthod,* Vol. 70, No.5, pp: 20-27

Bell, W.H., Gonzalez M. &, Samchukov M.L., et al., (1999) Intraoral widening and lengthening of the mandible in baboons by distraction osteogenesis. *J Oral Maxillofac Surg, Vol.* 57, No. 5, pp: 548-562

Blake, M. & Bibby K., (1998) Retention and stability: A review of the literature. *Am JOrthod Dentofacial Orthop Vol.*114, pp: 299-306

Braun, S., Bottrel A. & Legan H.L., (2002) Condylar displacement related to mandibular symhyseal distraction. *Am J Orthop Dentofacial Orthop,* Vol.121, pp: 162-165

Cano, J., Campo, J. & Moreno, L.A., et al., (2006) Osteogenic alveolar distraction: A review of the literature. *Oral Surg Oral Med Oral Pathol Oral Radiol Endod,* Vol.101, pp: 11-28

Chin, M. & Toth B.A., (1996) Distraction osteogenesis in maxillofacial surgery using internal devices: Review in five cases. *J Oral Maxillofac Surg,* Vol.54, pp: 45-53

Chin, M., (1999) Distraction osteogenesis for dental implants. *Atlas Oral Maxillofac Surg Clin North Am* Vol. 7, pp: 41–63

Codvilla, A., (1905) On the means of lengthening in the lower limbs, the muscles and tissues which are shortened through deformity. *Am J Orthop Surg,* Vol.2, pp: 353-369

Conley, R. & Legan H., (2003) Mandibular symphyseal distraction osteogenesis: diagnosis and treatment planning considerations. *Angle Orthod,Vol.* 73, pp: 3-11

Costantino, P.D., Shybut G. & Friedman C.D., et al. , (1990) Segmental mandibular regeneration by distraction osteogenesis. *Arch Otolaryngol Head Neck Surg,* Vol.116, pp: 535-545

Cricchio, G. & Lundgren S., (2003) Donor site morbidity in two different approaches to anterior iliac crest bone harvesting. *Clin Implant Dent Relat Res* Vol.5, No.3, pp:161-9

Del Santo, M., English J.D. & Wolford L.M., et al., (2002) Midsymphyseal distraction osteogenesis for correcting transverse mandibular discrepancies. *Am J Orthod Dentofacial Orthop,* Vol.121, pp: 629-638

Del Santo, M., Guerrero C.A. & Buschang P.H., et al., (2000) Long-term skeletal and dental effects of mandibular symphyseal distraction osteogenesis. *Am J Orthod Dentofacial Orthop* Vol.118, pp: 485–493

Duran, I., Malkoc S. & Iseri H., et al., (2006) Microscopic evaluation of mandibular symphyseal distraction. *Angle Orthod* Vol.76, pp: 369–374

El-Hakim I.E., Azim A.M. & El-Hassan M.F., et al. (2004). Preliminary investigation into theeffects of electrical stimulation on mandibular distraction osteogenesis in goats. Int J Oral Maxillofac Surg, Vol. 33, No.1, pp: 42-47

Froum, S., Cho S.C. & Rosenberg E. et al., (2002) Histological comparison of healing extraction sockets implanted with bioactive glass or demineralized freeze-dried bone allograft: a pilot study. *J Periodontol,* Vol.73, No.1, pp: 94-102

Gantous, A., Phillips J.H. & Catton P., et al., (1994) Distraction osteogenesis in the irradiated canine mandible. *Plast Reconstr Surg,* Vol. 93, pp: 164-170

Garrett, B.J., Caruso J.M. & Rungcharassaeng K, et al. (2008) Skeletal effects to the maxilla after rapid maxillary expansion assessed with cone-beam computed tomography. *Am J Orthod Dentofacial Orthop,* Vol. 134, pp: 8.e1-8.e11

Gerlach K.L. & Zahl C., (2003) Transversal palatal expansion using a palatal distractor. *J Orofac Orthop,* Vol. 64, pp: 443-449

Glassman, A.S., Nahigian S.J. & Medway J.M., et al., (1984) Conservative surgical orthodontic adult rapid palatal expansion: Sixteen cases. *Am J Orthod Dentofacial Orthop,* Vol.86, pp: 207–213

Gosain, A.K., Santoro T.D. & Havlik R.J. et al., (2002) Midface distraction following Le Fort III and monobloc osteotomies: problems and solutions. *Plast Reconstr Surg,* Vol.109, No. 6, pp: 1797-1808

Guerrero, C.A., (1990) Rapid mandibular expansion. *Rev Venez Orthod,* Vol.48, pp: 1-9

Guererero, C.A, Bell W.H. & Contasti G.I., et al., (1997) Mandibular widening by intraoral distraction osteogenesis. *Br J Oral Maxillofac Surg,* Vol.35, pp: 383-392

Guerrero, C.A., Bell W.H. & Contasti G.I., et al., (1999) Intraoral mandibular distraction osteogenesis. *Semin Orthod,* Vol. 5, pp: 35-40

Gunbay, T., Akay M.C. & Gunbay S., et al., (2008) Transpalatal distraction using bone-borne distractor: clinical observations and dental and skeletal changes. *J Oral Maxillofac Surg,* Vol. 66, pp: 2503-2514

Gunbay, T., Ozveri Koyuncu B. & Akay M.C. et al., (2008) Results and complications of alveolar distraction osteogenesis to enhance vertical bone height. *Oral Surg Oral Med Oral Pathol Oral Radiol Endod,* Vol.105, pp: e7-e13

Gunbay, T., Akay, M.C. & Aras A., et al. (2009) Effects of transmandibular symphyseal distraction on teeth, bone, and temporomandibular joint. *J Oral Maxillofac Surg,* Vol.67, No. 10, pp: 2254-2265

Haas, A.J., (1980) The treatment of maxillary deficiency by opening the mid-palatal suture. *Angle Orthod,* Vol. 50, pp: 189–217

Harper, R.P., Bell W.H. & Hinton R.J., et al., (1997) Reactive changes in the temporomandibular joint after mandibular midline osteodistraction. *Br J Oral Maxillofac Surg,* Vol. 35, pp: 20-25

Havlik, R. & Bartlett, S.P., (1994) Mandibular distraction lengthening in the severely hypoplastic mandible: A problematic case with tongue aplasia. J Craniofac Surg, Vol. 5, pp: 305

Herberger, R.J., (1981) Stability of mandibular intercuspid width after long periods of retention. *Angle Orthod,* Vol. 51, pp: 78-83

Ilizarov, G.A., (1971) Basic principles of transosseous compression and distraction osteosynthesis. *Orthop Travmatol Protez,* Vol. 32, pp: 7-15.

Ilizarov, G.A., (1988) The principles of the Ilizarov method. *Bull Hosp Jt Dis Orthop Inst.* 48:1-12.

Ilizarov, G.A., (1989a) The tension-stress effect on the genesis and growth of tissues. Part I. The influence of stability of fixation and soft-tissue preservation. *Clin Orthop Relat Res,* Vol. 238, pp: 249-281

Ilizarov, G.A., (1989b) The tension-stress effect on the genesis and growth of tissues: Part II. The influence of the rate and frequency of distraction. *Clin Orthop Relat Res,* Vol. 239, pp: 263-285

Imola, M.J., Hamlar D.D. & Thatcher G., et al., (2002) The versatility of distraction osteogenesis in craniofacial surgery. Int J Oral Maxillofac Surg, Vol. 34, No.4, pp: 357-363

Imola, M.J., Ducic Y. & Adelson R.T., (2008) The secondary correction of posttraumatic craniofacial deformities. *Otolaryngol Head Neck Surg*, Vol.39, No.5, pp: 654-660

Iseri, H. & Malkoc S., (2005) Long-term skeletal effects of mandibular symphyseal distraction osteogenesis. An implant study. *Eur J Orthod*, Vol. 27, pp : 512-517

Jovanovic, S.A., Schenk, R.K. & Orsini M., et al., (1995) Supracrestal bone formation around dental implants: an experimental dog study. *International Journal of Oral and Maxillofacial Implants*, Vol. 10, pp: 23–31

Karp, N.S., Thorne C.H. & McCarthy J.G., et al., (1990) Bone lengthening in the craniofacial skeleton. *Ann Plast Surg*, Vol. 24, No. 3, pp: 231-237

Karp, N.S., McCarthy J.G. & Schreiber J.S., et al., (1992) Membranous bone lengthening: a serial histological study. *Ann Plast Surg*, Vol. 29, pp: 2–7

Kewitt, G.F. & Van Sickels J.E., (1999) Long-term effect of mandibular midline distraction osteogenesis on the status of the temporomandibular joint, teeth, periodontal structures, and neurosensory function. *J Oral Maxillofac Surg*, Vol. 57, pp: 1419-1425

Koudstaal, M.J., Poort LJ. & van der Wal K.G.H., et al., (2005) Surgically assisted rapid maxillary expansion (SARME): a review of the literature. *Int J Oral Maxillofac Surg*, Vol. 34, pp: 709-714

Koudstaal, M.J., van der Wal K.G.H. & Wolvius E.B., et al., (2006) The Rotterdam Palatal Distractor: Introduction of the new bone-borne device and report of the pilot study. *Int J Oral Maxillofac Surg*, Vol.35, pp: 31–35

Krenkel, Ch. & Grunert I., (2007) A new callus distraction technique using the Endodistraction Implant in severely atrophic mandibles - long-term results of 18 patients. Press Conference, KRENKEL Endo-Distraction, Salzburg, Austria.

Little, R.M. & Riedel R.A. (1989) Postretention evaluation of stability and relapse-mandibular arches with generalized spacing. *Am J Orthod Dentofacial Orthop*,Vol. 95, No.1, pp: 37-41

Luchs, J,S., Stelnicki E.J. & Rowe N.M., et al., (1992) Molding of the regenerate in mandibular distraction: Part 1: Laboratory study. *J Craniofac Surg*, Vol. 13, No. 2, pp: 205-211

Martin, D.L., (1998) Transverse stability of multi-segmented Le Fort I expansion procedures(Master's thesis). Dallas: Baylor College of Dentistry

Matteini, C. & Mommaerts M.Y., (2001) Posterior transpalatal distraction with pterygoid disjunction: A short-term model study. *Am J Orthod Dentofacial Orthop*,Vol. 120, No. 5, pp: 498-502

McCarthy, J.G., Schrieber J. & Karp N, et al., (1992) Lengthening of the human mandible by gradual distraction. *Plast Reconstr Surg*, Vol.89, pp: 1-12

McCarthy, J.G., (1996) Distraction of the mandible and craniofacial skeleton. *J Craniomaxillofac Surg*, Vol. 24, pp: 193-199

McCarthy, J.G., Williams J.K. & Grayson B.H., (1998) Controlled multiplanar distraction of the mandible: device development and clinical application. *J Craniofac Surg*, Vol. 9,pp: 322-329

McNamara, J.A. & Brudon, W.L., (1993) Orthodontic and Orthopedic Treatment in the Mix Dentition. Ann Arbor, Mich: Neednam Press; pp: 171–178

Michieli, S. & Miotti, B., (1977) Lengthening of mandibular body by gradual surgical-orthodontic distraction. J Oral Surg, Vol. 35, pp: 187

Mommaerts, M.Y., (1999) Transpalatal distraction as a method of maxillary expansion. *Br J Oral Maxillofac Surg*, Vol. 37, No. 4, pp: 268-272

Mommaerts, M., Ali, N. & Correia, P., (2004a) The concept of bimaxillary transverse osteodistraction: a paradigm shift? *Mund Kiefer Gesichtschir*, Vol. 8, pp: 211-216

Mommaerts, M., Steyaert, L. & Polsbroek R., et al., (2004b) Correlation between ultrasound and radiographic data for assessment of symphyseal bony callus maturation after distraction. *Rev Stomatol Chir Maxillofac*, Vol. 105, pp: 19-22

Mommaerts, M.Y. & Vande Vannet B. (2004) Bimaxillary transverse distraction osteogenesis. *Ned Tijdschr Tandheelkd*, Vol. 111, pp: 40-43

Mommaerts, M., Polsbroek R. & Santler G., et al., (2005) Anterior transmandibular osteodistraction: clinical and model observations. *J Craniomaxillofac Surg*, Vol. 33, No. 5, pp: 318-325

Mommaerts, M.Y., Spaey Y.J.E. & Soares Correia P.E.G., et al. (2008) Morbidity related to transmandibular distraction osteogenesis for patients with developmental deformities. *J Craniomaxillofac Surg*, Vol. 36, No. 4, pp: 192-197

Mommaerts, M,Y., (2001) Bone anchoredintraora l device for transmandibular distraction. *Br J Oral Maxillofac Surg*, Vol. 39, pp: 8–12

Moss, J.P., (1968) Rapid expansion of the maxillary arch. II. Indications for rapid expansion. *J Pract Orthod*, Vol. 2, pp: 215–223

Mussa, R. & Smith J., (2003) Mandibular symphyseal distraction osteogenesis. A case report. *J Clin Orthod*, Vol. 37, pp: 13-18

Neyt, N., Mommaerts, M. & Abeloos J., et al., (2002) Problems, obstacles and complications in transpalatal distraction in non-congenital deformities. *J Craniomaxillofac Surg*, Vol. 30, pp: 139-143

Nkenke, E., Radespiel-Tröger, M. & Wiltfang J., et al., (2002) Morbidity of harvesting of retromolar bone grafts: A prospective study. *Clin Oral Implants Res*, Vol.13, No.5, pp: 514-21

Nocini, P.F., Albanese M. & Wangerin K. (2002) Distraction osteogenesis of the mandible: evaluation of callus distraction by B-scan ultrasonography. *Journal of Cranio-Maxillofacial Surgery*, Vol. 30, pp: 286–291

Orhan, M., Malkoc, S. & Usumez S. (2003) Mandibular symphyseal distraction and its geometrical evaluation: report of a case. *Angle Orthod*, Vol. 73, pp: 194-200

Palti, A., (2003) Primary stability of implants in the posterior maxilla with autogenous bone rings harvested in the mandible. *Dent Implantol Update*, Vol. 14, No. 9, pp: 65-71

Pensler, J.M., Goldberg D.P. & Lindell B., et al., (1995) Skeletal distraction of the hypoplastic mandible. Ann Plast Surg, Vol.134, No.2, pp: 130-136

Phatouros, A. & Goonewardene, M.S. (2008) Morphologic changes of the palate after rapid maxillary expansion: A 3-dimensional computed tomography evaluation. *Am J Orthod Dentofacial Orthop*, Vol. 134, pp: 117-124

Podesser, B., Williams, S. & Chrismani A.G., et al., (2007) Evaluation of the effects of rapid maxillary expansion in growing children using computer tomography scanning: A pilot study. *Eur J Orthod*, Vol. 29, pp: 37-44

Polley, J.W. & Figueroa A.A., (1998) Rigid external distraction: Its application in cleft maxillary deformities. *Plast Reconstr Surg*, Vol.102, pp: 1360–1372

Proffit, W.R., Turvey T.A. & Phillips C., (1996) Orthognathic surgery: A hierarchy of stability. Int J Adult Orthod Othognath Surg, Vol.11, pp: 191–204

Ramieri G.A., Spada M.C. & Austa M., et al. (2005) Transverse maxillary distraction with a bone-anchored appliance: dento-periodontal effects and clinical and radiological results. Int J Oral Maxillofac Surg, Vol.34, pp: 357–363

Samchukov, M.L., Cope, J.B. & Harper, R.P., et al., (1998). Biomechanical considerations ofmandibular lengthening and widening by gradual distraction using a computer model. *J Oral Maxillofac Surg*, Vol. 56, No. 1, pp: 51-59

Samchukov, M.L., Cope, J.B. Cherkashin A.M., (2001) The biomechanical effects of distraction device orientation during mandibular lengthening and widening. In:

Samchukov, M.L., Cope, J.B., Cherkashin, A.M. (Eds.), Craniofacial Distraction Osteogenesis. Mosby, St. Louis, pp. 131–146

Sasso, R.C., LeHuec, J,C. & Shaffrey, C., (2005) Spine Interbody Research Group. Iliac crest bone graft donor site pain after anterior lumbar interbody fusion: a prospective patient satisfaction outcome assessment. *J Spinal Disord Tech.* 18 Suppl: S77-81

Shetye, P.R., Davidson E.H. & Sorkin, M., et al., (2010). Evaluation of three surgical techniques for advancement of the midface in growing children with syndromic craniosynostosis. *Plast Reconstr Surg*, Vol.126, No.3, pp: 982-994

Simion, M., Trisi, P. & Piattelli, A., (1994) Vertical ridge augmentation using a membrane technique associated with osseointegrated implants. *International Journal of Periodontics and Restorative Dentistry, Vol.*14, pp: 497–511

Snyder, C.C., Levine, G,A. & Swanson H.M., et al., (1973) Mandibular lengthening by gradual distraction. Preliminary report. *Plast Reconstr Surg*, Vol.51, No.5, pp: 506-8

Suri, L & Taneja P., (2008) Surgically assisted rapid maxillary expansion. A literature review. *Am J Orthod Dentofacial Orthop*, Vol.133, pp: 290-302

Tae, K.C., Kang, K.W. & Kim, S.C., et al., (2006) Mandibular symphyseal distraction osteogenesis with stepwise osteotomy in adult skeletal class III patient. *Int J Oral Maxillofac Surg*, Vol. 35, pp: 556-558

Toth, B.A., Kim, J.W. & Chin, M., et al., (1998) Distraction osteogenesis and its application to the midface and bony orbit in craniosynostosis syndromes. *J Craniofac Surg*, Vol.9, No.2, pp: 100-113

Uckan, S., Haydar, S.G. & Dolanmaz, D., (2002) Alveolar distraction: analysis of 10 cases. *Oral Surg Oral Med Oral Pathol Oral Radiol Endod*, Vol. 94, pp: 561-565

Uckan, S., Guler, N.. & Arman, A,, et al., (2005). Mandibular midline distraction using asimple device. *Oral Surg Oral Med Oral Pathol Oral Radiol Endod*, Vol.100, pp: 85-91

Uckan, S., Guler, N. & Arman, A., et al., (2006) Mandibular midline distraction using a simple device.*Oral Surg Oral Med Oral Pathol Oral Radiol Endod*, Vol.101, pp:711-717

Vanarsdall, R.L., (1999) Transverse dimension and long-term stability. *Semin Orthod*, Vol.5, No.3, pp: 171-80

Vance, G.S., Greenwell, H. & Miller R.L., et al., (2004) Comparison of an allograft in anexperimental putty carrier and a bovine-derived xenograft used in ridgepreservation: a clinical and histologic study in humans. *Int J Oral Maxillofac Implants*, Vol. 19, No. 4, pp: 491-497

Vyas, R.M. & Jarrahy, R., (2009) Bone-borne palatal distraction to correct the constricted cleft maxilla. *J Craniofac Surg*, Vol. 20, pp: 733–736

Weil, T.S., Van Sickels, J.E. & Payne, C.J., (1997) Distraction osteogenesis for correction oftransverse mandibular deficiency: A preliminary report. *J Oral Maxillofac Surg*, Vol.55, pp: 953-960

8

Efficacy of Preoperative CT Imaging in Posterior Cervical Spine Surgery

Shiro Imagama and Naoki Ishiguro
Department of Orthopaedic Surgery,
Nagoya University Graduate School of Medicine
Japan

1. Introduction

The aging of society has increased the number of cases of cervical spine disorder. Improved surgery, including cervical laminoplasty for posterior decompression, has resulted in favorable outcomes in many cases (Hirabayashi et al. 1981, Kurokawa et al.1983). Instrumentation such as pedicle screws used in lumbar surgery has also been developed for treatment of cervical deformities caused by aging (Abumi et al.1994 & 1997). However, increased use of these surgical methods has also increased the risk of complications (Abumi et al.2000), which must be avoided to obtain good surgical results. Preoperative evaluation using CT imaging is important in cervical spine surgery, since this spine includes the spinal cord and vertebral artery, damage to which has the risk of tetraplegia or may be life threatening (unlike the cauda equina in the lumbar spine). The efficacy and key points of CT imaging for preventing postoperative complications in cervical spine surgery are discussed in this chapter.

2. Preoperative CT imaging in cervical spine surgery

2.1 Posterior decompression surgery (cervical laminoplasty)

2.1.1 Preoperative CT evaluation for safe laminoplasty procedures

Cervical laminoplasty is commonly performed for posterior decompression and gives favorable outcomes. This procedure is simple and effective, but preoperative CT evaluation is important for increasing safety and shortening the operative time. Laminoplasty can be performed using unilateral open door laminoplasty (Hirabayashi et al.1981) or French door laminoplasty (Kurokawa et al.1983). In both procedures, use of an air drill is common to make a gutter on the lamina. Thus, preoperative evaluation of the thickness and extent of sclerosis of the lamina on CT is helpful for making the gutter while avoiding intraoperative iatrogenic injury of the dura mater, nerve root or spinal cord by excessive use of the air drill (Fig.1A,B). Among the C3 to C7 laminae, those at C4 and C5 are generally thin. However, the thickness of each lamina varies with age, gender and disease, and therefore preoperative assessment of the thickness of the lamina is helpful for shortening the operative time. Careful and repeated evaluation of the residual lamina intraoperatively is also important to avoid excessive drilling.

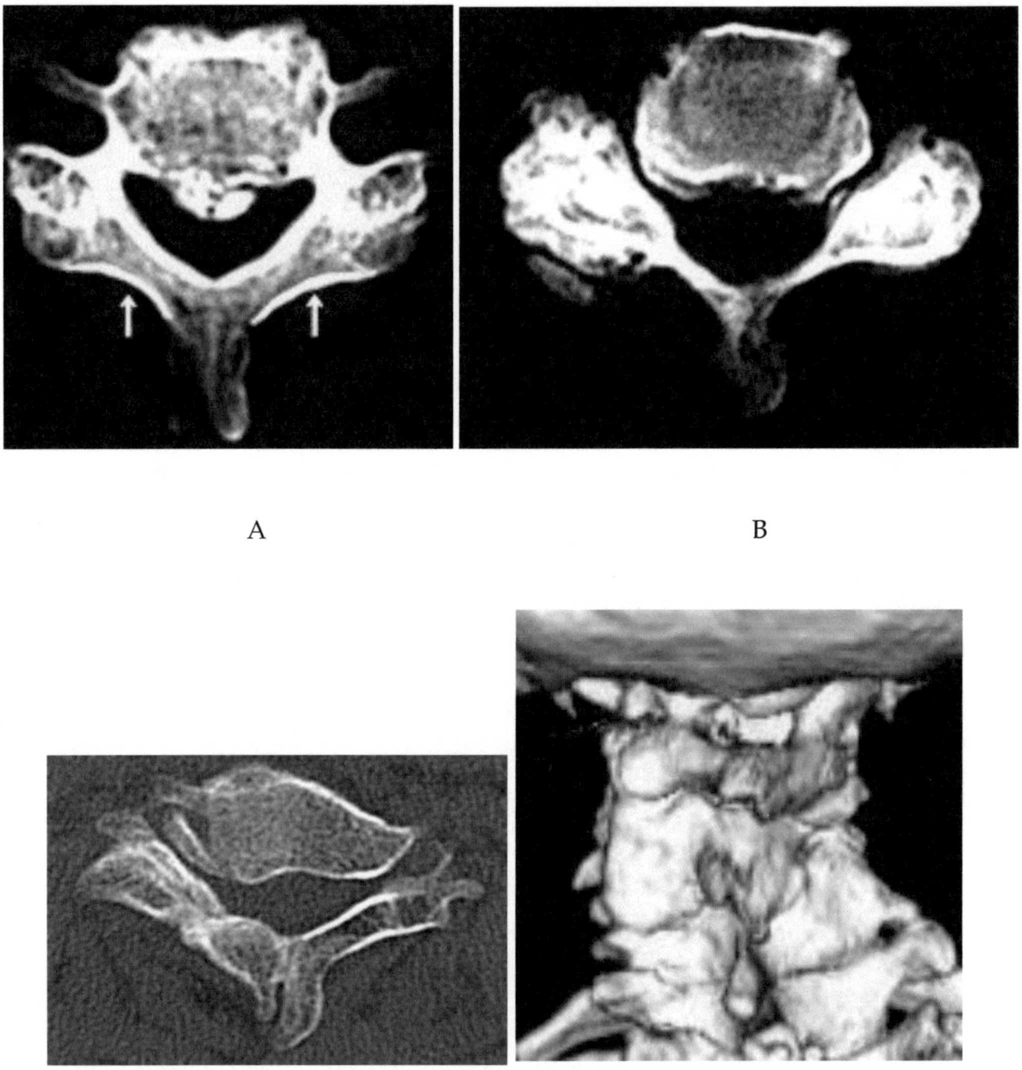

A B

C D

Fig. 1. **Preoperative CT findings.** A. Facet joints had little degeneration, which made it easy to determine the position of the gutter (arrow) B. Since the lamina in this patient was thin, care is required to avoid damage to the dura mater or spinal root during drilling. C, D. In a patient with Klippel-Feil syndrome, the lamina was thick and facet degeneration and fusion can be seen. Spontaneous bony fusion was clear on 3D CT.

Since the gutter is made only at the medial end of the facet joint in laminoplasty (Fig. 1A, arrow), it is important to avoid deformity or degenerative changes of the facet joint and lamina. In patients with cerebral palsy and Klippel-Feil syndrome, facet joints are often severely degenerated or may have undergone spontaneous fusion (Fig. 1C,1D). In these cases, it may be difficult to identify the position at which the gutter should be made without preoperative evaluation by CT. If the gutter is positioned too laterally, there is a risk of vertebral artery (VA) injury by drilling into the transverse foramen. 3DCT may also be useful for assessment of spontaneous bony fusion (Fig. 1D). Thus, comparison of preoperative CT images with intraoperative findings can avoid disorientation during surgery, while estimation of the lamina thickness on preoperative CT is helpful for use of the air drill.

2.1.2 CT evaluation for predicting a risk of C5 palsy after cervical laminoplasty

C5 palsy is a serious postoperative complication of laminoplasty that can cause paralysis in the upper extremities and severe pain. The incidence of C5 palsy after cervical laminoplasty has ranged from very low to 30% in previous reports(Satomi et al.1994, Wada et al.2001, Chiba et al.2002, Hasegawa et al.2007). C5 palsy has been recognized for 30 years, but preventive and therapeutic methods have yet to be established. Various aspects of the surgical procedure, pathology of the spinal cord, and impairment of the nerve root are implicated as causes of C5 palsy, but its low prevalence in most studies has prevented clarification of the pathology and resultant development of preventive methods.

In a multicenter study performed in 2010, we evaluated radiological findings in patients with C5 palsy (manual muscle test (MMT) score < 3) after cervical laminoplasty and searched for features on preoperative imaging that might help to predict its occurrence (Imagama et al.2010). We reviewed 1858 patients who had undergone cervical laminoplasty in institutes of the Nagoya Spine Group and identified 43 (2.3%) who developed C5 palsy with a MMT (MRC) grade of 0 to 2 in the deltoid, with or without involvement of the biceps, but without loss of muscular strength in any other muscles. These criteria ensured that only cases of definite C5 palsy were included in the analysis. The clinical features and radiological findings were compared for patients with (group P) and without (group C) C5 palsy, using results from plain radiographs, MRI and CT. In this chapter, we focus mainly on the CT findings, which included the width of the intervertebral foramen at C5 (Fig. 2A), the anterior protrusion of the superior articular process of C5 (Fig.2B), the presence of hinge dislodgement, and the position of the bony gutter (Fig. 2C).

CT images were acquired in the horizontal plane of the intervertebral disc. The width of the C5 intervertebral foramen was measured at its narrowest point and the anterior protrusion of the superior articular process of C5 was measured at its most prominent point. The gutter position was expressed as the ratio of the distance between the midline of the vertebral column at C5 and the medial point of the gutter relative to the distance between the midline of the vertebral column at C5 and the most medial part of the facet joint (Fig. 2C). The radiographic measurements (mm) of individual images were adjusted to give the actual length. A Mann-Whitney U test was used for statistical analysis, with $p < 0.05$ taken to indicate significance.

On CT measurements, a difference in width between the intervertebral foramina was found in 20 patients (47%), and in 16 (80%) the side of narrowing corresponded with the side that was paralyzed. In group P, the mean width of the intervertebral foramen was significantly less on the paralyzed side than on the normal side (1.6 *vs.* 2.1 mm, $p = 0.0043$) (Table 1, Fig. 3).

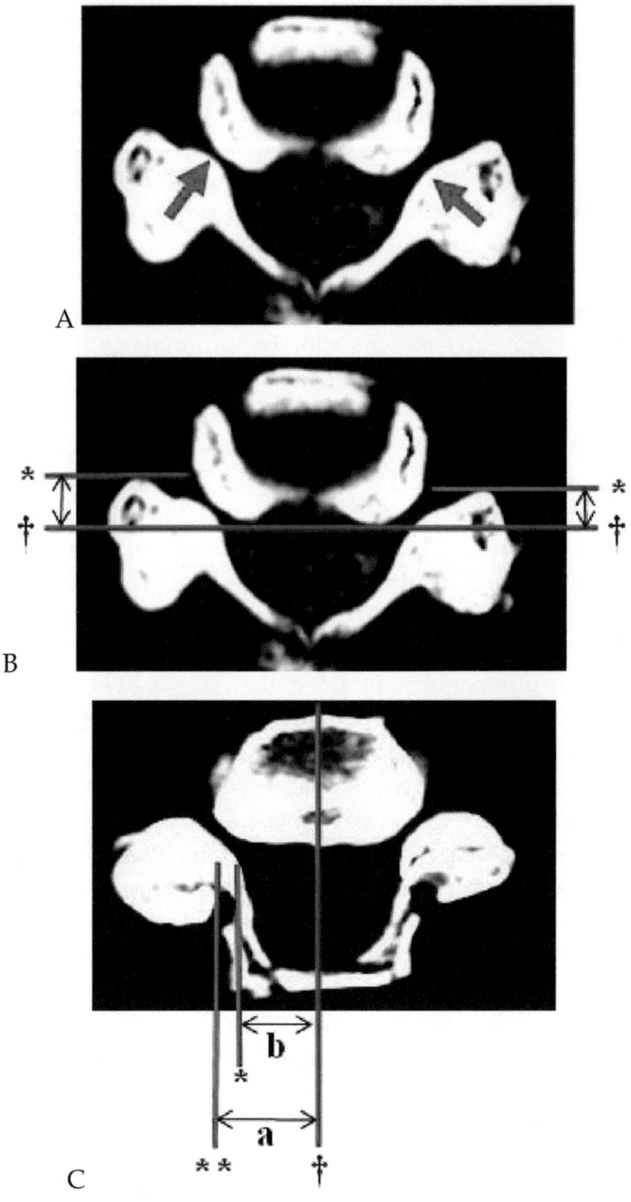

Fig. 2. **Radiological measurements by CT recorded bilaterally.** A) The width of the C5 foramen was measured at the narrowest point (arrow). B) Anterior protrusion of the C5 superior articular process (SAP) (double arrow). † indicates the posterior line of the vertebral column. * indicates the line corresponding to the most prominent site of the C5 SAP parallel to the posterior line of the vertebral column. C) The ratio of the width of the bony gutter and the facet joint, reflecting the position of the bony gutter. † indicates the midline of the vertebral column, * indicates the medial point of the bony gutter, ** indicates the medial point of the facet joint. These lines are vertical to the posterior line of the vertebral column. Distances were measured between † and ** (a), and between † and * (b), and then adjusted to give the actual length.

The mean anterior protrusion of the superior articular process of C5 was significantly greater on the paralyzed side than on the normal side (5.1 *vs.* 4.3 mm, $p = 0.029$). In group C, the mean width of the C5 intervertebral foramen (4.3 mm) was significantly greater and the degree of anterior protrusion of the superior articular process of C5 (3.5 mm) was significantly less than the respective values on the paralyzed or normal side in group P ($p < 0.0001$) (Table 1 and Fig. 4).

	C5 palsy	Control	p value
CT			
Width of the C5 intervertebral foramen (mm)			$p < 0.005$ [a]
Palsy side (C5 palsy) / right side (control)	1.6 ± 0.15	4.3 ± 0.13	$p < 0.0001$ [b]
Healthy side (C5 palsy) / left side (control)	2.1 ± 0.22	4.3 ± 0.15	$p < 0.0001$ [c]
Anterior protrusion of the C5 superior articular process (mm)			$p < 0.05$ [a]
palsy side (C5 palsy) / right side (control)	5.1 ± 0.38	3.5 ± 0.22	$p < 0.0001$ [b]
Healthy side (C5 palsy) / left side (control)	4.3 ± 0.39	3.5 ± 0.22	$p < 0.05$ [c]
Position of the bony gutter (%)			NS [a]
palsy side (C5 palsy) / right side (control)	85.4 ± 2.1	81.6 ± 2.0	NS [b]
Healthy side (C5 palsy) / left side (control)	85.6 ± 3.0	82.4 ± 1.6	NS [c]
MRI			
Number of compression levels	2.9 ± 0.16	2.7 ± 0.09	NS
Most compressive level (C3/4) (cases)	15 (35%)	27 (27%)	NS
HIA (cases)	33 / 43 (77%)	78 / 100 (78%)	NS
HIA level (C3/4) (cases)	8 (24%)	21 (27%)	NS
Focal HIA (cases)	29 (88%)	65 (83%)	NS
Linear HIA (cases)	4 (12%)	13 (17%)	NS
Posterior shift of the spinal cord (C4/5) (mm)	3.9 ± 0.27	3.0 ± 0.21	$p < 0.01$

*Values are given as means and the standard error of the mean.

[a] palsy side vs. healthy side; [b] palsy side vs. control; [c] healthy side vs. control

Table 1. Radiological assessment of the C5 palsy and control groups

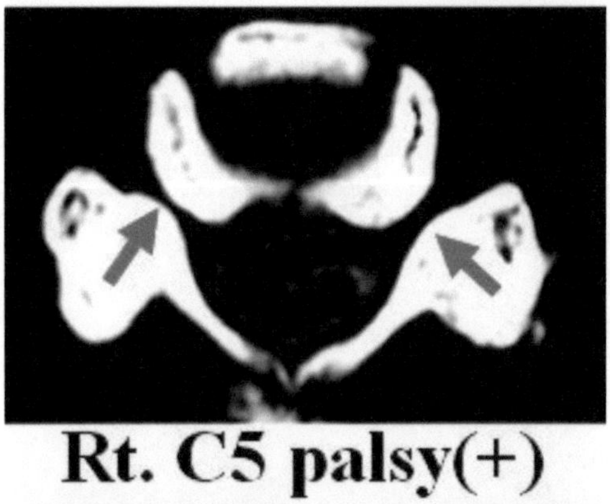

A

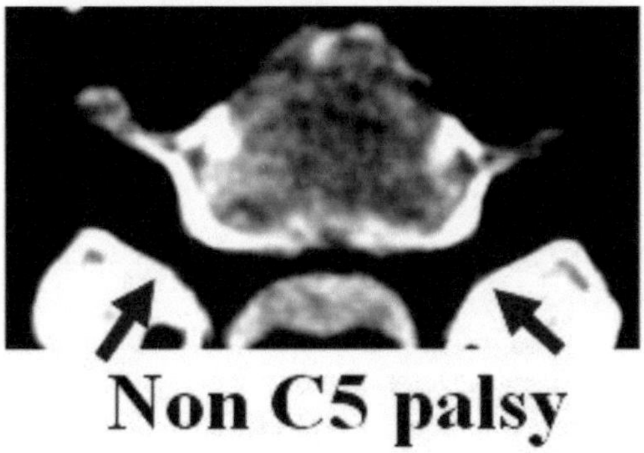

B

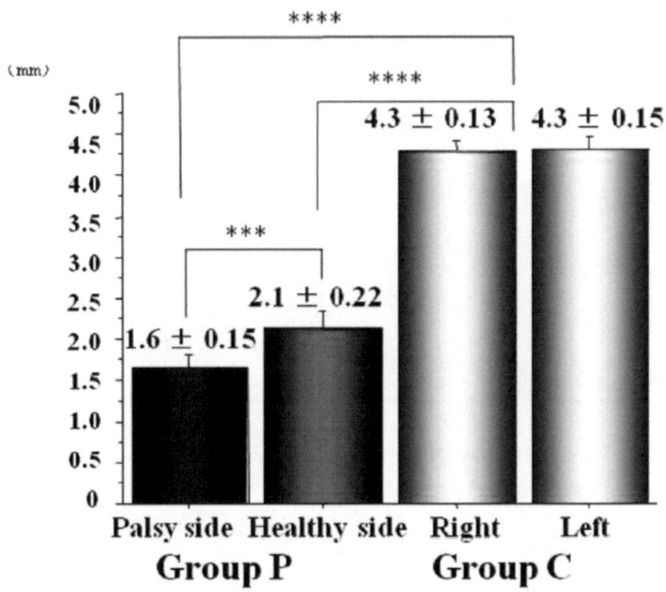

C

Fig. 3. **Width of the C5 intervertebral foramen.** The width was narrowest on the paralysis side (*** $p < 0.005$: palsy side *vs.* normal side, **** $p < 0.0001$ palsy side *vs.* control, **** $p < 0.0001$ normal side *vs.* control).

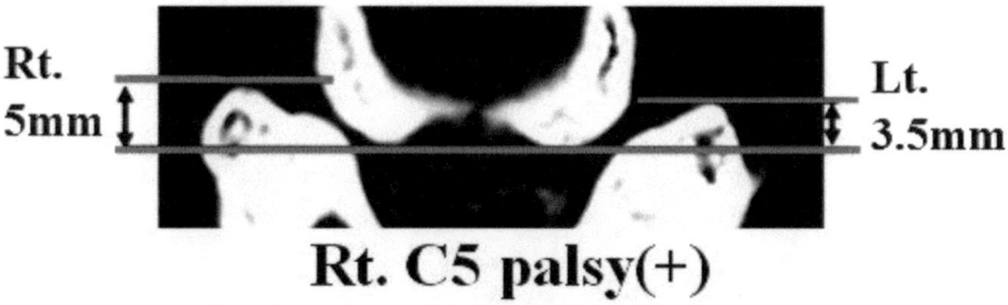

A

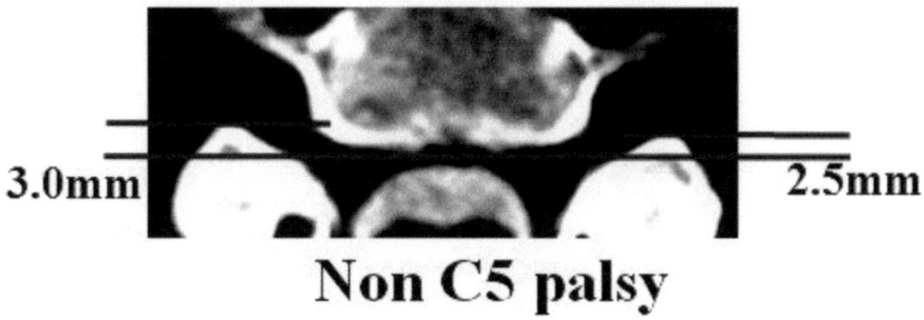

B

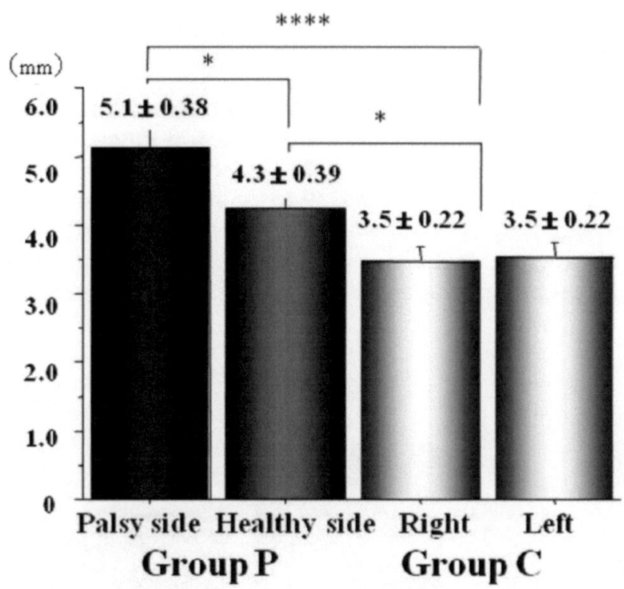

C

Fig. 4. **Anterior protrusion of the C5 superior articular process.** The protrusion was most prominent on the paralysis side (* $p < 0.05$: palsy side *vs.* normal side, **** $p < 0.0001$ palsy side *vs.* control; * $p < 0.05$ normal side *vs.* control).

In group P the ratios reflecting the position of the bony gutter were 85.4% on the paralyzed side and 85.6% on the normal side, whereas in group C these ratios were 81.6% on the right and 82.4% on the left side, with no significant effect on the development of C5 palsy (Table 1 and Fig. 5). There were no cases of dislodgement of the hinge.

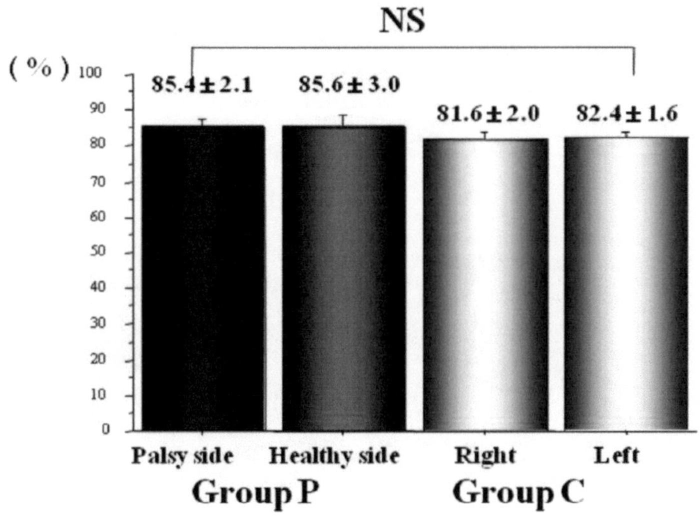

Fig. 5. **Position of the bony gutter.** In group P, the gutter tended to be more lateral than in group C, but there was no significant relationship between the position of the bony gutter and development of C5 palsy.

On MRI, there were no significant differences between the two groups in the number and location of the compressed levels, or in the prevalence and range of the high intensity area. However, the mean postoperative posterior shift of the spinal cord at C4-C5 was 3.9 mm (range: 0 to 7.5 mm) in group P and 3.0 mm (0 to 7.5 mm) in group C ($p = 0.0091$) (Table 1 and Fig. 6). On plain radiographs, there was no significant difference in the cervical lordotic angle, intervertebral angle, local kyphosis angle, cervical alignment, intervertebral instability or listhesis pre- and postoperatively between groups P and C.

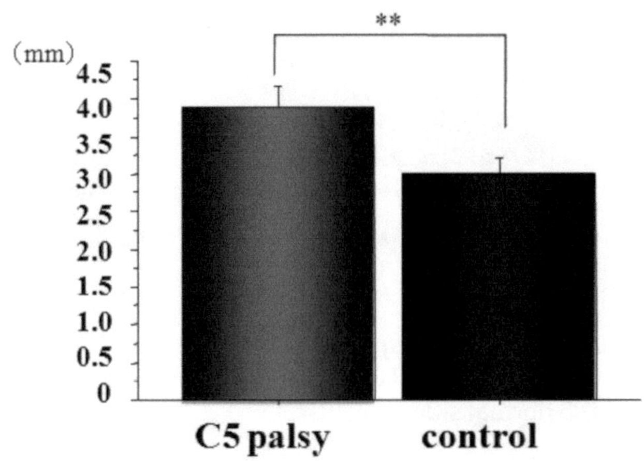

Fig. 6. **Posterior shift of the spinal cord on MRI.** The posterior shift was significantly greater in C5 palsy group (** $p < 0.01$).

These results provided the first imaging evidence of nerve root impairment of C5 palsy using CT and MRI in a multicenter comparative study. Tsuzuki et al. previously suggested that the pathology of C5 palsy includes impairment of the C5 nerve root, based on a demonstration in cadavers that impingement of the nerve root occurs inside the intervertebral joint with backward shifting of the spinal cord after laminoplasty (Tsuzuki et al. 1993). Furthermore, the superior articular process of C5 protrudes in a more anterior direction than those at other levels, the rootlets and root of C5 are shorter than those of other segments, and the C5 segment is usually the point at which the extent of posterior shift of the cord is greatest. These anatomical reasons may account for easier C5 nerve root impingement after laminoplasty. However, radiological evidence of nerve root impingement has not been obtained in previous studies because of the small number of cases and the mixing of patients with C5 palsy with those with paralyses of other nerves. In our study, the significantly greater posterior shift of the spinal cord on MRI in patients with C5 palsy indicated tethering of the nerve root, which might be made worse by the tendency of the bony gutter to adopt a more lateral position in these patients. The CT findings also support this argument. We also found that cases of C5 palsy accompanied by pain in the area of the C5 root accounted for about 80% of those in which root impairment was suspected clinically. This suggests that C5 palsy is more likely to be due to C5 root impairment than to spinal cord pathology.

We speculate that foraminotomy with laminoplasty may be useful for a case in which there is a risk of development of C5 palsy. A significant posterior shift of the spinal cord due to excessive expansion can easily lead to this lesion, and avoidance of tethering of the cord by excessive laminoplasty may prevent postoperative palsy of the C5 nerve root. Most cases of C5 palsy heal after conservative treatment; however, some severe cases do not recover and foraminotomy may be useful to treat patients with C5 palsy associated with severe pain or motor paralysis (MMT = 0 or 1), even after laminoplasty.

2.2 Instrumentation surgery for the posterior cervical spine

2.2.1 Screws in posterior cervical instrumentation

For most degenerative cervical diseases with myelopathy, cervical laminoplasty is sufficient for a good postoperative outcome. However, some patients with cervical kyphosis and/or cervical instability have poor clinical outcomes with posterior decompression surgery only (Abumi et al.1999). In most trauma cases, cervical spine fusion with instrumentation is required. Good correction and fusion can be achieved with instrumentation and this may give good long-term surgical results, even in patients with preoperative cervical spine deformity and cervical instability (Fig. 7A). Recently developed pedicle screws, lateral mass screws and laminar screws have contributed to attainment of strong fixation (Yukawa et al.2006) (Fig. 7B). However, vertebral arteries (VAs) are present in the transverse foramen of the cervical spine and injury to these arteries may cause serious postoperative complications with insertion of these screws. VA injury may increase intraoperative excessive bleeding or postoperative cerebellar infarction due to a thrombus, which may increase mortality. Therefore, careful preoperative evaluation of CT findings is very useful for surgical planning.

2.2.2 Preoperative CT evaluation of the VA for risk management in posterior cervical instrumentation surgery

There is a risk of VA injury when the lamina is exposed, especially at occipital-cervical junctions where the C1 posterior arch is deep and soft tissue is thick. In instrumentation

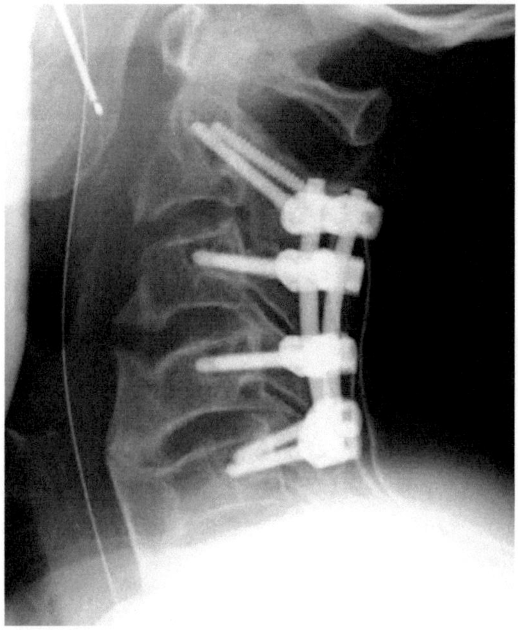

A

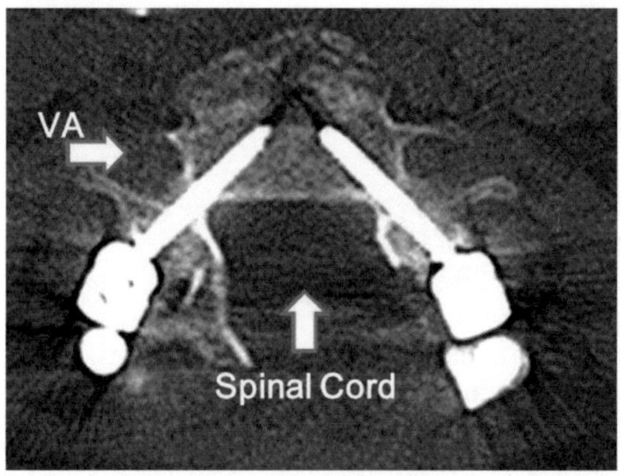

B

Fig. 7. **Posterior instrumentation surgery for the cervical spine.** A. Postoperative plain radiograph showing good fixation with cervical instrumentation. B. CT showing pedicle screw insertion at C4. A screw was safely placed within the pedicle without injury to the VA and spinal cord.

surgery, more working space for safety and exposure of soft tissue from the cervical spine are required. It is important to define the VA location preoperatively on CT, since the location of the VA varies in individuals. Contrast 3DCT is particularly effective for defining the relationship between the lamina and VA, compared to contrast MR angiography (Fig. 8). If soft tissue is exposed roughly without recognition of the variable VA location, this may lead to VA injury at a very early stage of surgery.

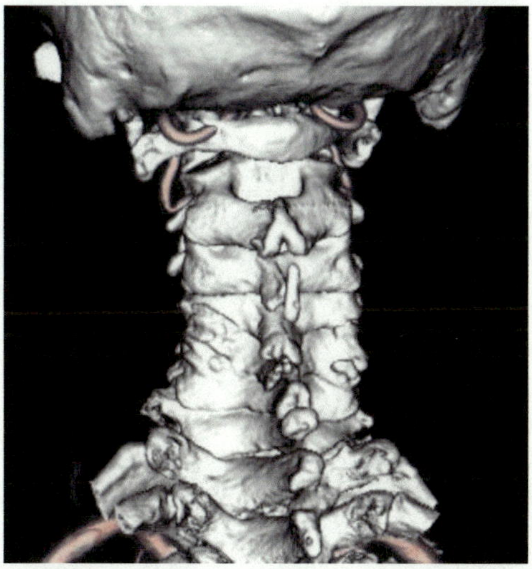

Fig. 8. **Preoperative contrast 3DCT**. 3DCT can be used to define the relationship between the lamina and VA. In this case, there is a risk of left VA injury. 3DCT also clearly revealed facet degeneration at left C4/5 and C5/6.

It is also important to consider anomalies in the C2 transverse foramen when inserting C2 pedicle screws. A high riding VA (a case in which the transverse foramen is located very close to the C2 pedicle) makes it difficult to insert C2 pedicle screws without a high risk of VA injury and the instrumentation should be changed in these cases. Multiplanar reconstruction CT (MPR-CT) images are useful to identify a high riding VA (Fig. 9).

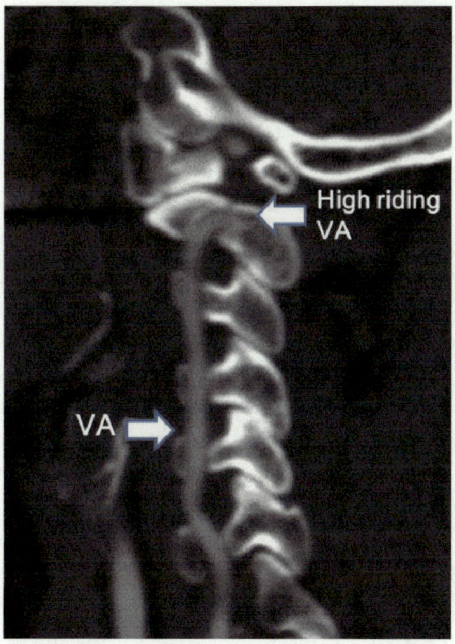

Fig. 9. **High riding VA on preoperative contrast MPR-CT.** This case had a high riding VA at C2 and insertion of a C2 pedicle screw was not performed to avoid VA injury.

For other cervical spine cases, CT findings of the size of the lateral mass and width of pedicles and laminae are very important for achieving successful posterior cervical spine fusion with screw fixation (Fig. 10).

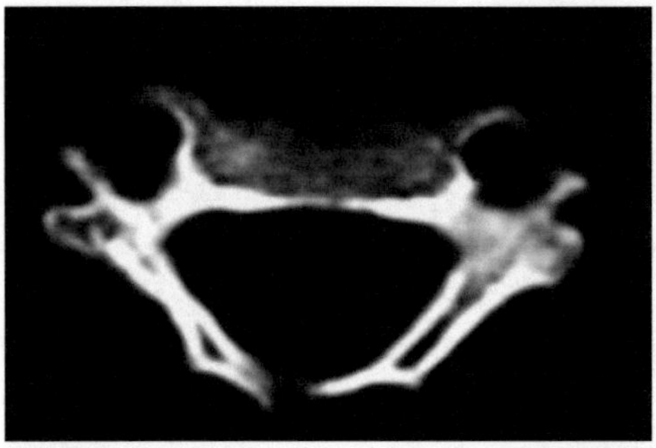

Fig. 10. **Preoperative evaluation of pedicle and lateral mass on CT**. This case had a narrow diameter of the right pedicle with bone sclerosis and a right small lateral mass was present.

For these reasons, evaluation of preoperative CT findings is important for choice of effective and safe anchors for successful cervical instrumentation surgery.

2.2.3 Prediction of the risk of C5 palsy after cervical instrumentation surgery

C5 palsy is also a concern after cervical instrumentation surgery. Several recent studies have shown an increased incidence of postoperative C5 palsy in cases treated with posterior decompression and instrumented fusion (Abumi et al.2000, Heller et al. 1995, Hojo et al. 2010), with one study showing a rate that was 11.6 times higher than that without instrumentation (Takemitsu et al. 2008). One cause of C5 palsy after instrumented corrective fusion may be iatrogenic foraminal stenosis following correction of cervical alignment. In use of instrumentation for cervical degenerative disease with kyphosis or instability, the aim is both decompression of the spinal cord and forward correction of cervical alignment to a lordotic position. In posterior fusion with instrumentation, the C5 intervertebral foramen may become stenotic after surgery, in addition to the anatomical disadvantages of C5 nerve root impingement after decompression surgery and the apex of cervical lordosis at C5. Therefore, it is important not to overcorrect the cervical deformity and to avoid a compression force between screws, with use of concomitant foraminotomy with instrumented cervical surgery for decompression of the nerve root.

It is difficult to define the appropriate extent of correction to avoid C5 palsy, but we believe that correction to the extent of the preoperative cervical alignment at the cervical extension position may be safe. The effect of foraminotomy for C5 palsy after instrumented cervical surgery is unclear. However, some risk factors for C5 palsy after instrumented cervical surgery were identified by colleagues at our hospital in a review of 84 patients who underwent posterior instrumented fusion using cervical pedicle screws for nontraumatic lesions (unpublished data). The pre- and postoperative width of the C5 intervertebral foramen on CT were significantly narrower in patients that did not develop C5 palsy and postoperative posterior shift of the spinal cord at C4-C5 tended to be greater in those with C5 palsy. These results suggest that concomitant foraminotomy with instrumented cervical spine surgery may be useful for preventing C5 palsy, especially in patients with a narrow C5 foramen preoperatively. Further investigations are needed to examine these issues.

3. Conclusion

In this chapter, we discussed the importance and efficacy of preoperative CT evaluation in posterior cervical spine surgery. Plain CT can reveal detailed bone information, while contrast CT shows the relationship between vascular elements, including the VA, and the spine. The indication of cervical posterior surgery has increased with aging of society and advances in cervical spine surgery. A good surgical outcome is likely in most cases, but preoperative evaluation is important for a good result and avoidance of complications, even in relatively simple procedures such as laminoplasty. There are still problems to resolve in cervical surgery, such as development of C5 palsy, but our CT findings suggest that preventive and therapeutic methods are possible. Thus, CT evaluation is valuable in posterior spine surgery. Further evaluation of the various types of CT imaging (plain, MPR, 3DCT, and contrast) is required to determine the appropriate methods for different types of surgery and disease.

4. Acknowledgement

We are grateful to all the staff of the Nagoya Spine Group for assistance with the multicenter study of C5 palsy.

5. References

Abumi K, et al. (1994) Transpedicular screw fixation for traumatic lesions of the middle and lower cervical spine: description of the techniques and preliminary report. *J Spinal Disord*;7:19-28.

Abumi K, Kaneda K. (1997) Pedicle screw fixation for nontraumatic lesions of the cervical spine. *Spine (Phila Pa 1976)*;22:1853-63.

Abumi K, et al. (1999) Correction of cervical kyphosis using pedicle screw fixation systems. *Spine (Phila Pa 1976)*;24:2389-96.

Abumi K, et al.(2000)Complications of pedicle screw fixation in reconstructive surgery of the cervical spine. *Spine (Phila Pa 1976)*;25:962-9.

Chiba K, et al. (2002) Segmental motor paralysis after expansive open-door laminoplasty. *Spine (Phila Pa 1976)*;27:2108-15.

Hasegawa K, Homma T, Chiba Y. (2007) Upper extremity palsy following cervical decompression surgery results from a transient spinal cord lesion. *Spine (Phila Pa 1976)*;32:E197-202.

Heller JG, Silcox DH, Sutterlin CE. (1995) Complications of posterior cervical plating. *Spine (Phila Pa 1976)*;20:2442-8.

Hirabayashi K, et al. (1981) Operative results and postoperative progression of ossification among patients with ossification of cervical posterior longitudinal ligament. *Spine (Phila Pa 1976)*;6:354-64.

Hojo Y, et al. (2010) A late neurological complication following posterior correction surgery of severe cervical kyphosis. *Eur Spine J*.in press.

Imagama S, et al.(2010) C5 palsy after cervical laminoplasty: a multicentre study. *J Bone Joint Surg Br*;92:393-400.

Kurokawa T, Tsuyama N, Tanaka H. (1982) Enlargement of spinal canal by the sagittal splitting of the spinous process. *Bessatsu SeikeiGeka*; 2:234-40.

Satomi K, et al. (1994) Long-term follow-up studies of open-door expansive laminoplasty for cervical stenotic myelopathy. *Spine (Phila Pa 1976)*;19:507-10.

Takemitsu M, et al. (2008) C5 nerve root palsy after cervical laminoplasty and posterior fusion with instrumentation. *J Spinal Disord Tech*;21:267-72.

Tsuzuki N, et al. (1993) Paralysis of the arm after posterior decompression of the cervical spinal cord. I. Anatomical investigation of the mechanism of paralysis. *Eur Spine J*;2:191-6.

Wada E, et al. (2001) Subtotal corpectomy versus laminoplasty for multilevel cervical spondylotic myelopathy: a long-term follow-up study over 10 years. *Spine (Phila Pa 1976)*;26:1443-7; discussion 8.

Yukawa Y, et al. (2006) Cervical pedicle screw fixation in 100 cases of unstable cervical injuries: pedicle axis views obtained using fluoroscopy. *J Neurosurg Spine*;5:488-93.

9

CT Scanning in Minor Head Injury

Saeed Shoar and Soheil Saadat
Sina Trauma Research Center
Tehran University of Medical Sciences
Iran

1. Introduction

Head injury is one of the most prevalent events accounting for about one million of emergency visits in US and UK annually. It occurs in over the 50% of traumatic patients and is the leading cause of death and disabilities in children and younger adults all over the world (Holmes, et al., 2006; Kraus & Nourjah, 1998; Langlois, et al., 2006).
Annually, traumatic brain injuries cause 435000 emergency department visits, 37000 hospital admissions, and 2685 deaths among children whose ages range from 0 to 14 in the USA (Jager et al., 2000; Langlois et al.,2004).
While there has been an increase in the number of CT performed for traumatic patients, particularly those with a suspected head injury, different studies have estimated the prevalence of significant intracranial lesions on a CT to be something between 0.7% and 20% (Bordignon & Arruda 2002, Holmes et al., 2006, Mower 2005, Stiell 2001). Because most of these patients have insignificant injuries requiring no specific therapy, some authorities are reluctant to advocate CT studies in all such patients. In contrast, other authorities, concerned with the potentially dramatic consequences of a missed finding, tend to encourage the liberal use of brain CT in such patients bringing an estimated 750 million $ cost for health system (Borczuk, 1995; Jeret et al., 1993; Schynoll et al., 1993); however, it has been reported that reduction in the number of patients complicated due to head trauma is happening as a result of better control of developing seizure or raised intracranial pressure (Klauber et al. 1989).
The majority of treated brain injuries are categorized as mild head injury (MHI) (Kraus & Nourjah,1988). While patients with moderate to severe head injury usually show obvious clinical signs, simplifying the decision to perform a head CT scan, there are controversies in the indications of CT scanning in MHI patients considering the fact that most of these patients represent minimal intracranial lesions, requiring no specific therapy (Shackford et al., 1992).
This chapter will recap the application of CT scanning in MHI patients in adults and children.

2. Minor head injury

The term "mild/minor head injury" was first described by Rimel and colleagues in 1981 (Rimel et al., 1981) as a head damage with rapid healing and not much severe post-traumatic complications. As the time past; however, more cases with fatal complications and further Sequelae due to MHI were detected. Between 6% to 21% of such patients develop intracranial lesions and 0.4% to 1% of them need neurosurgical intervention (Miller et al., 1997; af Geijerstam & Britton, 2003; Borg et al., 2004; Fabbri et al., 2004; Haydel, et al., 2000).

Having a minor nature of presentation in emergency admission, minor head injury is defined as a history of loss of consciousness < 15-20 minutes, amnesia < 1 hour, or disorientation in a conscious and talking patient, that is, one with Glasgow Coma Scale (GCS) of 13–15. These patients may experience fatigue, dizziness, difficulty in concentration and performing mental tasks, irritability, impairment of memory, insomnia and, decreased tolerance to stress, altogether referred to as ''post- concussional syndrome'' (PCS). Patients with "minimal head injury" may not experience an LOC or other neurological alteration (Stiell et al., 2005). Traumatic patients' visits start with determination of GCS in initial assessment. This scale is apparently correlated with severity of the damage happening inside the skull and beside; it can be measured with sufficient reliability by the health care providers (Menegazzi et al., 1993, Norwood et al., 2002). Therefore, GCS is a widely accepted measure of severity of neurological trauma.

There are variations in the definition of such injury; from a history of blunt head trauma on the initial emergency department evaluation with no experience of loss of consciousness or other neurologic deficits, to some more serious events causing higher impact on patient's alertness.

The incidence of hospital-treated patients with mild traumatic brain injury is something between 100 and 300 cases per 100,000 populations. Note, however, that much mild traumatic brain injury is not treated at hospitals, and the true population-based rate is probably more than 600 cases per 100,000 populations. The estimated number of patients with head trauma in the US ranges from 800,000 to 2 million cases annually. Of these cases, more than 80% are classified as minor head injuries (Cassidy et al., 2004).

3. CT scan in head trauma

Computed tomography (CT) is the modality of choice in trauma centers which helps rapid and accurate diagnosis of damages occurred to the head from a simple skull fracture to more serious lesions such as intracranial hematoma, hemorrhage, and brain contusions. From the emergence of CT scanning in medicine in 1970s, it has brought many benefits to patients. Quick diagnosis of ongoing intra cranial damage and the possible neurosurgical intervention afterward is the key to overcome life threatening events in head injured patients (Shackford et al., 1992; Stein & Ross, 1990, 1992). However, its overuse and the side effects of radiation on patients has been a concern. In 1990s, studies reported that positive findings in CTs performed during management of patients, did not exceed of 20% of traumatic cases (Stein & Ross, 1990; Harad & Kerstein 1992). However, the number of ordered CT scan increased by 120% and reached to 5.3% from the previous 2.4% in all emergency department visits. Currently in the US, 1 million patients with blunt head trauma undergo head CT scanning annually (Mc Caig & Burt 2001). This shows that CT has been increasingly overused in the past decade, while its diagnostic benefits have remained low.

CT scanning is generally repeated in order to follow traumatic patients and this increase the radiation concerns. Reporting the collective effective dose of radiation in CT scanning as 60% (2005-2006) in UK, 82% in USA, and 67% in Germany (2000-2005), it was showed that CT has been responsible for more than half of the radiation due to diagnostic imaging (Berrington De Gonzalex & Darby, 2004; Brix, 2009; Einstein, 2007; Hall & Brenner, 2008; Mettler, 2000).

Coming to the economic world, despite its wide spreading and explosive utilization, CT is an expensive modality in many countries (Katada, 2006). Besides its economic burden, additional benefits from mindful use of CT would include saving time, reducing overcrowding in the emergency, neurology, and radiology departments, decreased radiation, no more need for applying sedation in children, and preventing unnecessary transfers from departments without access to CT, like rural trauma centers, which in turn may harm critically ill patients.

4. The application of decision rules to order CT scanning

Prediction rules that help physicians to identify patients with clinically significant lesions on CT would reduce the number of scans performed and save millions of dollars in unnecessary scans. A 10% reduction in the number of scans ordered for minor head injury could result in a $20 million reduction in healthcare expenditures in the US (Haydel, 2005). In fact, it is rational to screen patients of mild head injury who have high risk factors to develop intracranial lesions which in turn affects the final result. Such risk factors include: amnesia, loss of consciousness, vomiting, possible skull fracture, history of coagulopathy or using anticoagulant, post-traumatic seizures, asymmetry in pupils, severe or increasing headache, focal neurological deficits, or multiple trauma (Dunning et al., 2004).

There are several decision rules that are developed to identify those MHI patients who will probably benefit from head CT scanning; from the earliest known "New Orleans Criteria (NOC)" in 2000, to recently defined CATCH rule (2010), for "Canadian Assessment of Tomography for Childhood Head injury". The other published decision rules include: "Canadian CT Head Rule (CCHR)", "CT in Head Injury Patients (CHIP) rule" , "Prediction of intracranial computed tomography findings in patients with minor head injury by using logistic regression" and "CATCH rule for Canadian Assessment of Tomography for Childhood Head injury" (Saadat et al., 2009; Smits et al., 2007; Stiell et al., 2001).

Being among the first prospectively designed decision rules, NOC and CCHR have been used extensively. These criteria are claimed to identify traumatic patients who need neurosurgical intervention after a minor head injury with 100% sensitivity; thus there is no need to perform CT scanning for MHI patients who do not represent sign and symptoms described in the decision rule. "New Orleans Criteria (NOC)" and "Canadian CT head rule (CCHR)" have been validated by Smith et al., in 2005 (smith et al., 2005). CT in head injury patients (CHIP) rule was developed by smith et al., after validation of NOC and CCHR.

It is clear that the highest possible sensitivity is required to avoid an unwanted neglect during emergency observation of MHI patients. In a survey carried out by Graham (Graham et al., 1998), more than half of the respondents among emergency physicians insisted on the necessity of a 100% sensitivity for the clinical decision guidelines which is aimed to be disseminated for ordering CT scan in mild head injury patients. However, the sensitivity and specificity that are reported in the original reports, fail to remain at the same level in other studies. Moreover, the external validity of the above mentioned decision rules are not exactly the same as they have included a specific group of MHI patients.

5. Indications of CT scan in minor head injury (MHI) patients

5.1 Miller's criteria, 1997

It was around 1997, when Miller et al. introduced almost the first clinical criteria to determine whether it could safely eliminate the need to send all the patients sustained a head trauma for head CT scanning (Miller et al., 1997).

They included all patients with a normal mental status, a history of LOC or amnesia, and who presented less than 2 hours after blunt head trauma to the emergency department. The patients included in Miller study were awake (i.e. having a GCS score of 15) at the time of presentation to the emergency department.

The positive outcome in CT scan included contusion, parenchymal hematoma, epidural hematoma, subdural hematoma, subarachnoid hemorrhage or a skull fracture.

The study sample size was 2143. They proposed that patients having one or more of the following signs or symptoms would need head CT scanning: severe headache, nausea, vomiting, and depressed skull fracture. While their criteria identified most of the minor head trauma patients with abnormal CT scan and all of those who need neurosurgical intervention, it reduced the number of performed head CT scans up to 61%.

5.2 New Orleans Criteria (NOC), 2000

The New Orleans Criteria (NOC) was introduced by Haydel et al. in 2000. They first developed their criteria by reviewing 520 MHI patients and then validated it by applying the criteria on other 909 patients.

They included all patients with a history of head injury, older than 3 years who presented within 24 hours to emergency department, and had a loss of consciousness with normal findings on a brief neurologic examination (normal cranial nerves and normal strength and sensation in the arms and legs) and a score of 15 on the Glasgow Coma Scale. Patients with previous CT, and no history of loss of consciousness (LOC) or amnesia were excluded.

The positive outcome included subdural, epidural, or parenchymal hematoma; subarachnoid hemorrhage; cerebral contusion; or depressed skull fracture.

The study sample size was 1429.

	Miller	**NOC**	**CCHR**	**Abdul Latip**	**NEXUS II**	**CHIP**	**Lee**	**Saadat**
Age group included	Adults and children	> 3	≥ 16	≥ 12	?	≥ 16	≥ 16	15-70
GCS included	15	15	13-15	13-15	15	13-14, 15 if accompanied by another risk factor	13-15	13-15
Was LOC necessary to be included in the study?	Yes	Yes	Yes	No	?	If there was no loss of GCS	No	No
CT scan performed for all patients?	Yes	Yes	No	?	No	According to the guideline §	?	Yes
Sample size	2143	520+909	3121	94	2100	3181	898	318
Included patients if MHI had occurred during the past:	2 h	24 h	24 h	?	?	24 h	12 h	12 h

? Not specifically described in the article

§ Twijnstra A, Brouwer O, Keyser A, Lanser J, Poels E, Rinkel G, et al. Guidelines for diagnosis and management of patients with minor head injury. Published in Dutch: Richtlijnen voor diagnostiek en behandeling van patie¨nten met een licht schedel-hersenletsel. Accessed at www.neurologie.nl/richtlijnen Accessed on 15 December 2006.

Table 1. Comparison of external validity of different criteria for brain CT scan in adulthood

The New Orleans Criteria consists of the following finding (Haydel et al., 2000):
1. Headache
2. Vomiting
3. Age more than 60
4. Drug or alcohol intoxication
5. Persistent antegrade amnesia (short- term memory deficit)
6. Visible trauma above the clavicle
7. Seizure

When using all the findings together, a 22% reduction would be anticipated to be achieved. The sensitivity and specificity of NOC was reported as 100% and 12.7%, respectively.

5.3 Canadian CT Head Rule (CCHR), 2001

Stiell et al. developed the Canadian CT Head Rule (CCHR) by studying 3121 MHI patients (stiell et al., 2001, 2005).

They included patients with a history of blunt trauma to the head resulting in witnessed loss of consciousness, definite amnesia, or witnessed disorientation; initial emergency department GCS score of 13 or greater; who were injured during the past 24 hours. They excluded the following patients: patients younger than 16 years old; minimal head injury (i.e., no loss of consciousness, amnesia, or disorientation); no clear history of trauma as the primary event (e.g., primary seizure or syncope); an obvious penetrating skull injury or obvious depressed fracture, had acute focal neurological deficit; had unstable vital signs associated with major trauma; had a seizure before assessment in the emergency department; had a bleeding disorder or used oral anticoagulants (i.e., coumadin); had returned for reassessment of the same head injury; or were pregnant.

The positive findings in the CT scan were defined in two categories: findings that necessitated neurological intervention and findings that indicated clinically important brain injury on CT. Need for neurological intervention was defined as either death within 7 days secondary to head injury or the need for any of the following procedures within 7 days: craniotomy, elevation of skull fracture, intracranial pressure monitoring, or intubation for head injury (shown on CT). Clinically important brain injury was defined as any acute brain finding revealed on CT which would normally require admission to hospital and neurological follow-up.

The following lesions were not considered a positive finding if the patient was neurologically intact: solitary contusion less than 5 mm in diameter; localized subarachnoid blood less than 1 mm thick; smear subdural hematoma less than 4 mm thick; isolated pneumocephaly, or closed depressed skull fracture not through the inner table.

Not all patients necessarily underwent CT scanning but based on the judgment of the treating physician.

CCHR is consisted of five high- risks and 2 medium- risks criteria. The high risk criteria are capable of detecting intracranial lesions that are severe enough to necessitate a neurological intervention, while medium risk criteria identify patients who probably have sustained brain injury (not necessarily requiring neurological intervention). According to CCHR, head CT scanning is only required for patients with minor head injuries (defined as witnessed loss of consciousness, definite amnesia, or witnessed disorientation in a patient with a GCS score of 13–15) with any one of the following criterion:

High risk (for neurological intervention)

1. GCS score < 15 at 2 hours after injury
2. Suspected open or depressed skull fracture
3. Any sign of basal skull fracture (hemotympanum, 'raccoon' eyes, cerebrospinal fluid otorrhoea/rhinorrhoea, Battle's sign)
4. Vomiting (at least, two episodes)
5. Age > 65 years

Medium risk (for brain injury on CT)

1. Amnesia before impact > 30 min
2. Dangerous mechanism of head trauma (motor vehicle crash to pedestrian, occupant ejected from motor vehicle, fall from height > 3 feet or five stairs).

The sensitivity and specificity of CCHR was reported as 100%and 50.6%- 65.6%, respectively.

5.4 Abdul Latip et al. , 2004

Abdul Latip et.al. conducted a cross-sectional study on 94 MHI patients who were 12 years old and above, with a history of a blow to the head, and a GCS score of 13–15. They excluded the cases of known medical illnesses, suffered from cerebrovascular diseases or intracranial pathology, those who were on anti-coagulant medication, had a previous history of brain surgery, or facial bone fracture.

The positive outcome findings in this study were as follows: extradural, subdural, subarachnoid, intraparenchymal or intraventricular hemorrhage, pneumocephalus, cerebral contusion, midline shift or depressed skull fracture and linear vault fracture.

According to this decision rule, patients with a GCS of 13 or 14 and any of the following signs or symptoms will benefit from CT scanning: vomiting, craniofacial injuries, abnormal CNS findings, involvement in non-motor vehicle accidents, having abnormal CNS examination, craniofacial injury or skull fracture. Patients with GCS of 15 who have a skull fracture are also eligible for CT scanning.

5.5 NEXUS II, 2005

National Emergency X-Radiography Utilization Study II (NEXUS II) was a prospective study performed as a multi center cohort on 13728 patients of blunt head trauma to design and validate a decision rule to detect those cases of head trauma which are at very low risk of developing intracranial injury in order to reduce the number of ordered CT scanning (Mower et al., 2002, 2005). Patients with a history of blunt head trauma referred to 21 participating center were included. They underwent head CT scanning based on the decision of the treating physician, not based on the study protocol.

The positive outcome findings were as follows: mass effect, signs of herniation, basal cistern compression or midline shift, substantial epidural or subdural hematomas (greater than 1.0 cm in width, or causing mass effect), substantial cerebral contusion, extensive subarachnoid hemorrhage, hemorrhage in the posterior fossa, intraventricular hemorrhage, bilateral hemorrhage of any type, depressed or diastatic skull fracture, pneumocephalus, diffuse cerebral edema, diffuse axonal injury.

The study sample size was 13728 but MHI patients were about 2100 cases.

The sensitivity of this decision rule to identify the intra cranial injury in MHI patients was 95.2% (92.2%–97.2%) and its specificity was 17.3% (16.5%- 18.0%).

According to this guideline, the head CT scanning is needed for the patients presenting any of the following signs and symptoms:

1. Evidence of significant skull fracture,
2. Scalp hematoma,
3. Neurologic deficit,
4. Altered level of alertness,
5. Abnormal behavior,
6. Coagulopathy,
7. Persistent vomiting,
8. Age of 65 years or more

5.6 CT in head injury patients (CHIP), 2007

Smiths et al., compared and validated NOC and CCHR in 2005 by a prospective cohort study on 3181 patients. They showed that NOC has a higher sensitivity for cranial neural traumatic lesions or clinically significant finding, when used in patients with a GCS score of 13-15; while CCHR had more power to detect patients requiring neurosurgical intervention and hence would reduce the number of CT scan performed (Smith et al., 2005).

Two years later, Smith et al., developed their decision rule named "CT in head injury patients (CHIP)"

They included patients aged 16 years old and more who presented within 24 hours of blunt injury to the head, with a GCS score of 13 to 14 or a GCS score of 15, with at least 1 of the following risk factors: history of loss of consciousness, short-term memory deficit, amnesia for the traumatic event, posttraumatic seizure, vomiting, severe headache, clinical evidence of intoxication with alcohol or drugs, use of anticoagulants or history of coagulopathy, external evidence of injury above the clavicles, and neurologic deficit.

The outcomes of interest were the intra cranial traumatic finding in CT scan (except for isolated linear skull fracture). The secondary outcome was need to neurosurgical intervention contingent to initial CT.

The study sample size was 3181.

According to CHIP criteria, a CT scanning is indicated if one major criterion or 2 minor criteria exist.

Major criteria were as follow:

1. Pedestrian or cyclist versus vehicle
2. Ejected from vehicle
3. Vomiting
4. Post- traumatic amnesia ≥4 h
5. Clinical signs of skull fracture (Any injury that suggests a skull fracture, such as palpable discontinuity of the skull, leakage of cerebrospinal fluid, raccoon eye bruising, and bleeding from the ear)
6. GCS score <15
7. GCS deterioration ≥2 points (1 hour after presentation)
8. Use of anticoagulant therapy
9. Posttraumatic seizure
10. Age ≥60 y

Minor criteria were as follows:

1. Fall from any elevation

2. Persistent antegrade amnesia (any deficit of short-term memory)
3. Posttraumatic amnesia of 2 to 4 h
4. Contusion of the skull
5. Neurologic deficit
6. Loss of consciousness
7. GCS deterioration of 1 point (1 hour after presentation)
8. Age of 40-60 years

CHIP prediction rule is of high sensitivity for selective use of CT in patients with minor head injury; it strongly identifies cases probable to have positive finding on CT and determines whether patients will need neurosurgery or not.

5.7 Lee et al. criteria, 2009

These criteria were developed based on a retrospective study on 898 MHI patients.

Patients aged 16 years and more, presented with a history of blunt head trauma, who had a GCS score of 13-15 (with or without LOC) and admitted to the hospital for more than 12 hours were included.

The positive outcome was defined as all intracranial post-traumatic hematoma or contusion, depressed fractures, traumatic subarachnoid hemorrhage, and pneumocephalus. Isolated linear skull fracture and initial diagnosis of chronic subdural hematoma were not considered as abnormal CT findings.

They identified four sub-groups of patients subject to minor head injury according to the possibility of developing post- traumatic complications:

Very low risk: GCS score of 15 having no history of LOC or headache;

Low risk: GCS score of 15 with LOC and/or headache;

Medium risk: GCS score of 15 with a skull fracture, neurological deficits or with one or more of the mentioned risk factors;

High risk: GCS score of 15 with abnormal CT findings and GCS score of 14 and 13.

Of these four divided sub- groups, CT scan was advised for all the head injured cases; very low and low risk factors may be discharged; while medium and high risk patients of minor head injury should be admitted for close observation due to the risk of deterioration; in addition, high risk cases should be treated as moderate head injured. Patients younger than 16 years old or those with penetrating head trauma and hospital admission in less than 12 hours had been excluded from this retrospective study.

5.8 Saadat et al., 2009

In a cohort study held in Tehran University of Medical Sciences in Iran in 2004, a statistical model was developed for predicting the occurrence of intracranial lesions in patients with MHI (Saadat et al., 2006). This study was ordered by Iranian ministry of health and medical education. It was intended to be considered by rural physicians as a guideline, to select the MHI patients that need to be referred for head CT scanning. The decision rule was more developed later, using larger sample size, and the final model was published in 2009 (Saadat et al, 2009). This decision rule was based on 318 patients with a history of blunt head trauma and a Glasgow Coma Scale (GCS) score ≥ 13 who had presented within 12 hours of trauma. Computed tomography findings that necessitated neurosurgical care (either observation or intervention) were considered as positive findings. This study considered broader intracranial findings on CT as an outcome measure including linear skull fracture as well as depressed, mastoid, comminuted, basilar, and sphenoid fracture; epidural, subdural, subarachnoid, intraparenchymal (including petechial), and intraventricular hemorrhage; brain contusion; pneumocephalus; and midline shift.

All MHI patients whose GCS score was 13–15, regardless of any other concomitant risk factors and LOC or amnesia, were included. Therefore, the results of this study could be applied to a broader spectrum of patients with minor head injury. The following patients were excluded from analysis: opium-addicted patients, those with concurrent major wounds or fractures that necessitated specialized care in a hospital, patients whose condition was unstable and who could not be safely transferred to the radiology department, patients suspected of malingering, and those patients who refused to participate in the study.

A logistic regression model was used to differentiate the subset of patients with minor head injury who may demonstrate intracranial lesions if they underwent brain CT scanning. According to this decision rule, MHI patients with 1 major criterion or 2 minor criteria need CT scanning and 13% of the cases represent positive intracranial lesion in head CT scan. A normal GCS score after a minor head injury did not guarantee the absence of significant neurological injury in this study, as 0.6% of such patients required neurosurgical intervention. The sensitivity and specify of this decision rule was reported as 100% and 46%, respectively. The criteria were as follows:

Major criteria:

1. GCS score < 14
2. Presence of the raccoon sign
3. Failure to remember the impact
4. Age > 65 years
5. Vomiting after impact

Minor criteria:

1. Scalp wound
2. GCS score < 15.

6. CT scanning in childhood

The indications of performing a CT in children are different from those applied in adults. This is partly due to the structure of skull and the neurological development of children. The concern with radiation to children is another reason for the difference of head CT scanning in childhood. It was estimated that the lifetime risk of cancer mortality, attributable to the ionizing radiation due to head CT scanning during the emergency admission, for a one-year-old child would be about 1 in 1500; while it is about 1 in 5000 for 10 years olds (Brenner et al., 2001). The national institute for Health and Clinical Excellence (NICE) has recommended immediate request for CT scan of head in children if there are any of the followings: Loss of consciousness lasting more than 5 minutes (witnessed), amnesia (antegrade or retrograde) lasting more than 5 minutes, abnormal drowsiness, three or more discrete episodes of vomiting, clinical suspicion of non-accidental injury, post-traumatic seizure but no history of epilepsy, GCS less than 14, or for a baby under 1 year GCS (pediatric) less than 15, on assessment in the emergency department, suspicion of open or depressed skull injury or tense fontanel, any sign of basal skull fracture (haemotympanum, 'panda' eyes, cerebrospinal fluid leakage from the ear or nose, Battle's sign), focal neurological deficit, if under 1 year, presence of bruise, swelling or laceration of more than 5 cm on the head, dangerous mechanism of injury (high-speed road traffic accident either as pedestrian, cyclist or vehicle occupant, fall from a height of greater than 3 m, high-speed injury from a projectile or an object). This guideline is not limited to MHI patients however. There are decision rules which recommend a set of findings in performing CT for children of traumatic cases when they are subjected to head trauma.

6.1 Children's head injury algorithm for the prediction of important clinical events (CHALICE); Dunning et al., 2006

This decision rule suggests a set of criteria based on history, physical examination findings and the mechanism of trauma to order a head CT scanning for MHI children. The criteria are as follows:

History

1. Witnessed LOC of >5 min duration
2. History of amnesia (either antegrade or retrograde) of >5 min duration
3. Abnormal drowsiness (defined as drowsiness in excess of that expected by the examining doctor)
4. ≥3 vomits after head injury (a vomit is defined as a single discrete episode of vomiting)
5. Suspicion of non accidental injury (defined as any suspicion of non accidental injury by the examining doctor)
6. Seizure after head injury in a patient who has no history of epilepsy

Examination

7. GCS less than 14, or GCS less than 15 if the patient is younger than one year old
8. Suspicion of penetrating or depressed skull injury or tense fontanel
9. Sign of basal skull fracture (defined as evidence of blood or cerebrospinal fluid leakage from the ear or nose and panda eyes)
10. Battle's sign, haemotympanum, facial crepitus or serious facial injury)
11. Positive focal neurological sign (defined as any focal neurological sign, including motor, sensory, coordination or reflex abnormality)
12. Presence of bruise, swelling or laceration >5 cm if the patient is younger than one year old

Mechanism

13. High-speed road traffic accident either as a pedestrian, cyclist or occupant (defined as accident with speed >40 m/h or 64 km/h)
14. Fall of more than 3 meters in height
15. High-speed injury from a projectile or an object

A CT scan is required if any of the above criteria are present

6.2 Canadian Assessment of Tomography for Childhood Head (CATCH), 2010

It was the name that Osmond et al. gave to their clinical decision rule for the use of computed tomography in children with minor head injury.

They included children aging between 0-16 years old, subject to blunt head trauma within 24 hours, with a GCS score of 13 to 15, with loss of consciousness, disorientation, amnesia, persistent irritability or vomiting. Exclusion was done if the cases were of obvious penetrating injury or depressed skull fracture, acute focal neurologic deficits, chronic

developmental delay generally, suspected child abuse leading to such head trauma, and if they were referred for reassessment of previously treated head injury.
They studied 3866 cases and examined 2043 cases by CT scanning.
According to this decision rule a head CT scan is necessary if the child has a minor head trauma (defined as head injury within the past 24 hours associated with loss of consciousness, amnesia, disorientation, persistent vomiting (more than one episode) or persistent irritability (in a child under two years of age) in a patient with GCS score of 13 - 15) and one of the following criteria:

1. GCS score lower than 15 two hours post trauma
2. Possible open or depressed skull fracture
3. Irritability
4. Worsening headache

The above signs and symptoms identify patients with ***High risk*** in whom neurosurgery intervention is unavoidable
The following criteria are indication for CT scanning as well and they identify patients with ***Medium risk*** in whom brain injury on CT scanning (not necessarily requiring neurological intervention) is probable:

5. "Raccoon" eyes, otorrhea or rhinorrhea of cerebrospinal fluid, hemotympanum, Battle's sign or other signs suggesting basal skull fracture
6. Large and boggy hematoma of the scalp
7. Dangerous mechanism of injury (e.g. fall from > 3 ft [91 cm] or higher than 5 stairs, or motor cycle rider with no helmet)

The Sensitivity and specificity of this decision rule was reported 100% and 70.2%, respectively. When all these seven risk factors were considered, 51.9% of patients would be eligible for CT scanning.

7. Conclusion

There are several decision rules published in the literature. Adherence to a decision rule will result in uniformity in ordering CT scan. However, there are considerations on selection of a decision rule:

- *External validity:* The study subjects enrolled in different studies have not been totally similar. The inclusion/exclusion criteria used in the specific study, determines its external validity, that is, what population of patients will benefit from that specific decision rule. For example, Miller's criteria and NOC are developed based on patients who had presented with a GCS score of 15 and a history of LOC, while patients studied for CCHR, CHIP, Lee et al and Saadat et al included patients with GCS 13 and more. Therefore, Miller's and NOC criteria may not be generalizable to patients who are presented with a GCS score of 13-14. Similarly, while Saadat et al criteria are applicable to patients with and without LOC, this may not be the case with the decision rules that excluded patients who do not represent with LOC.

  On the other hand, a wide inclusion criteria may affect the internal validity of a study; therefore, a decision rule that is developed based on a heterogeneous group of patients may be less reliable than criteria that are developed by focusing on a homogenous, well defined group of patients. It is best applicable however, to the same defined group of patients.

- *Positive outcome:* CCHR excluded patients with obvious depressed skull fracture while NEXUS II considered depressed skull fracture as a positive outcome. Isolated linear skull fracture was not considered a positive outcome in CHIP criteria and Lee et al study, but it was considered so in Abdul Latip et al. study.
  While adopting a decision rule, one should note the capabilities of the health facility setting to manage the consequences of a missed lesion. If a neurosurgeon is available in the health facility, then missing a lesion that could be safely managed later, may not be that serious. On the other hand, if management of a missed lesion is not possible in the given health facility, it would be better to adhere to decision rules that are designed to detect a wide range of outcomes.
- *Age group:* NOC included patients 3 years and older while CCHR, CHIP, Lee et al and Saadat et al included patients 16 years and older and Abdul Latip et al. included patients aged 12 and more. Therefore, these latter criteria should not be applied to children.
  Almost all published criteria are developed based on the assumption that the predictive power of the decision rules is the same across the age groups included in the study. While this remains to be studied specifically, equal distribution of cases in the study group may promise similar predictive value in all ages. This is of special importance in the case of elderly patients.
- *Sample size:* as a rule, the larger sample size is expected to give a more reliable prediction rule, provided that a reasonable proportion of cases represent positive outcome. Therefore, among the studies that have prepared CT scan from all the included patients, a greater sample size results in better prediction rule.
- *Inter-rater agreement:* the criteria will be used by different practicing physicians. They may have different perception from a single criterion. For example, the inter-observer agreement of physicians on the CCHR criteria is reported to be higher than NOC (stiell e. al. 2005).
  The inter-observer reliability of physicians should be measured and considered before adopting a specific decision rule.
- *Sensitivity and specificity:* The sensitivity and specificity of decision rules are described by their authors; however, the external validation studies generally provide less promising estimates. The higher sensitivity will result in less risk of missing a positive case. Generally, the higher sensitivity means less specificity that in turn results in less reduction of unnecessary CT scans. One should take in mind that these indices should be interpreted in conjunction with the "Positive outcome definition" of a specific study. A decision rule may appear more sensitive simply because it did not mean to detect some intracranial outcomes that another decision rule intended to do so.
  In external validation studies, CCHR and the NOC provided with similarly high sensitivity to detect serious neurological outcomes in MHI patients with GCS =15 ; however, the specificity of the CCHR was higher than the NOC. Therefore, application of the CCHR would result in lower use of CT imaging (stiell e. al. 2005). In patients aged 1 to 20 years, the sensitivity of NOC was reported higher than NEXUS II and CCHR. The specificity of CCHR was higher than NEXUS II and it was higher than NOC.
- *To order or not to order?* While decision rules are developed to reduce unnecessary CT scanning, they are more reliable when used to detect the patients who need a CT rather than exclude a patient from scanning. The reason is the limited number of positive cases

that the models are based on them. Note that deriving a decision rule is different from fitting a model for a cause-effect relationship. Both the indications used in decision rules and the intracranial lesions are results of another cause, the trauma. The statistical models just try to find visible signs and symptoms that are indicative of intracranial injury and there is no guarantee that there is no lesion if none of the visible signs or symptoms is present.

In some of the above mentioned studies, all patients did not undergo CT scanning but based on the judgment of the treating physician. If all patients are not studied by CT scan, there is no guarantee that they did not benefit from CT scanning. In fact, this limits the advantage of big sample size of NEXUS II study as it included the large number of patients whom physicians decided to order CT. Validity of this criteria for MHI patients who did not undergo CT scan is to be studied.

8. Future studies

There is need for further studies to cover the following issues:

- The optimal time of the first CT scanning in MHI patients needs to be studied. The predictive value of a single CT may depend on the time elapsed since the trauma. This needs to be studied specifically.
- A single CT scan may not reveal any significant intracranial finding; however, clinicians may order another brain scan according to the clinical presentations of the patient. The optimum time interval that is required to pass before re-ordering a CT scan needs to be studied.
- There is variability in the positive outcome definition. Medical centers need to assure detection of some important intracranial lesions. The important lesion may not mean the same for different settings (e.g. rural clinics versus different levels of trauma centers).

9. References

NICE. Head injury: Triage, assessment, investigation and early management of head injury in infants, children and adults [online]. Available at: http://www.nice.org.uk

Abdul Latip L.S., Ahmad Alias N.A., Ariff aR., et al. (2004). CT scan in minor head injury: a guide for rural doctors. J Clin Neurosci, Vol. 11, No. 8, (Nov), pp 835-839, ISSN 0967-5868 (Print)

Af Geijerstam J.L. & Britton M. (2003). Mild head injury - mortality and complication rate: meta-analysis of findings in a systematic literature review. Acta Neurochir (Wien), Vol. 145, No. 10, (Oct), pp 843-850; discussion 850, ISSN 0001-6268 (Print)

Berrington De Gonzalez A. & Darby S. (2004). Risk of cancer from diagnostic X-rays: estimates for the UK and 14 other countries. Lancet, Vol. 363, No. 9406, (Jan 31), pp 345-351, ISSN 1474-547X (Electronic)

Borczuk P. (1995). Predictors of intracranial injury in patients with mild head trauma. Ann Emerg Med, Vol. 25, No. 6, (Jun), pp 731-736, ISSN 0196-0644 (Print)

Bordignon K.C. & Arruda W.O. (2002). CT scan findings in mild head trauma: a series of 2,000 patients. Arq Neuropsiquiatr, Vol. 60, No. 2-A, (Jun), pp 204-210, ISSN 0004-282X (Print)

Borg J., Holm L., Cassidy J.D., et al. (2004). Diagnostic procedures in mild traumatic brain injury: results of the WHO Collaborating Centre Task Force on Mild Traumatic Brain Injury. J Rehabil Med, Vol. No. 43 Suppl, (Feb), pp 61-75, ISSN 1650-1977 (Print)

Brenner D., Elliston C., Hall E., et al. (2001). Estimated risks of radiation-induced fatal cancer from pediatric CT. AJR Am J Roentgenol, Vol. 176, No. 2, (Feb), pp 289-296, ISSN 0361-803X (Print)

Brix G., Nissen-Meyer S., Lechel U., et al. (2009). Radiation exposures of cancer patients from medical X-rays: how relevant are they for individual patients and population exposure? Eur J Radiol, Vol. 72, No. 2, (Nov), pp 342-347, ISSN 1872-7727 (Electronic)

Cassidy J.D., Carroll L.J., Peloso P.M., et al. (2004). Incidence, risk factors and prevention of mild traumatic brain injury: results of the WHO Collaborating Centre Task Force on Mild Traumatic Brain Injury. J Rehabil Med, Vol. No. 43 Suppl, (Feb), pp 28-60, ISSN 1650-1977 (Print)

Dunning J., Batchelor J., Stratford-Smith P., et al. (2004). A meta-analysis of variables that predict significant intracranial injury in minor head trauma. Archives of Disease in Childhood, Vol. 89, No. 7, (July 1, 2004), pp 653-659, 1468-2044 (Electronic)

Dunning J., Daly J.P., Lomas J.P., et al. (2006). Derivation of the children's head injury algorithm for the prediction of important clinical events decision rule for head injury in children. Arch Dis Child, Vol. 91, No. 11, (Nov), pp 885-891, ISSN 1468-2044 (Electronic)

Einstein aJ., Henzlova M. J.& Rajagopalan S. (2007). Estimating risk of cancer associated with radiation exposure from 64-slice computed tomography coronary angiography. JAMA, Vol. 298, No. 3, (Jul 18), pp 317-323, ISSN 1538-3598 (Electronic)

Fabbri A., Servadei F., Marchesini G., et al. (2004). Prospective validation of a proposal for diagnosis and management of patients attending the emergency department for mild head injury. J Neurol Neurosurg Psychiatry, Vol. 75, No. 3, (Mar), pp 410-416, ISSN 0022-3050 (Print)

Graham I.D., Stiell I.G., Laupacis A., et al. (1998). Emergency Physicians' Attitudes toward and Use of Clinical Decision Rules for Radiography. Academic Emergency Medicine, Vol. 5, No. 2, pp 134-140, ISSN 1553-2712

Hall E.J. & Brenner D.J. (2008). Cancer risks from diagnostic radiology. Br J Radiol, Vol. 81, No. 965, (May), pp 362-378, ISSN 1748-880X (Electronic)

Harad F.T. & Kerstein M.D. (1992). Inadequacy of bedside clinical indicators in identifying significant intracranial injury in trauma patients. J Trauma, Vol. 32, No. 3, (Mar), pp 359-361; discussion 361-353, ISSN 0022-5282 (Print)

Haydel M.J. (2005). Clinical decision instruments for CT scanning in minor head injury. JAMA, Vol. 294, No. 12, (Sep 28), pp 1551-1553, ISSN 1538-3598 (Electronic)

Haydel M.J., Preston C.A., Mills T.J., et al. (2000). Indications for computed tomography in patients with minor head injury. N Engl J Med, Vol. 343, No. 2, (Jul 13), pp 100-105, ISSN 0028-4793 (Print)

Holmes J.F., Hendey G.W., Oman J.A., et al. (2006). Epidemiology of blunt head injury victims undergoing ED cranial computed tomographic scanning. Am J Emerg Med, Vol. 24, No. 2, (Mar), pp 167-173, ISSN 0735-6757 (Print)

Jager T.E., Weiss H.B., Coben J.H., et al. (2000). Traumatic Brain Injuries Evaluated in U.S. Emergency Departments, 1992-1994. Academic Emergency Medicine, Vol. 7, No. 2, pp 134-140, ISSN 1553-2712

Jeret J.S, Mandell M., Anziska B., et al. (1993). Clinical predictors of abnormality disclosed by computed tomography after mild head trauma. Neurosurgery, Vol. 32, No. 1, (Jan), pp 9-15; discussion 15-16, ISSN 0148-396X (Print)

Katada K. (2006). [CT radiation exposure in Japan: analysis of social factors]. Nippon Hoshasen Gijutsu Gakkai Zasshi, Vol. 62, No. 5, (May 20), pp 649-656, ISSN 0369-4305 (Print)

Klauber M.R., Marshall L.F., Luerssen T.G., et al. (1989). Determinants of head injury mortality: importance of the low risk patient. Neurosurgery, Vol. 24, No. 1, (Jan), pp 31-36, ISSN 0148-396X (Print)

Kraus J.F. & Nourjah P. (1988). The epidemiology of mild, uncomplicated brain injury. J Trauma, Vol. 28, No. 12, (Dec), pp 1637-1643, ISSN 0022-5282 (Print)

Langlois Ja., Rutland-Brown W. & Ke. T. (2006). Traumatic Brain Injury in the United States: Emergency Department Visits, Hospitalizations, and Deaths. Centers for Disease Control and Prevention, National Center for Injury Prevention and Control

Langlois Ja., Rutland-Brown W. & Ke. T. (2004). Traumatic Brain Injury in the United States: Emergency Department Visits, Hospitalizations, and Deaths. Centers for Disease Control and Prevention, National Center for Injury Prevention and Control

Lee Y.B. & Kwon S.J. (2009). A more detailed classification of mild head injury in adults and treatment guidelines. J Korean Neurosurg Soc, Vol. 46, No. 5, (Nov), pp 451-458, ISSN 1598-7876 (Electronic)

Mccaig L.F. & Burt C.W. (2001). National Hospital Ambulatory Medical Care Survey: 1999 emergency department summary. Adv Data, Vol. No. 320, (Jun 25), pp 1-34, ISSN 0147-3956 (Print)

Menegazzi J.J., Davis E.A., Sucov aN., et al. (1993). Reliability of the Glasgow Coma Scale when used by emergency physicians and paramedics. J Trauma, Vol. 34, No. 1, (Jan), pp 46-48, ISSN 0022-5282 (Print)

Mettler Fa, Jr.Wiest, P.W., Locken J.A., et al. (2000). CT scanning: patterns of use and dose. J Radiol Prot, Vol. 20, No. 4, (Dec), pp 353-359, ISSN 0952-4746 (Print)

Miller E.C., Holmes J.F. & Derlet R.W. (1997). Utilizing clinical factors to reduce head CT scan ordering for minor head trauma patients. J Emerg Med, Vol. 15, No. 4, (Jul-Aug), pp 453-457, ISSN 0736-4679 (Print)

Mower W.R., Hoffman J.R., Herbert M., et al. (2002). Developing a clinical decision instrument to rule out intracranial injuries in patients with minor head trauma: methodology of the NEXUS II investigation. Ann Emerg Med, Vol. 40, No. 5, (Nov), pp 505-514, ISSN 0196-0644 (Print)

Mower W.R., Hoffman J.R., Herbert M., et al. (2005). Developing a decision instrument to guide computed tomographic imaging of blunt head injury patients. J Trauma, Vol. 59, No. 4, (Oct), pp 954-959, ISSN 0022-5282 (Print)

Norwood S.H., Mcauley C.E., Berne J.D., et al. (2002). A prehospital glasgow coma scale score < or = 14 accurately predicts the need for full trauma team activation and patient hospitalization after motor vehicle collisions. J Trauma, Vol. 53, No. 3, (Sep), pp 503-507, ISSN 0022-5282 (Print)

Osmond M.H., Klassen T.P., Wells G.A., et al. (2010). CATCH: a clinical decision rule for the use of computed tomography in children with minor head injury. CMAJ, Vol. 182, No. 4, (Mar 9), pp 341-348, ISSN 1488-2329 (Electronic)

Rimel R.W., Giordani B., Barth J.T., et al. (1981). Disability caused by minor head injury. Neurosurgery, Vol. 9, No. 3, (Sep), pp 221-228, ISSN 0148-396X (Print)

Saadat S., Ghodsi S.M., Holakouei Naeini K., et al. (2006). A statistical model for predicting the occurrence of intracranial lesions in patients with mild head trauma. PAYESH JULY, Vol. 5, No. 3, pp 193-200

Saadat S., Ghodsi S.M., Naieni K.H., et al. (2009). Prediction of intracranial computed tomography findings in patients with minor head injury by using logistic regression. J Neurosurg, Vol. 111, No. 4, (Oct), pp 688-694, ISSN 1933-0693 (Electronic)

Schynoll W., Overton D., Krome R., et al. (1993). A prospective study to identify high-yield criteria associated with acute intracranial computed tomography findings in head-injured patients. Am J Emerg Med, Vol. 11, No. 4, (Jul), pp 321-326, ISSN 0735-6757 (Print)

Shackford S.R., Wald S.L., Ross S.E., et al. (1992). The clinical utility of computed tomographic scanning and neurologic examination in the management of patients with minor head injuries. J Trauma, Vol. 33, No. 3, (Sep), pp 385-394, ISSN 0022-5282 (Print)

Smits M., Dippel D.W., De Haan G.G., et al. (2005). External validation of the Canadian CT Head Rule and the New Orleans Criteria for CT scanning in patients with minor head injury.JAMA, Vol. 294, No. 12, (Sep 28), pp 1519-1525, ISSN 1538-3598 (Electronic)

Smits M., Dippel D.W., Steyerberg E.W., et al. (2007). Predicting intracranial traumatic findings on computed tomography in patients with minor head injury: the CHIP prediction rule. Ann Intern Med, Vol. 146, No. 6, (Mar 20), pp 397-405, ISSN 1539-3704 (Electronic)

Stein S.C. & Ross S.E. (1990). The value of computed tomographic scans in patients with low-risk head injuries. Neurosurgery, Vol. 26, No. 4, (Apr), pp 638-640, ISSN 0148-396X (Print)

Stein S.C. & Ross S.E. (1992). Minor head injury: a proposed strategy for emergency management. Ann Emerg Med, Vol. 22, No. 7, (Jul), pp 1193-1196, ISSN 0196-0644 (Print)

Stiell I.G., Clement C.M., Rowe B.H., et al. (2005). Comparison of the Canadian CT Head Rule and the New Orleans Criteria in patients with minor head injury. JAMA, Vol. 294, No. 12, (Sep 28), pp 1511-1518, ISSN 1538-3598 (Electronic)

Stiell I.G., Lesiuk H., Wells G.A, et al. (2001). Canadian CT head rule study for patients with minor head injury: methodology for phase II (validation and economic analysis). Ann Emerg Med, Vol. 38, No. 3, (Sep), pp 317-322, ISSN 0196-0644 (Print)

Stiell I.G., Lesiuk H., Wells G.A., et al. (2001). The Canadian CT Head Rule Study for patients with minor head injury: rationale, objectives, and methodology for phase I (derivation). Ann Emerg Med, Vol. 38, No. 2, (Aug), pp 160-169, ISSN 0196-0644 (Print)

Stiell I.G., Wells G.A.,Vandemheen K., et al. (2001). The Canadian CT Head Rule for patients with minor head injury. Lancet, Vol. 357, No. 9266, (May 5), pp 1391-1396, ISSN 0140-6736 (Print)

10

Routine CT- Chest in Primary Evaluation of the Major Blunt Trauma Patients; Pros and Cons

Abdel-Mohsen M. Hamad
Department of Cardiothoracic Surgery, Tanta University,Tanta, Egypt

1. Introduction

Trauma is a major worldwide public health problem and it is one of the leading causes of death in both industrialized and developing countries. Injuries of the thorax are a major cause of morbidity and mortality in blunt trauma patients. Approximately 20% of trauma-related deaths are attributable to chest injuries (LoCicero and Mattox, 1989).

In trauma patients, a clear history is rarely available as most patients are confused, unconscious or even anesthetized and the clinical findings have been shown to be equivocal or misleading in 20–50% of victims of blunt polytrauma (Poletti et al., 2002).

Consequently, radiology plays a major role in evaluation of the trauma patient.

The Advanced Trauma Life Support (ATLS 2004) course recommended performing the plain film radiography of the chest, abdomen, and cervical spine in all the blunt trauma patients. Nowadays, Chest computed tomography (CCT) is being used with increasing frequency in the evaluation of blunt chest trauma. CCT frequently detects injuries not seen on routine initial chest x-ray (CxR) (occult findings). However, in the vast majority of patients the impact of these findings on patient management is debatable (Blostein et al., 1997, Hamad and regal, 2010).

CT is used primarily to assess for traumatic aortic injuries but also has been shown to be useful in the evaluation of skeletal, pulmonary, airway, and diaphragmatic injuries.

2. Chest wall injuries

Rib fractures are the most common finding after blunt chest trauma with an incidence reported up to 40%. Chest radiography is routinely used to assist in the diagnosis of rib fractures, even though it has limited sensitivity. it is even more insensitive in showing costochondral fractures. CT is the most sensitive technique for imaging rib fractures, since it can help to determine the site and number of fractures and, more importantly, provide information regarding any associated injuries (Primak and Collins, 2002).

Sternal fractures are found in 8–10% of blunt chest traumas and it is a marker of a high-energy trauma. The most common site of the sternal fractures is approximately 2 cm down from the manubrio-sternal joint. Sternal fracture usually cannot be diagnosed on frontal chest radiographs, whereas the lateral projections can detect it with high sensitivity. Spiral

CT, with sagittal and coronal reformations, should be the examination of choice in the suspicion of sternal fracture, as it identifies with high accuracy both the fracture, especially that with minimal dislocation, and the associated lesions.

Thoracic spine fractures account for 16% to 30% of all spine fractures. These fractures are usually difficult to detect on routine chest radiographs, especially those located in the upper portion. CT is much more sensitive for diagnosing thoracic spine fractures and is the imaging modality of choice. In addition to soft tissue and lung windows, chest CT scans in the trauma patient also should be viewed in bone windows for skeletal injuries. The most common fractures of the thoracic spine are anterior wedge compression fractures and burst fractures, most of which occur near the thoracolumbar junction (Meyer, 1992). If a thoracic spine fracture is suspected on either plain radiographs or chest CT, a dedicated thoracic spine CT at the level in question should be obtained with sagittal and coronal reconstructions to determine the type of fracture and to assess its stability.

3. Pleural space injuries

Pneumothorax, an air collection in the pleural space occurs in approximately 30% to 40% of cases of blunt trauma (Sariego et al., 1993). The diagnosis of pneumothorax is important whatever it is small because they may enlarge and progress to tension pneumothorax particularly if the patient undergoes mechanical ventilation or general anesthesia (Enderson et al., 1993). In supine position, pleural air will rise to the most nondependent portion of the thorax, which is the anterior, caudal aspect of the pleural space in the supine patient. Radiographic signs of pneumothorax in the supine trauma patient include 1) the deep sulcus sign, which is a deep, lucent costophrenic sulcus, 2) a relative increase in lucency at the affected lung base, and 3) the double diaphragm sign, which is created by the interfaces between the ventral and dorsal portions of the pneumothorax with the anterior and posterior aspects of the hemidiaphragm. CT is more sensitive for detecting pneumothorax than radiography, particularly in the supine patient. Pneumothoraces that are not apparent on the supine chest radiograph have been shown on CT in 10% to 50% of patients with head and blunt abdominal trauma (Wolfman et al., 1993).

It is generally safe to observe a stable patient with an occult pneumothorax, the situation is more controversial when the patient udergoes PPV. In a randomized study of treatment of occult pneumothorax with or without tube thoracostomy regardless of presence or absence of PPV, there was no difference in the incidence of respiratory distress or the need for emergent tube thoracostomy in either group suggesting that size progression of occult pneumothorax is unrelated to PPV (Brazel et al., 1999).

Pneumomediastinum in blunt trauma, the most common cause of pneumomediastinum is from rupture of the alveoli caused by a sudden increase in intra-alveolar pressure. The air then tracks centripetally through the pulmonary interstitium into the mediastinum ("Macklin effect"). On plain radiographs and CT, pneumomediastinum is diagnosed when air is seen outlining mediastinal soft tissue structures and the parietal pleura. The continuous diaphragm sign may be seen when air is present between the pericardium and the diaphragm.

4. Lung parenchymal injuries

Pulmonary contusion is defined as focal parenchymal injury with edema and alveolar and interstitial hemorrhage. It is reported in 17%-70% of blunt traumas cases, it is usually seen adjacent to solid structures like vertebrae, ribs, the liver, and the heart (Gavelli et al., 2002). In chest radiographs, lung contusion appears within the first 6-8 hours following trauma as non-segmental, non-lobar, peripheral, and in the form of increased density (Kerns et al., 1990). It is more likely to detect contusions with thoracic CT than with chest radiography (Schild et al., 1989).

Pulmonary laceration is defined as the disruption of alveolar spaces with formation of a cavity filled with blood or air, and may occur from penetrating trauma or from shearing forces associated with blunt trauma. It is difficult to detect lacerations with chest radiography as they usually overlap accompanying contusion areas. On CT, pulmonary laceration is characterized by air collections within an area of consolidation. CT detects far more lacerations; in one study of 85 patients with pulmonary laceration, 99 lacerations were present on CT, but only 5 were seen radiographically (Wagner et al., 1988). Pulmonary hematoma results from complete filling of a laceration cavity with blood. Hematomas are seen as well-defined, spherical or oval, homogenous increased densities, both with thoracic CT and chest radiography. A traumatic pneumatocele is a completely air-filled cystic space after either acute laceration or complete resolution of a pulmonary hematoma. The radiographic sequelae of pulmonary laceration may persist for months or years (Mirvis et al., 1992).

5. Tracheobronchial injury

Tracheobronchial ruptures due to thoracic trauma are relatively rare, reported in 0.4–1.5% of patients in clinical series of major blunt thoracic trauma. More than 80% of bronchial injuries occur in the main bronchi within 2.5 cm of the carina, with the right side more commonly than the left side (Euathrongchit et al., 2006). Common but nonspecific radiographic findings of tracheobronchial injury are pneumothorax, pneumomediastinum, and subcutaneous emphysema. More specific findings of tracheobronchial injury include persistent pneumothorax after adequate chest tube placement, collapse of the lung away from the hilum ("fallen lung sign"), and overdistension or herniation of the endotracheal balloon. Helical CT with sagittal and coronal reconstructions is more sensitive and specific than radiography (Unger et al., 1989; Wintermark et al., 2001).

6. Esophageal injury

Esophageal rupture is extremely rare as a complication of blunt trauma (1/1000 cases of blunt chest trauma). However it must be excluded in any case of mediastinal penetrating trauma. Radiographic signs are not specific and include persistent cervical and mediastinal emphysema, pleural fluid, and abnormal mediastinal contour caused by leakage of fluids, hematoma, or mediastinitis (Rivas et al., 2003). CT findings include the radiographic findings, as well as mediastinal fluid and extraluminal enteric contrast.

7. Diaphragmatic injury

Diaphragmatic injuries occur in approximately 1% to 8% of blunt trauma cases (Boulanger et al., 1993). Most injuries occur in the posterolateral portion of the left hemidiaphragm (Worthy et al., 1995). Chest radiographic findings of diaphragmatic injury depend mainly on herniation of hollow viscus into the thorax, and abnormal course of the nasogastric tube. The most common finding of diaphragmatic injury on CT is abrupt discontinuity of the diaphragm. Other CT findings include herniation of abdominal contents into the thorax and constriction of bowel at the herniation site ("collar sign"). The sensitivity of axial CT for diaphragmatic tears ranges between 70% and 90%, and the specificity is approximately 90% (Murray et al., 1996). Pitfalls in diagnosing diaphragmatic tears on CT occur when intraabdominal blood or hemothorax obscures the diaphragm. Also, small incidental diaphragmatic defects are often identified, particularly in older patients.

8. Aortic injury

Diagnosis of acute aortic injury is critical. The frontal chest radiograph is the initial study for the evaluation of aortic injury. The greatest utility of chest radiography is not in diagnosing aortic injury, however, but in excluding it. Normal chest radiograph has a 98% negative predictive value (Pretre et al., 1997). Radiographic findings that may indicate mediastinal hematoma include mediastinal widening, abnormal contour or indistinctness of the aortic knob, apical pleural cap, rightward deviation of the nasogastric tube within the esophagus, rightward deviation of the trachea, downward displacement of the left main stem bronchus, and thickening of the right paratracheal stripe. However, mediastinal widening due to mediastinal hematoma is not specific for aortic injury and can be caused by other injuries such as sternal fractures, thoracic spine fractures, venous injury, or great vessel injury.

According to initial chest radiograph findings, and level of clinical suspicion, further workup for aortic injury may be necessary. For a long time aortography has been considered the gold standard for diagnosing aortic injury. More recently several studies have evaluated the use of contrast-enhanced helical CT as a screening and diagnostic modality and recommended CT for routine evaluation (Mirvis and Shanmuganathan 2007). The chest CT scan performed for possible aortic injury is evaluated for direct evidence of a tear, including abnormal aortic contour, pseudoaneurysm, intimal flap, active extravasation of contrast, or abrupt tapering of the descending aorta relative to the ascending aorta ("pseudocoarctation"). Prospective studies with helical CCT for the evaluation of blunt aortic injury (BAI) shows comparable sensitivity (100% vs. 92%) and negative predictive value (NPV) (100% vs. 97%) when compared to aortography, but performed poorly by comparison in regards to specificity (83% vs. 99%) (Fabian et al., 1998).

9. Comment

While conventional X-rays still play an important role as the primary screening method, CT imaging has become an integral part of the trauma screening and resuscitation phase.

In general, The CCT is superior to routine screening CxR with regard to sternal, rib and spine fractures, lung lacerations and contusions, pneumothorax, hemothorax, heart, pericardium, aorta and diaphragm (Guerrero-Lopez et al., 2000, Rivas et al., 2003). However, it is not clear whether CT chest should be used in the general blunt trauma population routinely or on selective basis.

Several authors reported the detection of clinically significant findings more frequently on CCT in 'high risk' blunt trauma admissions, These patients included but were not limited to high-speed motor vehicle collisions, >15 foot falls, pedestrian versus motor vehicle collisions, patients with any sign of thoracic trauma on physical examination or any mediastinal abnormalities on CxR (Demetriades et al., 1998; Exadaktylos et al., 2001). A significant number of these patients (14–65%) can have a completely normal CxR (Trupka et al., 1997; Demetriades et al., 1998; Exadaktylos et al., 2001; Plurad et al., 2007).

The lethality of the occult injury defines the urgency and pertinence of subsequent clinical action. For example, the finding of an aortic or great vessel injury or spine fracture would mandate critical management or diagnostic manoeuvres, while the diagnosis of an occult pneumothorax may not (Brazel et al., 1999).

Therefore, use of CCT in Selected patients can lead to significant changes in patient management (18– 41%) (Trupka et al., 1997; Guerrero-Lopez et al., 2000; Renton, 2003; Salim et al., 2006; Deunk et al., 2007) while application of CCT more liberally results in little consequential intervention overall (Blostein and Hodgeman, 1997; Plurad et al., 2007; Wisbach et al., 2007) based on these occult diagnoses.

On the other hand, others argue that the higher discovery of injuries with CT is of questionable clinical significance at great costs. For example, it has previously been shown that occult pneumothoraces can be treated expectantly, even with positive pressure ventilation (Guerrero-Lopez et al., 2000; Brazel et al., 1999). Also, The significance of occult rib fractures, hemothorax, or contusion is also questionable because hemothoraces may resolve without intervention (Poole et al., 1993) and there is no treatment for the vast majority of rib fractures other than pain management. The increased use of CCT for blunt trauma, presumably for the diagnosis BAI, has not resulted in a significant increase in detection overall. It can also be questioned as to whether all occult BAIs needs to be treated, because this probably was the case before the evolution of the CCT (Plurad et al., 2007).

The question is, when should CT be used in the general blunt trauma population? Should we scan selectively if clinical examination or plain radiography is abnormal or should we use a lower threshold and scan on a routine basis?

On trying to answer this question, Brink et al., tested a number of risk factors (age ≥55 years, abnormal chest PE, altered sensorium, abnormal thoracic spine PE, abnormal chest and thoracic spine CR, abnormal abdominal US or pelvic CR, Hb<6 and BE < −3 mmol/l.) as independent predictors of positive findings on chest CT in high-energy blunt trauma patients. Presence of any of these criteria can predict presence of chest injuries on CT with a sensitivity of 95%. However, they reported that if these positive predictors were implemented as scanning indications, 5% of all patients with chest injuries on CT would not be identified. This implies that the chance of missing injuries of the chest remains 13% in the low-risk patients if these patients do not undergo chest CT (Brink et al., 2010).

The liberal use of CT scanning is not without concerns; in addition to the cost issue, radiation exposure, time loss and isolation of patient from medical care are important drawbacks.

There is a general consensus that the current levels of CT radiation may be associated with an increased risk of cancer. The effective radiation dose to all organs from a single full-body CT examination is 12 to 16 milli-Sieverts (mSv). Considering that studies of Japanese atomic bomb survivors who received only 5–150 mSv dose have increased risk of cancer, it is reasonable to assume that the risk of cancer from CCT exposure is small but real. Even the lowest dose in the exposed atomic-bomb survivor population (range, 5-50 mSv; mean, 20 mSv) is associated with an increased cancer mortality risk. This risk is more important in children (Kalra et al., 2004; Brenner et al., 2007; Huda 2007).

In most trauma centers, the CT scanner is located outside of the trauma resuscitation bay, even in a different department of the hospital. This requires patient transportation and isolation from the ER team; this potentially influences the decision to perform CT imaging on a patient-to-patient basis.

In Amsterdam, the Academic Medical Center recently introduced a moveable CT scanner in the trauma room itself (Fung Kon Jin et al., 2008). The aim of this concept is the elimination of patient transfer for CT imaging with subsequent shorter time(79 min. in comparison to 105 min before) until completion of diagnostic imaging in patients requiring CT imaging. Moreover patients in Amsterdam can be treated during CT imaging this progress can encourage ER team to incorporate CT imaging during the initial trauma evaluation thus favoring the decision to go for diagnostic accuracy over immediately performing emergency surgery with Less than optimal insights in the potential injuries of the trauma patient.

On the extreme side, some institutions in Europe have reported their experience with full body CT imaging prior to physical examination by the trauma team in their effort to reduce time (Weninger et al., 2007).

Multiple trauma presentations at the same moment undoubtedly influence the overall time needed for complete radiological evaluation, especially when CT imaging is required. Fung Kon Jin et al in a high-volume level-1 trauma center, reported that complete radiological workup, including CT scanning, of a stable trauma patient is completed in a median of 114 min. Patients that are more severely injured (ISS > 15) were transported faster to CT, resulting in faster diagnostic imaging (Fung Kon Jin et al., 2008).

10. References

American College of Surgeons Committee on Trauma. (2004). ATLS advanced trauma life support program for doctors. American College of Surgeons: Chicago, IL.

Blostein PA, Hodgman CG. (1997). Computed tomography of the chest in blunt thoracic trauma: results of a prospective study. *J Trauma* 43:13–8.

Boulanger BR, Milzman DP, Rosati C, Rodriquez A. (1993). A comparison of right and left blunt traumatic diaphragmatic rupture. J Trauma 35:255–60.

Brazel KJ, Stafford RE, Weigelt JA, et al. (1999). Treatment of occult pneumothoraces from blunt trauma. *J Trauma* 46:987–991.

Brenner DJ, Elliston CD. (2004). Estimated radiation risks potentially associated with full-body CT screening. *Radiology* 232:735-738.

Brink M, Deunk J, Dekker HM, Edwards MJ, Kool DR, van Vugt AB, van Kuijk C, Blickman JG. (2010). Criteria for the selective use of chest computed tomography in blunt trauma patients. *Eur Radiol* 20(4):818-28.

Brink M, Deunk J, Dekker HM, et al. (2008). Added value of routine chest MDCT after blunt trauma: evaluation of additional findings and impact on patient management. *Am J Roentgenol* 190:1591-8..

Demetriades D, Gomez H, Velmahos G, et al. (1998). Routine helical computed tomographic evaluation of the mediastinum in high risk blunt trauma patients. *Arch Surg* 133:1084 -1088.

Deunk J, Dekker HM, Brink M, van Vugt R, Edwards MJ, van Vugt AB. (2007). The value of indicated computed tomography scan of the chest and abdomen in addition to the conventional radiologic work-up for blunt trauma patients. *J Trauma* 63(4):757-63.

Enderson BL, Abdalla R, Frame SB, et al. (1993). Tube thoracostomy for occult pneumothorax: a prospective randomized study of its use. *J Trauma* 35:726–9.

Euathrongchit J, Thoongsuwan N, Stern EJ. (2006). Nonvascular mediastinal trauma. *Radiol Clin North Am* 44:251–258.

Exadaktylos AK, Sclabas G, Schmid SW, et al. (2001). Do we really need routine computed tomographic scanning in the primary evaluation of blunt chest trauma in patients with "normal" chest radiograph? *J Trauma* 51:1173–1176.

Fabian TC, David KA, Gavant ML, et al. (1998). Prospective study of blunt aortic injury. *Ann Surg* 227: 666–77.

Fung Kon Jin PH, van Geene AR, Linnau KF, Jurkovich GJ, Ponsen KJ, Goslings JC. (2009). Time factors associated with CT scan usage in trauma patients. *Eur J Radiol* 72(1):134-8.

Fung Kon Jin PHP, Goslings JC, Ponsen KJ, et al. (2008). Assessment of a new Trauma Workflow Concept Implementing a Sliding CT Scanner in the Trauma Room: the Effect onWorkup Times. *J Trauma* 64(5):1320–6.

Gavelli G, Canini R, Bertaccini P, et al. (2002). Traumatic injuries: imaging of thoracic injuries. *Eur Radiol* 12:1273–1294.

Guerrero-Lopez F, Vazquez-Mata G, Cazar- Romero PP, Fernandez-Mondejar E, Guayo-Hoyos E, Linde-Valverde CM. (2000). Evaluation of the utility of computed tomography in the initial assessment of the critical care patient with chest trauma. *Crit Care Med* 28:1370–1375.

Hamad AM, Regal M. (2009). Is Routine Spiral CT-Chest Justified in Evaluation of the Major Blunt Trauma Patients? *Eur J Trauma* 35:31-4.

Huda W. (2007). Radiation doses and risks in chest computed tomography examinations. *Proc Am Thorac Soc* 4: 316-20.

Kalra MK, Maher MM, Rizzo S, et al. (2004). Radiation exposure from chest CT: Issues and strategies. *J Korean Med Sci* 19:159-166.

Kerns SR, Gay SB. (1990). CT of blunt chest trauma. *Am J Roentgenol* 154:55–60.

LoCicero III J and Mattox KL. (1989). Epidemiology of chest trauma. *Surg Clin North Am* 69:15–9.

Meyer S. (1992). Thoracic spine trauma. *Semin Roentgenol* 27:254–61.

Mirvis SE, Shanmuganathan K. (2007). Diagnosis of blunt traumatic aortic injury: still a nemesis. *Eur J Radiol* 64:27–40.

Mirvis SE, Templeton P. (1992). Imaging in acute thoracic trauma. *Semin Roentgenol* 27:184–210.

Murray JG, Gaoili E, Gruden JF, et al. (1996). Acute rupture of the diaphragm due to blunt trauma: diagnostic sensitivity and specificity of CT. *Am J Roentgenol* 166:1035–9.

Plurad D, Green D, Demetriades D, et al. (2007). The increasing use of chest computed tomography for trauma: is it being overutilized? *J Trauma* 62:631-5.

Poletti PA, Wintermark M, Schnyder P, Becker CD. (2002). Traumatic injuries: the role of imaging inthemanagement of the polytrauma victim (conservative expectation). *Eur Radiol* 12:969–78.

Poole GV, Morgan DB, Crenston PE, et al. (1993). Computed tomography in the management of blunt thoracic trauma. *J Trauma* 35:296 –302.

Pretre R and Chilcott M. (1997). Blunt trauma to the heart and great vessels. *N Engl J Med* 336:626–632.

Primak SL and Collins J. (2002). Blunt nonaortic chest trauma: radiographic and CT findings. *Emergency Radiology* 9:5-12.

Renton J. (2003). Should helical CT scanning of the thoracic cavity replace the conventional chest x-ray as a primary assessment tool in pediatric trauma? An efficacy and cost analysis. *J Pediatr Surg* 8:793–797.

Rivas LA, Fishman JE, Munera F, et al. (2003). Multislice CT in thoracic trauma. *Radiol Clin North Am* 41:599-616.

Salim A, Sangthong B, Martin M, et al. (2006). Whole body imaging in blunt multisystem trauma patients without obvious signs of injury. *Arch Surg* 141:468–475.

Sariego J, Borwn JL, Matsumoto T, Kerstein MD. (1993). Predictors of pulmonary complications in blunt chest trauma. *Int Surg* 78:320–3.

Schild HH, Strunk H, Weber W, et al. (1989). Pulmonary contusion CT vs plain radiograms. *J Comput Assist Tomogr* 13:417–420.

Trupka A, Waydhas C, Hallfeldt K, et al. (1997). Value of thoracic computed tomography in the first assessment of severely injured patients with blunt chest trauma: results of a prospective study. *J Trauma* 43:405– 412.

Unger JM, Schuchmann GG, Grossmann JE, et al. (1989). Tears of the trachea and main bronchi caused by blunt trauma: Radiologic findings. *AJR* 153:1175–80.

Wagner RB, Crawford Jr. WO Schimpf PP. (1988). Classification of parenchymal injuries of the lung. *Radiology* 167:77–82.

Weninger P, Mauritz W, Fridrich P, et al. (2007). Emergency room management of patients with blunt major trauma: evaluation of the multislice computed tomography protocol exemplified by an urban trauma center. J Trauma 62(3):584–91.

Wintermark M, Schnyder P, Wicky S. (2001). Blunt traumatic rupture of a mainstem bronchus: spiral CT demonstration of the "fallen lung" sign. *Eur Radiol* 11:409-411.

Wisbach GG, Sise MJ, Sack DI, et al. (2007). What is the role of chest x-ray in the initial assessment of stable trauma patients? *J Trauma* 62:74-8.

Wolfman NT, Gilpin JW, Bechtold RE, et al. (1993). Occult pneumothorax in patients with abdominal trauma: CT studies. *J Comput Assist Tomogr* 17:56–9.

Worthy SA, Kang EY, Hartman TE, Kwong JS, Mayo JR, Müller NL. (1995). Diaphragmatic rupture: CT findings in 11 patients. Radiology 194:885–8.

Part 3

3D Modelling

11

Influence of End-Plates on Biomechanical Response of the Human Lumbosacral Segment

Vincenzo Moramarco[1], Claudia Macchia[1],
Carmine Pappalettere[1] and Amaya Pérez del Palomar[2]
[1]*Politecnico di Bari, Dipartimento di Ingegneria Meccanica e Gestionale*
[2]*Universidad de Zaragoza, Departamento de Ingenieria Mecanica*
[1]*Italy*
[2]*Spain*

1. Introduction

Diseases of lumbar spine and associated diseases of the intervertebral disc are a major focus of contemporary spinal care. Low back pain, in fact, is becoming in the recent years one of the most diffuse chronic pathologies and represents one of the highest direct and indirect costs for national welfare. It can affect for years the patient with obvious disabling consequences and many times without a complete explanation of the causes (Devor & Tal, 2009).

Some clinical studies (Latorraca & Forni Niccolai Gamba, 2004) showed that the greatest proportion (about 90%) of spinal diseases, like lumbar hernias, is located in the lumbar spine segment. Recent investigations based on clinical-radiological observations pointed out those rachidian affections such as lumbar and sciatic pains that in the worst cases last for years with very invalidating effects on the patient mainly depending on disk-vertebral insufficiency caused by degenerative phenomena. At the same time, in absence of pathological disease, daily activities, lifting stationary work postures, heavy physical work and vibrations are factors that contribute to low back disorders (Natarajan et al., 2004).

Usually, orthopaedic therapy is essentially based on the experience of the surgeon who predicts the best solution for each patient. Using mathematical models and computer simulations could potentially be an important tool to support clinical decisions in order to predict the appearance and evolution of spine pathologies, for preoperative planning and implant design.

The present work is focused on the analysis of the lumbar spine with the aim of studying the influence and the roles that the different components of the spine play on its biomechanical response.

In particular the presence of the cartilagineous endplates separating the soft tissues of the intervertebral disc from the strong bone of the vertebrae will be studied.

The endplates, in fact, are demonstrated to perform a double function in the global response of the spine respectively mechanically "protecting" the discs from a direct contact with the vertebrae avoiding the disc to bulge axially under compression and, at the same time, acting as the favourite nutrients transport route for the same discs. The endplates also absorb the

considerable hydrostatic pressure that results from mechanical loading of the spine (Broberg, 1983).
Although the cartilaginous end-plates (CEP) play a great role in the biomechanics of the intervertebral discs (Adams & Roughley, 2006), most authors (Eberlein et al., 2004; Rohlmann et al., 2006; Moramarco et al., 2010) did not consider the presence of the CEP in their models or simulated it using the same mechanical properties of the annulus fibrosus (Zander et al., 2009).
In order to understand the influence of the CEP in the modelling of the lumbar spine segment two accurate computational models, with and without CEP, of the whole lumbosacral spinal unit (L1-S1) of the human rachis, based on CT-scan imaging and experimental data, were built and their mechanical response under static loading was compared.

2. Model

The lumbar spine is the most caudal part of the articulated vertebral column and it normally supports the highest mechanical loads. In a person who does not carry extra weight, the lumbar structure bears at least 55% of the total body mass (Noailly, 2009). In particular the lumbar spine is composed of five vertebrae and the sacrum, a large, triangular bone, that consists of five vertebrae fused together. Between each vertebra there is a disc that serves to cushion the vertebrae and connect them together in a flexible way. The disc and the surface of the vertebrae are separated by a cartilaginous endplate which is the interface that avoids the direct contact between the two components above mentioned.
An accurate FE computational model of the complete L1-S1 segment of the human rachis of a real patient, based on CT-scan imaging and experimental data, has been built in order to simulate the non-linear behaviour of the rachis measured in vitro. In particular with the aim of studying the mechanical role of the cartilaginous endplates, two models, differing exclusively in the presence of the endplates, will be presented.

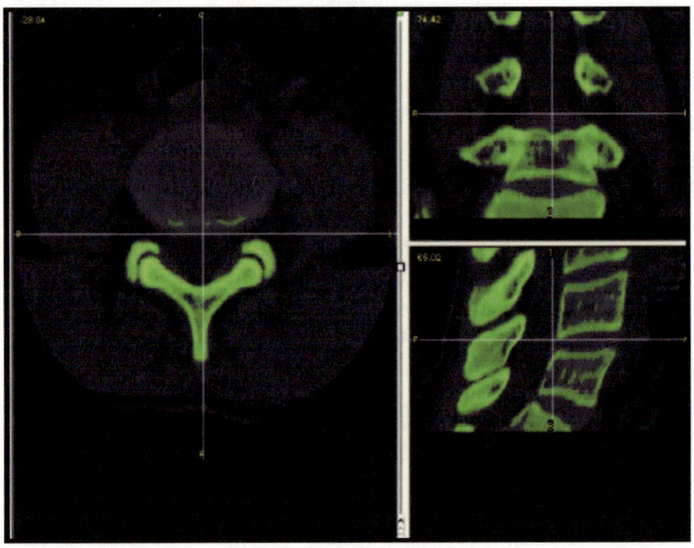

Fig. 1. CT data scan of the human lumbosacral region.

2.1 Vertebrae geometry definition

To reconstruct the FE model of the healthy lumbar segment, CT scan data of a subject with no current spinal pathology consisting of 101 slides each of 0.90 mm were used (Fig. 1).

The reconstruction of three-dimensional models of the vertebrae was performed using the software Mimics® 10.0 by Materialise Inc, in particular the domain boundary of each vertebra was created individually, using the built-in module MedCAD® available in the software application.

For this, it is essential to define the edges of the vertebra separating them from the bottom of the initial image. This is done initially relying on the different gray value of the CT image, a different gray level indicates a different density of the object in the image, so it is possible to define a threshold level that separates the parts of interest from the background. All pixels with a grey level higher than the threshold are considered part of the vertebra. In this case the upper threshold level was set to 1200 of the Hounsfield scale while the lower level to 200 (Fig. 2).

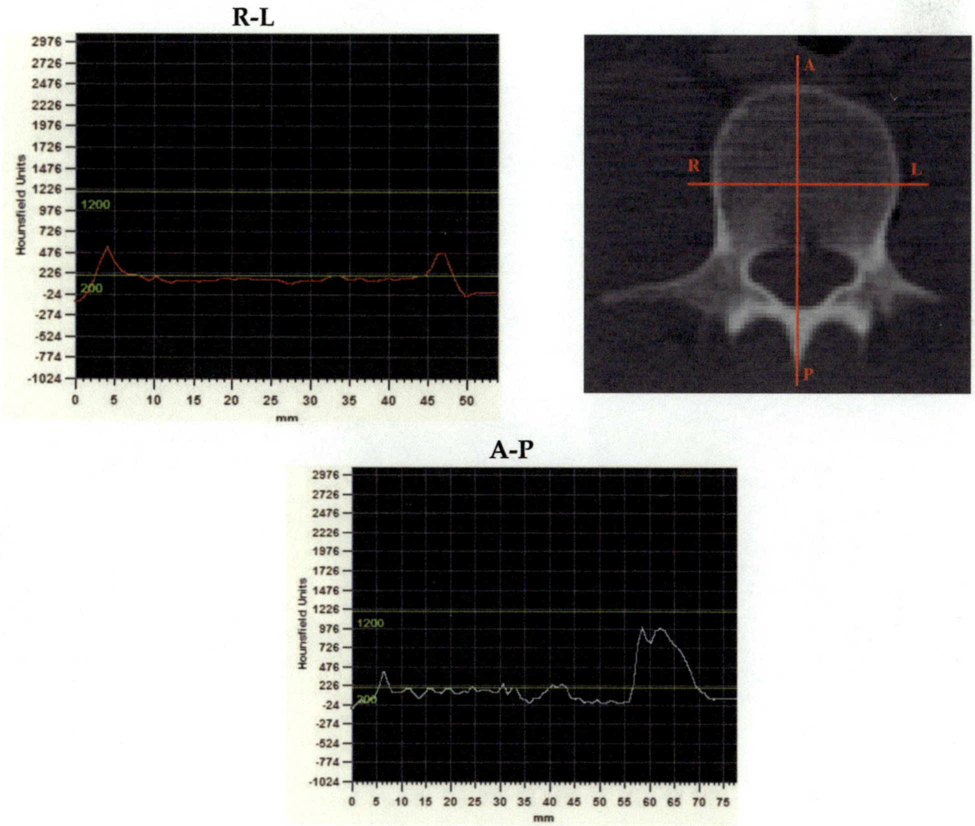

Fig. 2. An example of the anterior-posterior (A-P) and right-left (R-L) Hounsfield scale profiles.

The pixels selected in all the slides and in all three planes (sagittal, transverse end axial) of the CT file are joined together using the so-called "mask".
An example of "mask" in which the threshold was set in order to select the areas of the bone is shown in green in Fig.1. In the same figure it is evident that selecting the single vertebra is not possible and that there are cavities in the mask.
For this reason after creating the mask on the different gray levels the masks of the single vertebrae must be created and adjusted in order to obtain a refined mask which allows the software to calculate the three-dimensional model of the single vertebra (Fig 3).
In order to preserve the original geometry as well as possible no smoothing operations were carried out on the surfaces.
The 3D models thus obtained can be converted into formats readable from other softwares, such as those for the finite element analysis (FE).
In our case the models of individual vertebrae of the lumbar-sacral segment L1-S1 were exported in the *.inp format readable by the commercial FE software ABAQUS® which will be used later to carry out the numerical simulations.

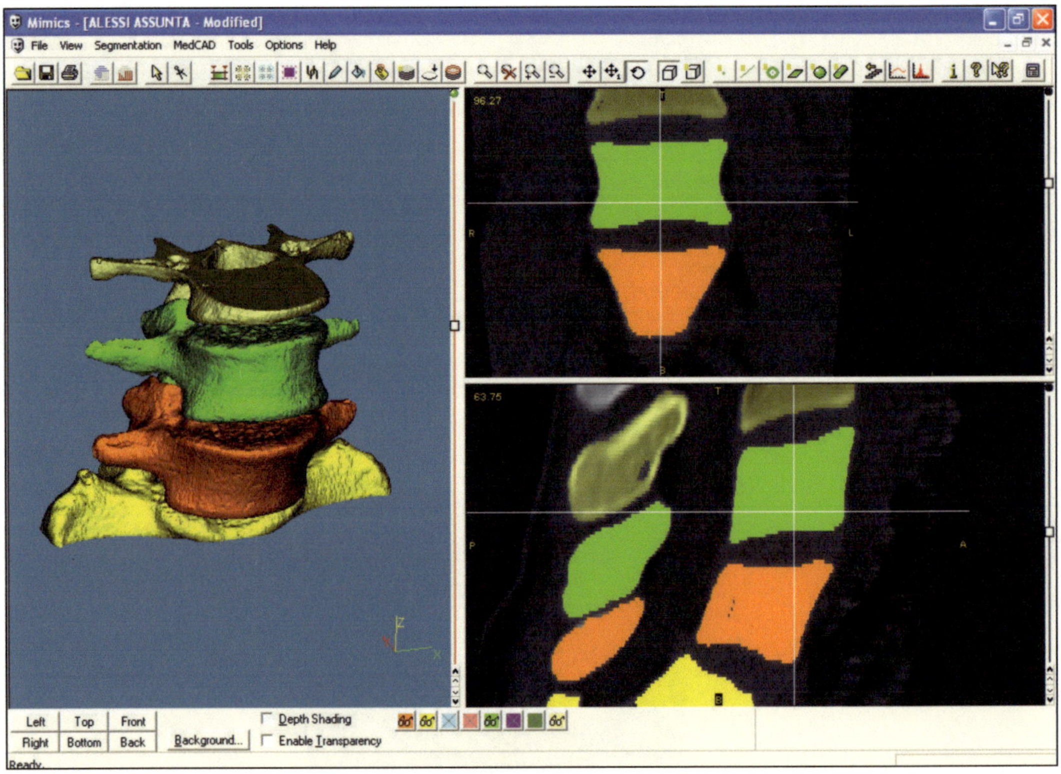

Fig. 3. Domain boundary creation with Mimics®.

Then, the vertebrae were discretized using surface triangular 3-nodes elements and reassembled preserving the original positions. The single vertebrae were imported in ABAQUS where they were assembled to create the complete model of the lumbar spine having the same geometry of the real one obtained with CT scan (Fig. 4).

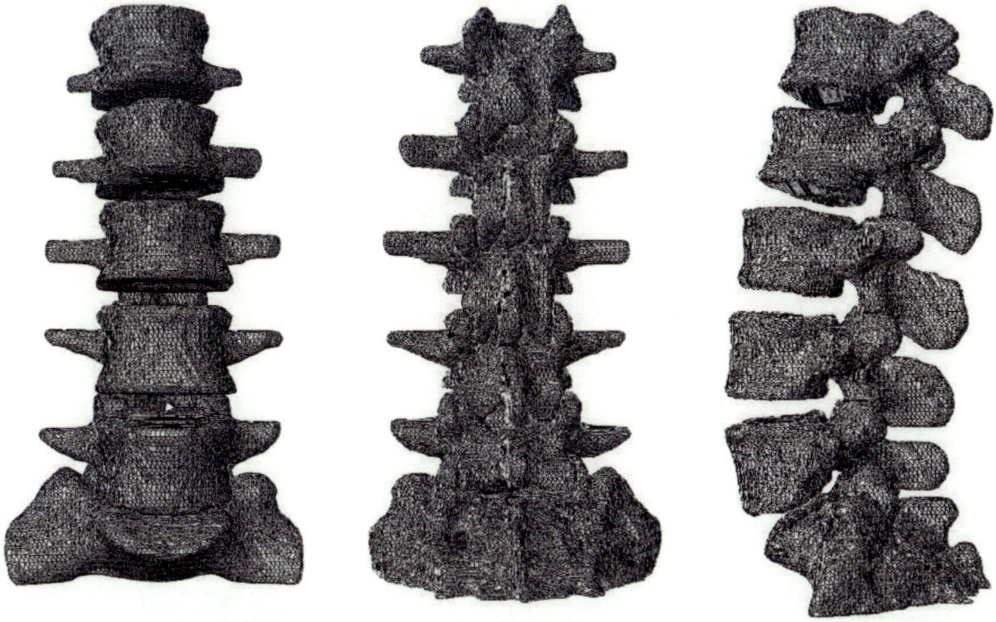

(a) (b) (c)

Fig. 4. Front (a), back (b) and lateral (c) view of the discretized lumbosacral segment of the human rachis.

2.2 Intervertebral disc (IVD) geometry definition

The intervertebral discs were modelled with deformable elements. The soft tissues, unlike the tissues characterized by high density as the bone, are not directly visible in a normal CT scan. For this reason the creation of the disc has been based not only on the CT data but also on anatomical studies present in literature.

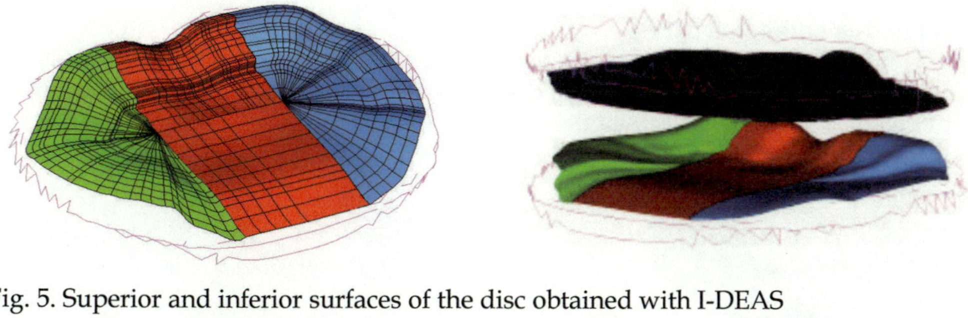

Fig. 5. Superior and inferior surfaces of the disc obtained with I-DEAS

The upper and the lower surfaces of each disc were defined using the surface of the vertebrae above and below respectively. The software I-Deas 9 (Altair Computing Inc.) (Structural Dynamics Research Corporation, 1993) was used to generate these surfaces (Fig 5.).
Then, using Cubit 10.1 (Leland, 2001), the volume domain was generated and the annulus fibrosus and the nucleus pulposus were drawn so that volumetric ratio was 3:7 like reported in Goto et al. (2002). The domain was discretized with 8-node hexahedral elements. Figure 6

shows the intervertebral disc as it has been obtained in CUBIT. Two zones, the nucleus pulposus and the annulus fibrosus can be distinguished.

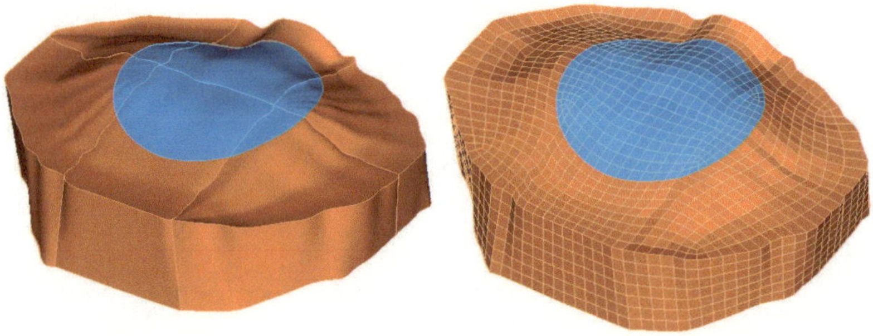

(a) (b)

Fig. 6. Intervertebral disc obtained in CUBIT 10.1: before (a) and after (b) meshing

Finally all disc meshes were adjusted to the related vertebrae surfaces in order to obtain a perfect continuity and to remove interferences between the bodies (Fig. 7).

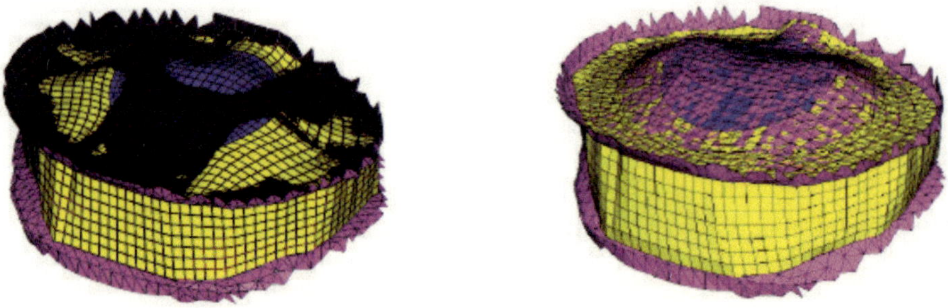

(a) (b)

Fig. 7. L4-L5 intervertebral disc volume definition: bodies interferences removal

2.3 Cartilaginous endplates (CEP)

The cartilaginous endplate, being considered as a part of the soft intervertebral disc, has been constructed using the surfaces of each disc. In this way the geometry and the condition of non-interference with the surfaces of the vertebrae were respected.

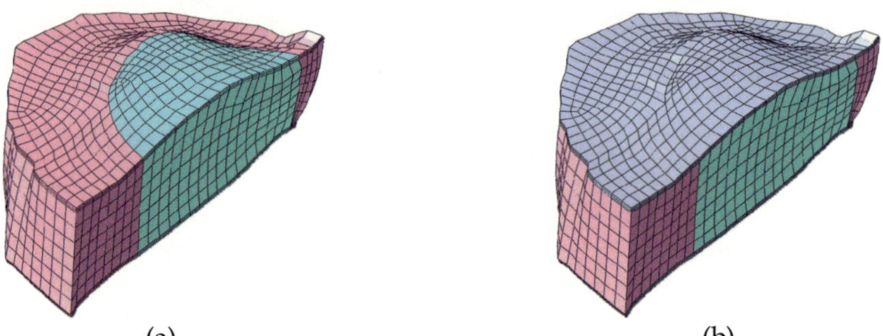

(a) (b)

Fig. 8. Intervertebral disc without (a) and with (b) endplate

In particular each endplate has been carried out with two layers, each with 0.5 mm thick and characterized as a linear elastic material.
The elastic response of the cartilaginous endplates is purely isotropic. Only tensile stress is sustained by the one-dimensional collagen fibres (Eberlein et al., 2001).

2.4 The whole model of the lumbosacral segment L1-S1

The whole model was assembled using ABAQUS CAE 6.8. The relative position of all parts, the geometry and the natural curvature of the spine were preserved. The ligaments, anterior longitudinal (ALL), posterior longitudinal (PLL), intertransverse (ITL), flavum (LF), capsular (JC), interspinous (ISL) and supraspinous (SSL) were added.

Ligament	E_1 [MPa]	E_2 [MPa]	ε_{12}	Elements	Area [mm²]
ALL	7.8	20.0	0.12	5	32.4
PLL	1.0	2.0	0.11	5	5.2
LF	1.5	1.9	0.062	3	84.2
ITL	10.0	59.0	0.18	4	1.8
SSL	3.0	5.0	0.20	3	25.2
Ligament	**Spine Level**	**Area [mm²]**	**Poisson's Ratio v**	**Elements**	**Stiffness *k* [N/mm]**
JC	L1-L2	43.8	0.4	6	42.5
	L2-L3				33.9
	L3-L4				32.3
	L4-L5				30.6
	L5-S1				29.9
ISL	L1-L2	35.1	0.4	6	10.0
	L2-L3				9.6
	L3-L4				18.1
	L4-L5				8.7
	L5-S1				16.3

Table 1. Lumbar ligaments properties (Pintar et al., 1992; Chazal et al., 1985; Goel et al.,1995; Goto et al., 2003).

Since they are able to response only at traction loads, they were modelled as tension only nonlinear truss elements with the features described in the table below.
The finite element model was formed of six vertebrae, from the L1 to the S1, and five intervertebral discs interposed between them. The ligaments were placed in the model so that the natural configuration was respected.
The model contains 128793 elements, in particular 46887 hexaedrical 8-nodes elements (C3D8) for the nucleus, the annulus and the endplates, 73016 rigid elements (R3D3) to simulate bone behaviour and 180 truss (T3D2) elements for the ligaments.
Contact constrain was activated between the facets of the posterior processes using 30 GAP elements. Gap elements allow the nodes to be in contact (gap closed) or separated (gap

open) with respect to particular directions and separation conditions. The whole model with all its component is shown in Fig. 9.
In all conducted FE simulations bones were modelled as rigid bodies; in fact, they are much stiffer than the soft tissues present in the model and their deformation can be consider negligible in comparison with those undergone by the latter.

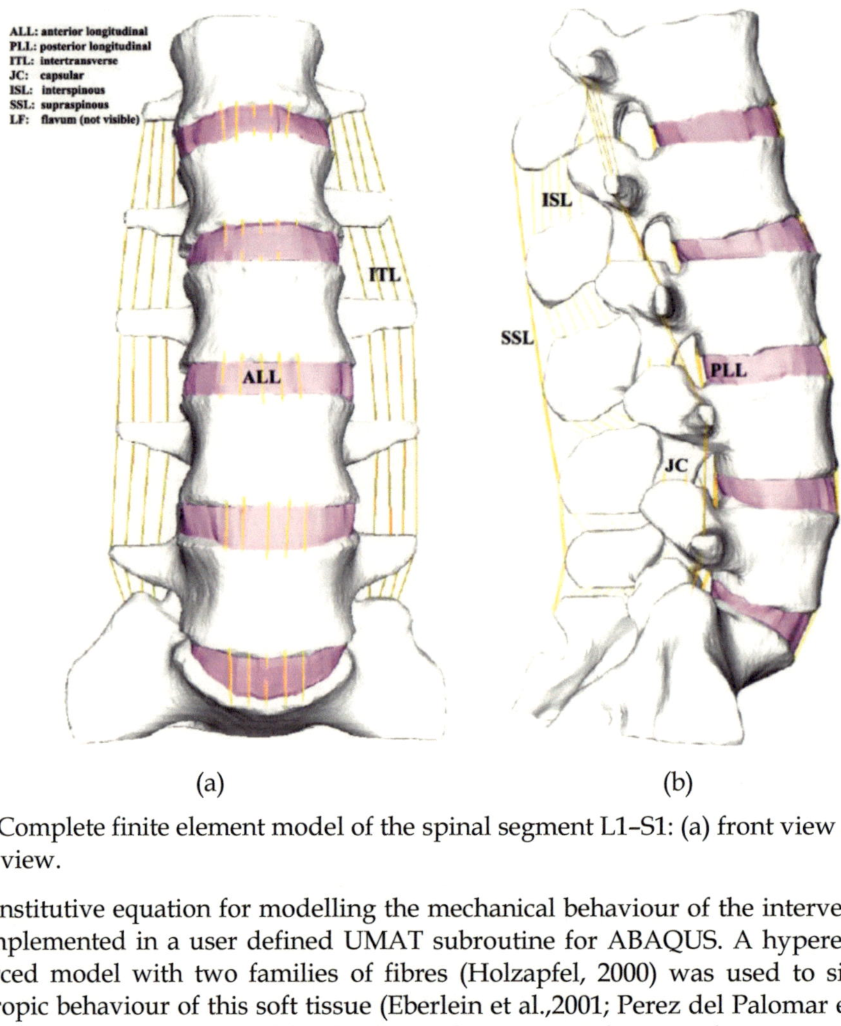

Fig. 9. Complete finite element model of the spinal segment L1–S1: (a) front view and (b) lateral view.

The constitutive equation for modelling the mechanical behaviour of the intervertebral disc was implemented in a user defined UMAT subroutine for ABAQUS. A hyperelastic fibre-reinforced model with two families of fibres (Holzapfel, 2000) was used to simulate the anisotropic behaviour of this soft tissue (Eberlein et al.,2001; Perez del Palomar et al., 2008). The strain energy function used for this hyperelastic material is given by

$$\begin{aligned}\Psi &= C_{10}(\bar{I}_1-3)+C_{01}(\bar{I}_2-3)+C_{20}(\bar{I}_1-3)^2+C_{02}(\bar{I}_2-3)^2\\ &+C_{11}(\bar{I}_1-3)(\bar{I}_2-3)+\frac{K_1}{2K_2}\left\{\exp\left[K_2(\bar{I}_4-1)^2\right]-1\right\}\\ &+\frac{K_1}{2K_2}\left\{\exp\left[K_2(\bar{I}_6-1)^2\right]-1\right\}+\frac{1}{D}(J-1)^2\end{aligned} \quad (1)$$

where Cij are material constants related to the ground substance, K_1 and K_2 are the parameters which identify the exponential behaviour due to the presence of collagen fibres of both families (note that here to simplify the model, the same response was assumed for both families) and D identifies the tissue incompressibility modulus. The invariants are defined as:

$$\overline{I_1} = tr\overline{C} \qquad \overline{I} = \frac{1}{2}\left[\left(tr\overline{C}\right)^2 - tr\left(\overline{C}\right)^2\right] \tag{2}$$

$$\overline{I_4} = a^D \cdot \overline{Ca^D} \qquad \overline{I} = b^D \cdot \overline{C}b^D$$

where a^D is the unitary vector defining the orientation of the first family of fibers, b^D the direction of the second family both in the reference configuration and $\overline{C}$ is the modified right Green strain tensor:

$$\overline{C} = \overline{F}^T\overline{F} \qquad \text{with} \qquad \overline{F} = J^{\frac{1}{3}}F \tag{3}$$

being F the deformation gradient and J = det(F).

Each family of fibres was placed circumferentially around the nucleus with an orientation of ±30° with respect to the disc plain (Goel et al.,1995). The values of the elastic constants were determined using the stress-strain response under a traction axial load for a specimen with two families of fibres, placed at ±30°. The theoretical model behaviour was fitted to experimental data presented by Ebara et al. (1996) using MatLab v.7.1. It can be observed (Fig. 10) how the resultant curve can be considered a good average fit of experimental data of the whole annulus.. Moreover the magnitude of the found values for the material constants was in the range of the available data in the literature (Ebara et al., 1996; Eberlein et al., 2001; Zander et al., 2009).

To define the nucleus pulposus it was considered that the behaviour of this part was isotropic and almost incompressible, so it was modelled as a hyperelastic Neo- Hookean material with material constants C_{10} = 0.16 MPa and D = 0.024 MPa (Perez del Palomar et al., 2008). Contact constrain was activated between the facets of the posterior processes using GAP elements. Table2 sums up all mechanical and element type properties of the model.

Component	Notes	Element type	Material constants
End-plates	Linear elastic	C3D8	E=20MPa, v=0.4
Bone	Rigid body	R3D3	
Nucleus Pulposus	Hyperelastic neo-Hookean	C3D8	C_1 =0.16 MPa D =0.024 MPa^{-1}
Annulus Fibrosus	Hyperelastic fibred-reinforced material	C3D8	C_{10} =0.1 MPa C_{20} =2.5 MPa K_1 = 1.8 MPa K_2 = 11 D = 0.306 MPa^{-1} a = ±30°
Posterior processes contact		GAP	

Table 2. Material properties in the finite element model (Moramarco et al., 2010)

3. Numerical analysis

In order to study the influence of the cartilaginous endplates on the biomechanical response of the lumbo-sacral segment, two distinct models reproducing the lumbar rachis were created. The behaviour of a complete model provided of six vertebrae, five discs and two endplates for each disc was compared with a model identical to the previous but without endplates.

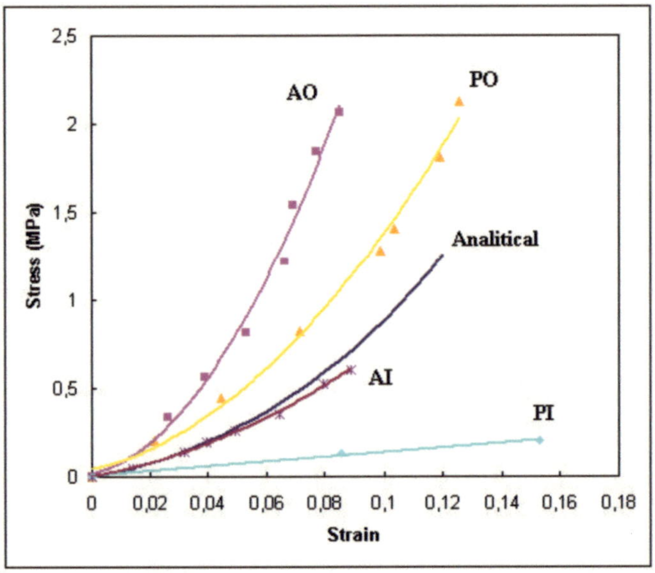

Fig. 10. Comparison between experimental data, measured by Ebara et al. (1996), and the analytical curve using our constants (AO=anterior outer annulus ; PO=posterior outer annulus; AI=anterior inner annulus; PI=posterior inner annulus)

The exact mechanical role of the endplates has not been described satisfactorily in literature. In this section we will show that the presence of the endplate acting as an interface between the vertebral bodies and the discs (Kramer 2009) is important to reduce the stresses in the disc when the spine is loaded.

3.1 Boundary conditions

To demonstrate the goodness of this model the in vitro tests performed by Panjabi et al. (1994) were reproduced *in silico* under similar conditions. The proposed test includes the study of a sample of whole fresh-frozen human cadaveric lumbosacral-spine specimens in which muscles and soft tissues, except ligaments, were removed.

The lower lumbar vertebra of each specimens obtained was fixed to the test table while the loads were applied to the most cephalic (the first or second lumbar) vertebra. The vertebrae were unconstrained, to allow natural physiological movements of the spine to occur in response to the applied load (Panjabi et al., 1994).

In the experimental test the specimens were loaded by pure flexion and extension moments both of 10 Nm, applied incrementally to the most cephalic vertebra by equal and opposing forces generated by pneumatic actuators. Throughout the testing, a compressive pre-load of 100 N was applied along the longitudinal axis of the specimen (Panjabi et al., 1994).

The numerical model implemented was tested under the same load and boundary conditions proposed in the experimental experience in order to validate the model and numerically prove the nonlinear behaviour of the model in the entire flexion-extension range of the movement (Fig. 11).

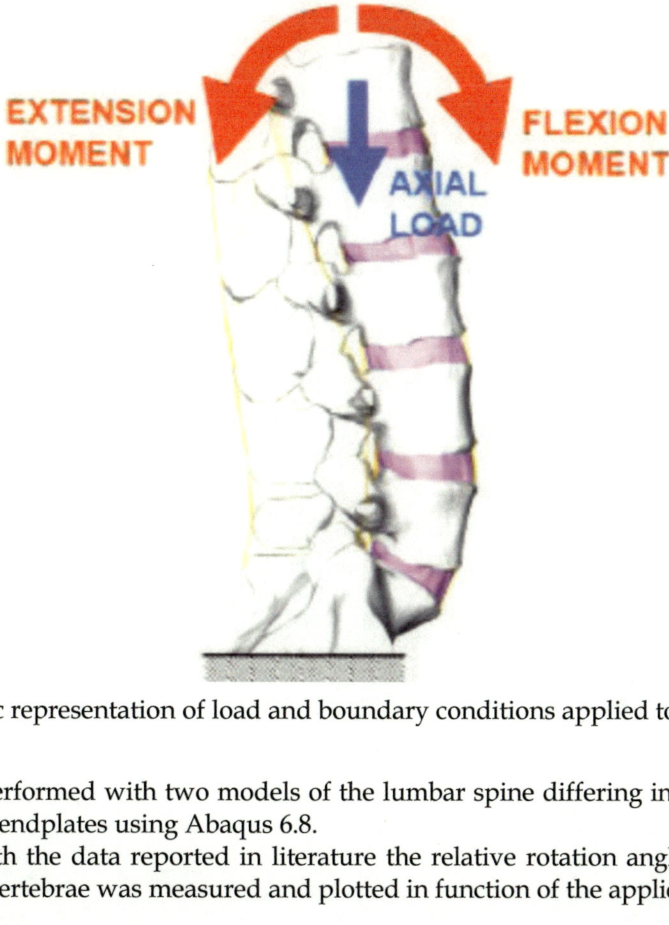

Fig. 11. Schematic representation of load and boundary conditions applied to the numerical model.

The tests were performed with two models of the lumbar spine differing in the presence of the cartilaginous endplates using Abaqus 6.8.
In agreement with the data reported in literature the relative rotation angle between each pair of adjacent vertebrae was measured and plotted in function of the applied moment.

3.2 Cinematic response comparison

Figure 12 shows the comparison between the experimental results and the values obtained in the numerical simulations relative to the models with and without endplates.
Firstly, analyzing the numerical results, it is possible to state that the model presents a good agreement with the experimental data with the numerical curve falling within the experimental standard deviation interval.
The results show that the presence of the CEP permits to obtain a grater no-linearity of the spine response but a small decrease of the predicted ROM in flexion.
In particular in extension the curves representing the rotation angles for the numerical model displays a good concordance with the experimental ones especially for L1-L2, L2-L3 and L5-S1 segments. The curves for the model with endplates follow with a very small error the trend of the experimental results.

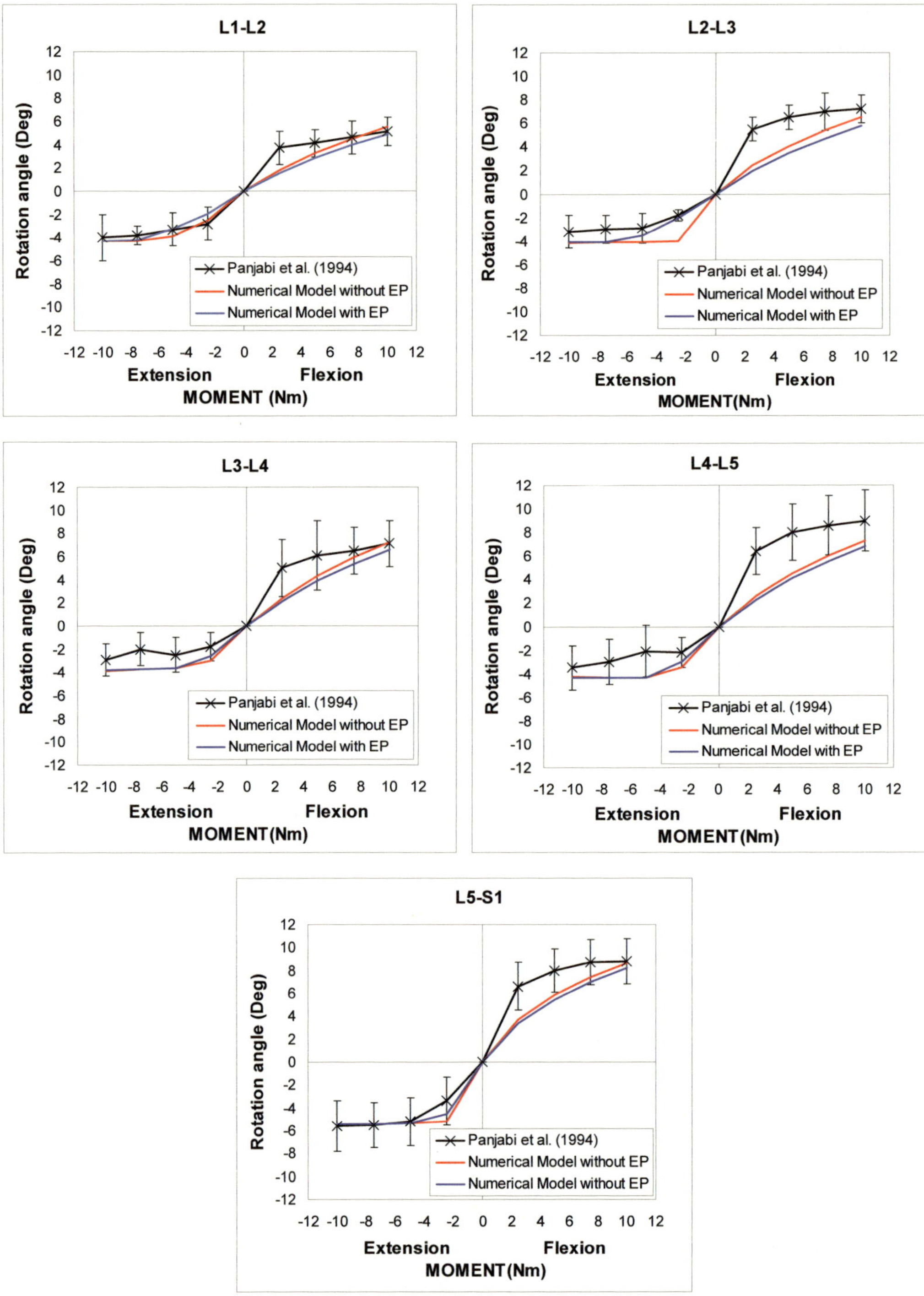

Fig. 12. Comparison between the relative rotation angle under flexion-extension moment predicted by the FE model and that measured by Panjabi et al. (1994).

In particular for the L2-L3 segment is evident a remarkable difference between the two numerical models in analysis showing a great improvement in the results obtained. The maximum deviation from the experimental results obtained in the model with endplates in this segment is in the range of 0.9° while the model without endplates shows a maximum error of 2°. In flexion the two numerical models do not show a noticeable difference. The curves are similar with slightly higher rotation angles for the model without endplates. The maximum difference encountered between the numerical models is obtained at L2-L3 level with a deviation of 0.7°.

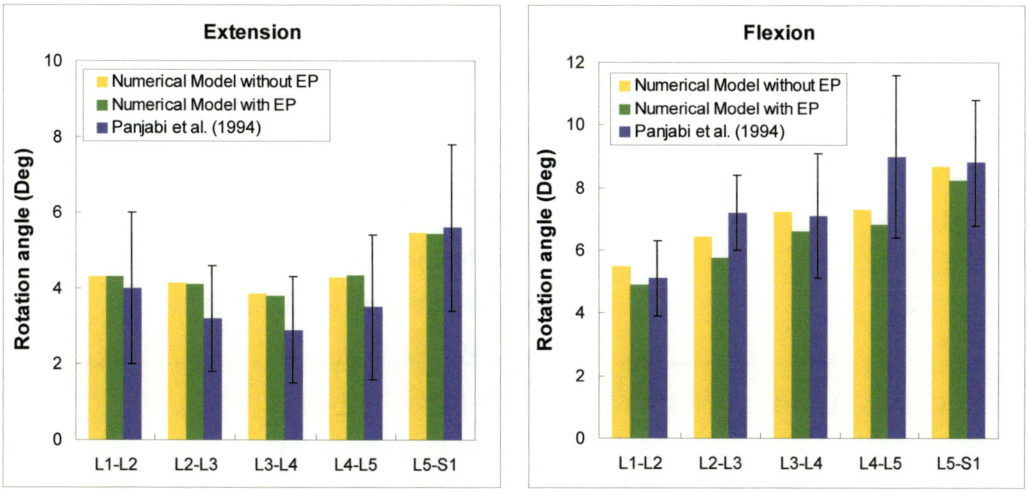

(a) (b)

Fig. 13. Maximum relative rotation angle measured with the numerical model with endplates and without endplates compared with the experimental results (M.M. Panjabi 1994) for an extension (a) and a flexion (b) test.

In Fig.13 the maximum (flexion) and the minimum (extension) relative rotation angles obtained in the two analysis are shown and compared with the experimental results. The correspondence with the experimental values is almost perfect in extension for the L5-S1 segment in which we obtain for the complete model (with endplates) a maximum rotation of 5.4° against the 5.6° calculated in the experimental analysis. The agreement is good also at L1-L2 level in which we obtain a value of 4.3° against the experimental value of 4°. In flexion the segment L1-L2 shows the best results with an error of 0.2° between the numerical and experimental. As stated before the model without endplates shows higher rotation values in flexion. According to experimental data, there is clearly increasing motion moving inferiorly from the level between the first and second lumbar vertebrae to that between the fifth lumbar and first sacral vertebra. The ROM for the maximum flexion moment of the segments L5-S1, in fact, results substantially higher than for the other segments.

All the considerations made so far are confirmed in Fig. 14 in which the relative rotations between the five vertebrae are represented. In fact, comparing the ROM for a 10 Nm flexo-extension moment, it is possible to remark that the three models have the same distribution of the ROM between all the different segments with the curves of the numerical model perfectly falling within the standard deviation interval.

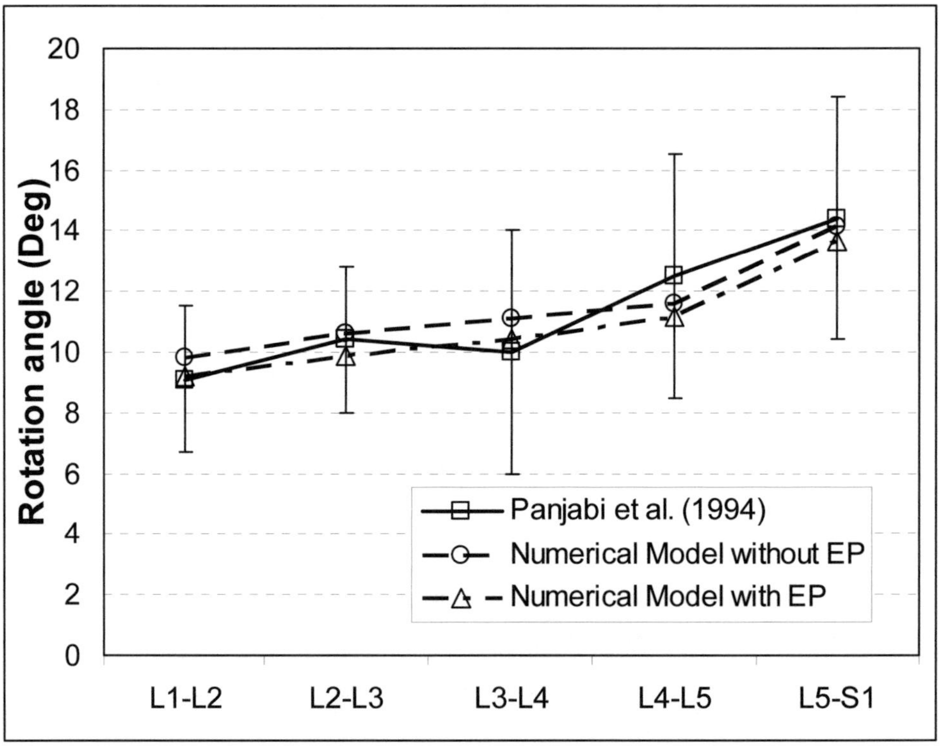

Fig. 14. Comparison between the relative rotation angles under a 10 Nm flexo-extension moment predicted by the FE models and that measured by Panjabi et al (1994).

3.3 Stress result comparison

In subjects not afflicted with bone tissue related pathologies, disc injury within physiological load represents one of the main causes of the alteration of the spine behaviour and, therefore, pain. In particular, the interface between intervertebral discs and vertebral surfaces represents the most critical region for the onset of spinal diseases. Moreover, some recent studies (Costi et al., 2007; Wilson et al., 2003) showed how the shear effects are dominant in disc tissue failures. For these reasons, it was considered interesting to plot, for the more stressed disc, in Panjabi configuration (Panjabi et al 1994), the maps of the maximum shear stress for flexion and extension moments and to compare the distributions for the two models, with and without endplates, in order to underline how the presence of the endplates allow the reduction of the stress condition in the intervertebral disk.

The results for the flexion moment (Fig. 15) indicate that the greater values of the stresses were located at L5-S1 levels just in the interfaces between disc and vertebrae across the posterior and posterolateral zone for both models but the model without CEP reach stress level 1.5 times grater.

A similar result was obtained for the extension moment load case. In fact, the model without EP shows a grater average stress values in comparison with the model with EP (Fig 16).

Finally the stress responses of the two models, as expected, highlight that the most risky load condition corresponds to the flexion moment. In this case, in fact, the maximum stress values is 31 MPa compared to a value of 4 MPa calculated in the extension test.

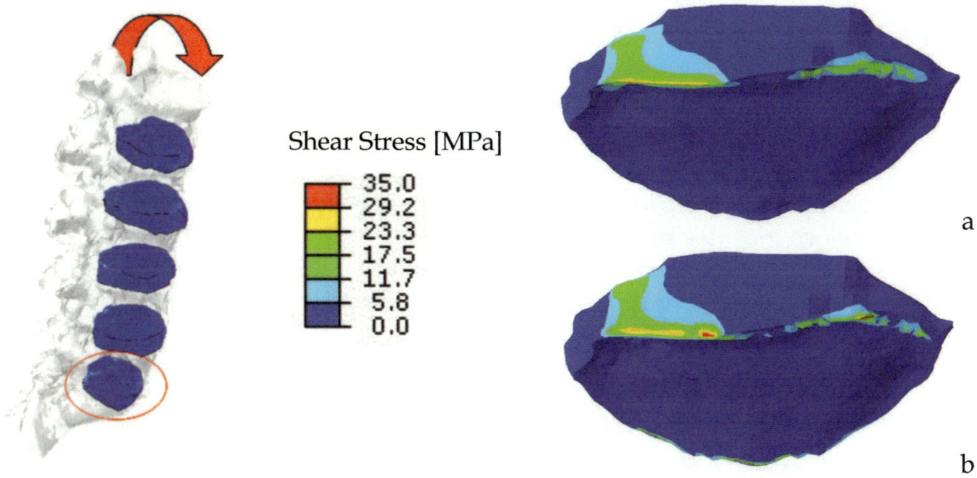

Fig. 15. Maximum shear stress distribution under a 10 Nm flexion moment for disc L5–S1: with (a) and without endplates (b).

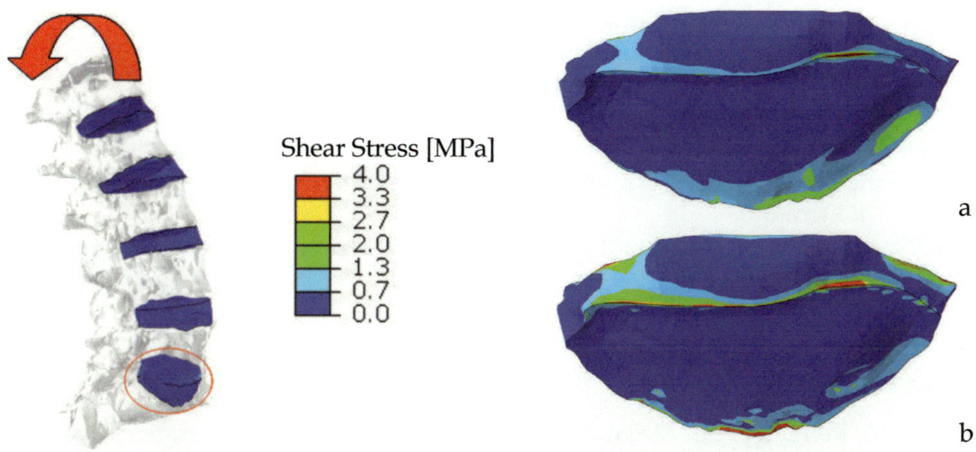

Fig. 16. Maximum shear stress distribution under a 10 Nm extension moment for disc L5–S1: with (a) and without endplates (b).

4. Conclusion

With the aim of understanding the influence of the CEP in the modelling of the lumbar spine segment two numerical models of the lumbar rachis, differing exclusively in the presence of the cartilaginous endplates, were created and compared.

The complete model could be considered a valid numerical representation of the three-dimensional load-displacement behaviour of the human lumbosacral spine at almost all vertebral levels. The FE model, infact, presents some interesting similarities with the informations about the spine known by literature. First of all the spinal behaviour in extension and in flexion is non linear and asymmetric in agreement with literature. The average highest ROM for each segment in flexion (6.5°) is usually much bigger than in extension (-4.3°). Furthermore while in extension the maximum rotation value has little variation between upper (-5.4° for L5-S1 level) and lower (-3.8° for L3-L4) segments, in flexion this range is much bigger from 4.9°, in L1-L2, to 8.3°, in L5-S1.

In particular the created models were used to study of the influence of the presence of the endplates on the mechanical response of the lumbar rachis under static loading.

Each intervertebral disc, in fact, is surrounded with two cartilagineous layers that constitute the interface between the discs and the vertebral bodies.

The analysis of the results allowed us to demonstrate the great importance of the endplates. Firstly the reduction of the stress and strain ranges to which the discs are subjected demonstrates the ability of the endplates to perform a sort of protection for the disc avoiding the direct contact between the soft tissue of the disc and the hard bone of the vertebrae.

At the same time their presence determined significant changes in the relative rotation between each couple of vertebrae, as stated in the first section of the analysis of the obtained results.

The model with endplates is able to follow more accurately the trend of experimental curves.

Moreover a perfect coincidence between numerical and experimental results is not possible due to all the variables involved in this kind of problems.

First of all we have to consider that the behaviour of human tissues, here univocally characterized, is affected by a series of factors including, for example, the age, the alimentation, the lifestyle of the subject; in addition the geometry of the rachis, that changes for all subjects, certainly influences its mechanical response under load. For this reason we can state that the behaviour of this numerical model qualitatively responds to the reported values present in literature.

Consequently the created model could be considered as a a valuable tool for the study and mechanical analysis of the lumbar segment in the perspective of using it as a support for clinical analysis.

6. References

Adams, M.A. & Roughley, P.J. (2006). What is intervertebral disc degeneration, and what causes it? *Spine*, Vol.31, No. 18, (August 2006), pp. 2151-2161, ISSN 1528-1159

Broberg, K. B. (1983). On the mechanical behaviour of the intervertebral disc. *Spine*, Vol.8, No.2, (March 1983), pp. 151–165, ISSN 1528-1159

Chazal, J. ; Tanguy, A. ; Bouges, M. ; Gaurel, G. ; Escande, G.; Guillot, M. & Vanneuville, G. (1985). Biomechanical properties of spinal ligaments and an histological study of the supraspinal ligament in traction. *Journal of Biomechanics*, Vol.18, No.3, (March 1985),pp. 167-176, ISSN 0021-9290

Costi, J.J.; Stokes, I.A.; Gardner Morse, M.; Laible, J.P.; Scoffone, H.M. & Iatridis, J.C. (2007). Direct measurement of intervertebral disc maximum shear strain in six degrees of freedom: Motion that place disc tissue at risk injury. *Journal of Biomechanics*, Vol.40, No.11, (October 2007), pp. 2457-2466, ISSN 0021-9290

Devor, M. & Tal, M. (2009). What causes low back pain? *Pain*, Vol.142, No.1-2, (March 2009), pp. 11-12, ISSN 0304-3959

Ebara, S., Iatridis, J.C., Setton, L.A., Foster, R.J., Mow, V.C., Weidenbaum, M., 1996. Tensile properties of nondegenerate human lumbar annulus fibrosus. *Spine*, Vol.21, No.4, (February 1996), pp. 452-461, ISSN 0362-2436

Eberlein, R.; Holzapfel, G.A. & Schulze-Bauer, C.A.J. (2001). An anisotropic model for annulus tissue and enhanced finite element analysis of intact lumbar disc bodies. *Computer Methods in Biomechanic and Biomedical Engeeniering*, Vol.4, No.3, (March 2001), pp 209-229, ISSN 1476-8259

Eberlein, R.; Holzapfel, G. & Fröhlich, M. (2004). Multi-segment FEA of the human lumbar spine including the heterogeneity of the annulus fibrosus. *Computational Mechanics*, Vol.34, No.2, (July 2004) pp.147-163, ISSN 1432-0924

Goel, V.K.; Monroe, T.; Gilbertson, L.G. & Brinckmann, P. (1995). Interlaminar shear stresses and laminae separation in a disc. *Spine*, Vol.20, No.6, (March 1995), pp. 689-698, ISSN 0362-2436

Goto, K.; Tajima, N.; Chosa, E.; Totoribe, K.; Kuroki, H.; Arizumi, Y. & Arai, T. (2002). Mechanical analysis of the lumbar vertebrae in the three-dimensional finite element method moments in which intradiscal pressure in the nucleus pulposus was used to establish the model. *Journal of Orthopaedic Science*, Vol.7, No.2, (March 2002), pp. 243-246, ISSN 1436-2023

Goto, K.; Tajima, N.; Chosa, E.; Totoribe, K.; Shinichiro, S. & Kuroki, H. (2003). Effect of lumbar spinal fusion on the orther lumbar intervertebral levels (three dimensional finite element analyses). *Journal of Orthopaedic Science*, Vol.8, No.4, (July 2003), pp. 577-584, ISSN 1436-2023

Latorraca, A. & Forni Niccolai Gamba, C. (2004). Analysis on 149 consecutive cases of intervertebral disc prolepses operated with microendoscopic (MetrX) technique. *Reumatismo*, Vol.56, No.1, (Marzo 2004), pp. 31-35, ISSN 0048-7449

Markolf, K.L. & Morris, J.M. (1974). The structural components of the vertebral disc. A study of their contribution to the ability of the disc to withstand compressive force. *The Journal of Bone and Joint Surgery Am.*, Vol.56, No.4, (June 1974), pp. 675-687, ISSN 0021-9355

Moramarco, V.; Pérez Del Palomar, A.; Pappalettere, C. & Doblaré, M (2010). An accurate validation of a computational model of a human lumbosacral segment. *Journal of Biomechanics*, Vol.43, No.2, (Jenuary 2010), pp. 334-342, ISSN 0021-9290

Natarajan, R.N.; Williams, J.R. & Andersson, G.B.J. (2004). Recent advances in analytical modelling of lumbar disc degeneration. *Spine*, Vol.29, No.23, (December 2004), pp. 2733-2741 ISSN 1528-1159

Noailly, J. (2009). *Model developments for in silico studies of the lumbar spine biomechanics*, PhD Thesis, Technical University of Catalonia, Barcelona, Spain

Panjabi, M.M.; Oxland, T.R.; Yamamoto, I. & Crisco, J.J. (1994). Mechanical behaviour of the human lumbar and lumbosacral spine as shown by three dimensional load-displacement curves. *The Journal of Bone and Joint Surgery Am.*, Vol.76, No.3, (March 1994), pp. 413-424, ISSN 0021-9355

Pérez del Palomar, A.; Calvo, B. & Doblaré M. (2008). An accurate finite elements model of the cervical spine under quasi-static loading. *Journal of Biomechanics*, Vol.41, No.3, (January 2008), pp. 523-531, ISSN 0021-9290

Pintar, F.A.; Yoganandam, N.; Myers, T.; Elhagediab, A. & Sances Jr., A. (1992). Biomechanical properties of human lumbar spine ligaments. *Journal of Biomechanics*, Vol.25, No.11, (November 1992), pp. 1351-1356, ISSN 0021-9290

Rohlmann, A.; Bauer, L.; Zander, T.; Bergmann, G. & Wilke, H.J. (2006). Determination of trunk muscle forces for flexion and extension by using a validated finite element model of the lumbar spine and measured in vivo data. *Journal of Biomechanics*, Vol.39, No.6, (January 2006), pp.981-9, ISSN 0021-9290

Wilson, W.; van Rietbergen, B.; van Donkelaar, C.C. & Huiskes, R. (2003). Pathways of load induced cartilage damage causing cartilage degeneration in knee after meniscectomy. *Journal of Biomechanics*, Vol.36, No., (June 2003), pp. 845-851, ISSN 0021-9290

Zander, T.; Rohlmann, A. & Bergmann, G. (2009). Influence of different artificial disc kinematics on spine biomechanics. *Clinical biomechanics*, Vol.24, No.2, (February 2009), pp. 135-142, ISSN 0268-0033

12

Computer-Assisted Visualization of Central Lung Tumours Based on 3-Dimensional Reconstruction

S. Limmer[1], C. Stöcker[2], V. Dicken[2], S. Kraß[2], H. Wolken[1] and P. Kujath[1]
[1]*Department of Surgery, University of Luebeck Medical School,Luebeck,*
[2]*Fraunhofer MEVIS, Bremen,*
[1,2]*Germany*

1. Introduction

Each year, lung cancer is diagnosed in approximately 1.4 million people world-wide. There are approx. 205,000 new cases in the USA and approx. 345,000 in Europe [Cancer Atlas of the Federal Republic of Germany]. US researchers at the Centers for Disease Control and Prevention [CDC] expect the number of deaths to continue to rise as an immediate consequence of smoking. During the 20th Century, tobacco consumption caused about 100 million deaths, and this number is estimated at about one billion deaths world—wide for the 21st Century [CDC].
Axial 2-D computed tomography (CT) of the thorax is the accepted and established standard method used in pre-operative morphological imaging diagnosis in patients with central benign or malignant lung tumours. Tumour size, infiltration of central structures or segmental relatedness are the decisive parameters that the surgeon can derive in variable quality from 2-dimensional images, in order to assess the technical operability and the extent of the resection. However, the availability and quality of CTs vary greatly from one hospital to the next. The surgeon is thus often given print-outs on paper of a CT with 5 mm slices. Comprehensive coverage across the board with multi-slice detector CT (MSDCT) with 1mm slices and the possibility of interactive observation by the operator is, however, not yet available. Improved imaging and image-processing is crucial to the further optimization of pre-operative risk assessment, especially with reference to population development in industrialized nations. Multimorbid patients, patients with severe obstructive or restrictive diseases of the respiratory tract, as well as patients of advanced age, often limit the - actually required - tactical oncological extent of resection due to a post-operative lung function that is too low. Demands must therefore be made for a best-possible pre-operative localization and functional diagnostics, also with reference to the constant rise in patient age for the corresponding co-morbidities.

2. 3-D visualization in modern clinical practice

The pre-operative assessment of a malignant lung tumour, its anatomical and topographical position, the final extent of the tumour and the possibility of infiltration of central

mediastinal structures or of the thoracic wall are of central importance to the thoracic surgeon undertaking the treatment. The (technical) operability of a patient is ultimately determined to a large degree based on the imaging, in combination with the lung capacity and the concomitant co-morbidities (functional operability).
Based on digital CT data, a precise 3-dimensional reconstruction of lung tumours, the tumour position, blood supply and the relationship to the bronchial system was developed within an research project of Fraunhofer MEVIS together with about 20 german hospitals for lung surgery (funded by the german society for research, DFG PE 199/20-1) and could serve as a new basis for pre-operative risk assessment. Different approaches for computer assistance in image based surgery planning were assessed within that large research cooperation. Can an improved pre-operative risk assessment be achieved through animated 3-D imaging, analogous to cardiac surgery? And how can the high-risk group of patients with a central lung tumour benefit from this? The following question were focus of that part of research, that was conducted at the University Hospital Lübeck: The aims of our research were to evaluate the use of computer-assisted reformatting and visualization using specially adapted software with reference to risk assessment and surgical strategy in patients with a central lung tumour [Limmer et al. 2010].
Within the framework of pre-operative imaging, two main application areas make use of in this computer-assisted approach: On the one hand, the computer-assisted extraction of quantitative diagnostic parameters, such as the estimation of lung emphysema portions which help to make predictions of post-operative lung function impairment possible through objectivation and expansion of the pre-operative imaging diagnostics. On the other hand, the computer-assisted approach should help the surgeon to plan surgery as precisely as is possible [Huenerbein M et al. 2003]. Computer-assisted planning based on images is the clinical standard today in the areas of neurosurgery as well as in operations on the locomotor apparatus [Tormenti MJ et al. 2010]. Radiation therapy also uses a computer-assisted approach with specially adapted software to achieve a precise radiation localization and optimized doses during stereotactic irradiation of tumours - under suppression of respiratory excursions [Alexander E 2001; Jolesz FA 2005]. The computer-assisted approach during surgical interventions on parenchymatous organs is currently the focus of interdisciplinary research conducted by collaboration between the fields of surgery, radiology and information technology. A central problem is that the pre-operative data cannot simply be transferred to the site of the operation due to organ movement and deformation. Furthermore, the pre-operative diagnostic data cannot be matched to the intra-operative situation using osseous landmarks [Grenacher L et al. 2005]. Concepts in the computer-assisted planning of surgery have been successfully driven forward in recent years, especially in the field of hepatic surgery [Lang H et al. 2005; Oldhafer KJ et al. 1999; Bornik A. et al. 2006]. The aims were to reduce the risks of surgery through pre-operative identification of structures that are at risk, as well as through predictions and minimization of the functional impairment to portions of tissue due to inadequate blood supply or backflow in the case of surgically induced disorders in the vascular system. The development of computer-assisted intra-operative support through suitable navigation systems and recording procedures for soft tissue surgery has been a focus of research for many years (BMBF funded project FUSION - Future Environment for Gentle Liver Surgery Using Image-Guided Planning and Intra-Operative Navigation [FUSION]). The research

conducted by the University Hospital Luebeck in the field of navigated hepatic surgery is worthy of particular mention here [Hildebrand et al. 2007 und 2009].

3. Computer assistance for thoracic surgery planning

Standard risk assessment in thoracic surgery is based on conventional imaging techniques like x-ray and CT. In exceptional cases, additional examinations are carried out using, e.g., MRT, PET, SPECT or US. The oncological requirements (curative therapeutic approach), on the one hand, and the patient's technical and functional prerequisites, on the other, must be balanced individually for each patient. While the computer-assisted approach to the planning of thoracic surgical interventions is the aim of the current research, other questions pertaining to CT-assisted pulmonary diagnostics have already been answered. Rigorous quantification and visualization methods already exist for screening and early recognition of bronchial carcinomas, planning of biopsies, radiological monitoring of chemotherapy for lung metastases, quantification of parenchyma in lung function disorders, or embolism diagnostics. The researchers that specialize in medical applications at Fraunhofer MEVIS - Institute for Medical Image Computing, Bremen, develop prototypic software applications for the reconstruction, quantification and visualization of thoracic CT data, with the aim of supporting the planning of thoracic surgery in cases where complex resections are required in oncological lung patients [Dicken et al. 2005, Stoecker et al. 2009]. Methods and algorithms have been developed in close collaboration with about 20 german hospitals for lung surgery, to facilitate the delimitation of anatomical structures and pathologies in high-resolution CT data on the lungs.

Results, conducted by the University Hospital Luebeck from a 3-D reconstruction dating from 2005 revealed reformatting and visualization that was still highly simplified and the user modules for interactive use had also not yet been developed. The technical feasibility and a 3-dimensional reconstruction were initially evaluated and validated on 9 patients in a first exploratory phase between December 2005 and February 2006. These patients were characterized by a great diversity as possible with reference to age, tumour genesis, primary tumour/relapse, tumour localization or infiltration of extra-thoracic / mediastinal structures. The original CT and the reconstructed data sets for a 54-year-old patient with bilateral lung metastases derived from a uterine leiomyosarcoma are shown below as an example (Fig. 3.1 and Fig. 3.2). In addition to the simplified screen shots, the coarse grid of the reformatting is of particular note.

Over the course of the years, a computer-assisted approach was developed that allowed automatic segmentation of the lungs, the branching structures of the bronchial tree as far as the subsegmental level and interactive segmentation of the pulmonary blood supply. The method of reformatting and 3-D visualization has also proved to be robust in cases of central tumour localization with potential tumour invasion of larger vessels or central mediastinal structures. The differentiation of the lobes of the lungs is carried out automatically, the approximation of the individual lung segments is also possible with some manual interaction. The segmentation masks of the delimited regions form the basis for a quantitative analysis of functional CT data, such as lung volumes, emphysema index or mean lung density. The portion of the lung requiring resection can be calculated prior to surgery using this instrument and the expected post-operative loss of function can be approximated.

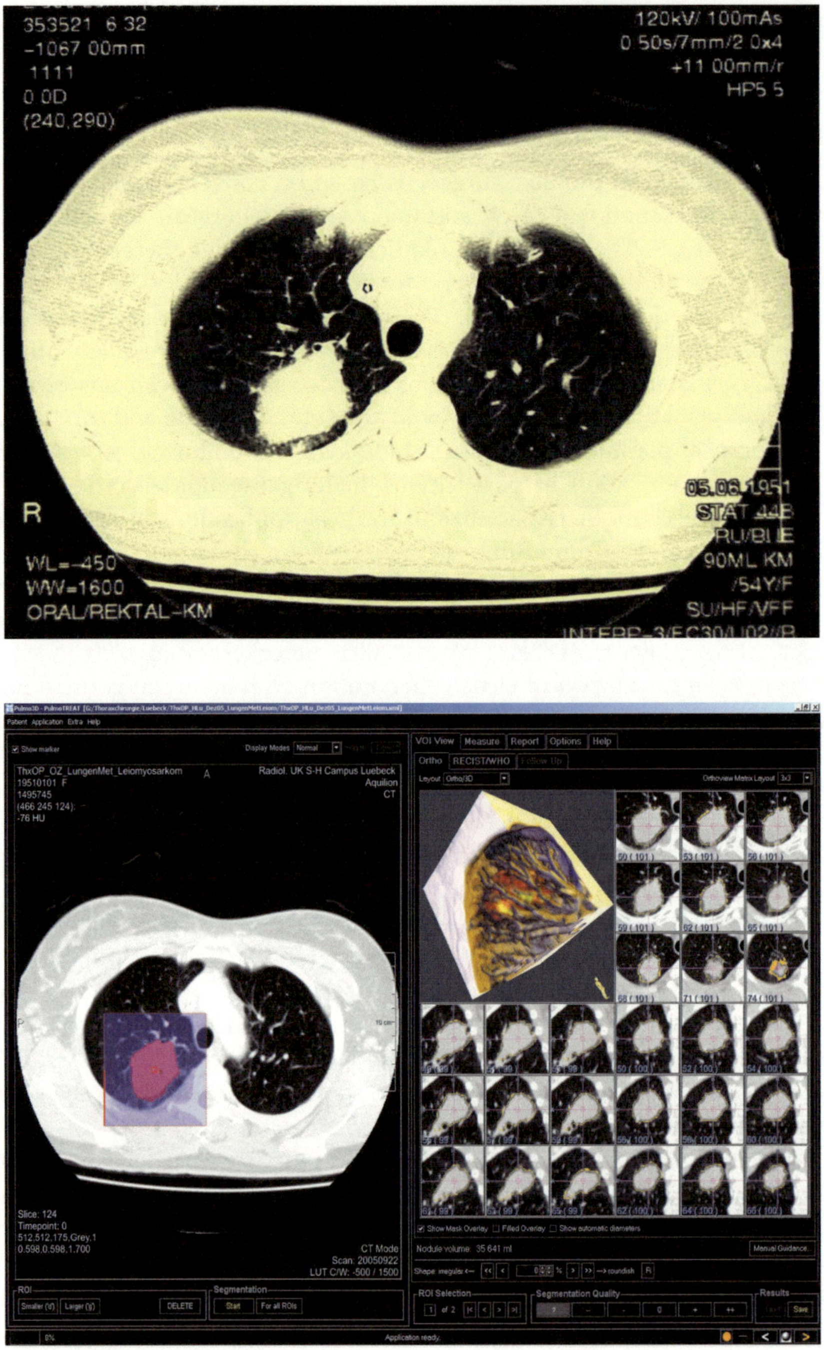

Fig. 3.1 Axial CT of a 54-year-old patient with bilateral lung metastases. As an example, the largest metastasis is shown in the right left upper lobe of the lung (left). Reformatting and volumetric evaluation of the metastasis (right image).

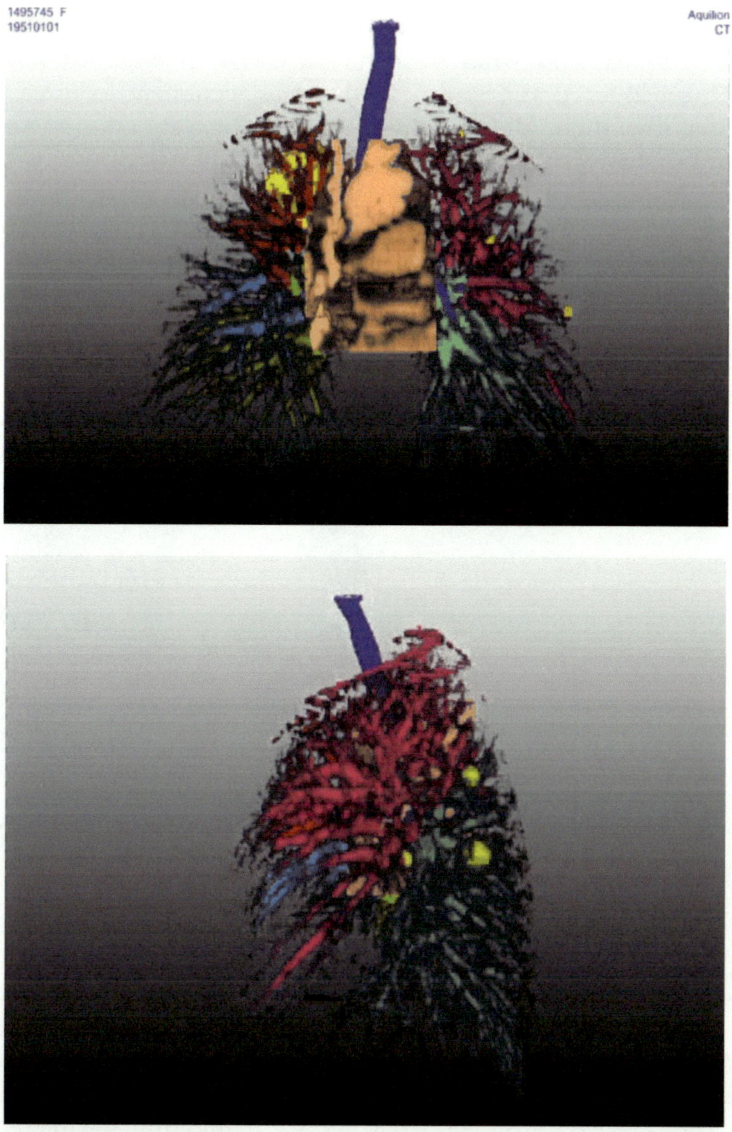

Fig. 3.2 Animated 3-D reconstruction of the axial CT images (3.1). Ventral (left) and left-lateral (right) view. The lobes of the lungs are coloured selectively, the bronchial tree is blue, lung metastases are coloured yellow.

Conventional methods (multiplanar reformatting, volume rendering) can be complemented by colour coding and anatomical reformatting of the data [Dicken et al. 2003], i.e., the data are not depicted on flat sections, but based on their distance to the pleura. This means that more superficial changes, e.g., pleural mesotheliomas, defects in the thoracic wall or osseous changes in the bony thorax can be depicted in a way that resembles the surgical situation (Fig. 3.3). Volumetric and metric calculations permit a precise statement on tumour thickness or distance of the tumour from its surrounding structures (thoracic wall). Furthermore, 3-D visualizations of the hilum of the lung or of regions around the lesions can be produced, in order to depict the morphological and topographical relationship of the tumour to the bronchial and vascular tree with colour coding. All pulmonary areas, including emphysematous portions, can be depicted separately in three dimensions in variable detail and resolution. All 3-D scenes can be interactively rotated or enlarged by the observer and set to obtain an optimum view.

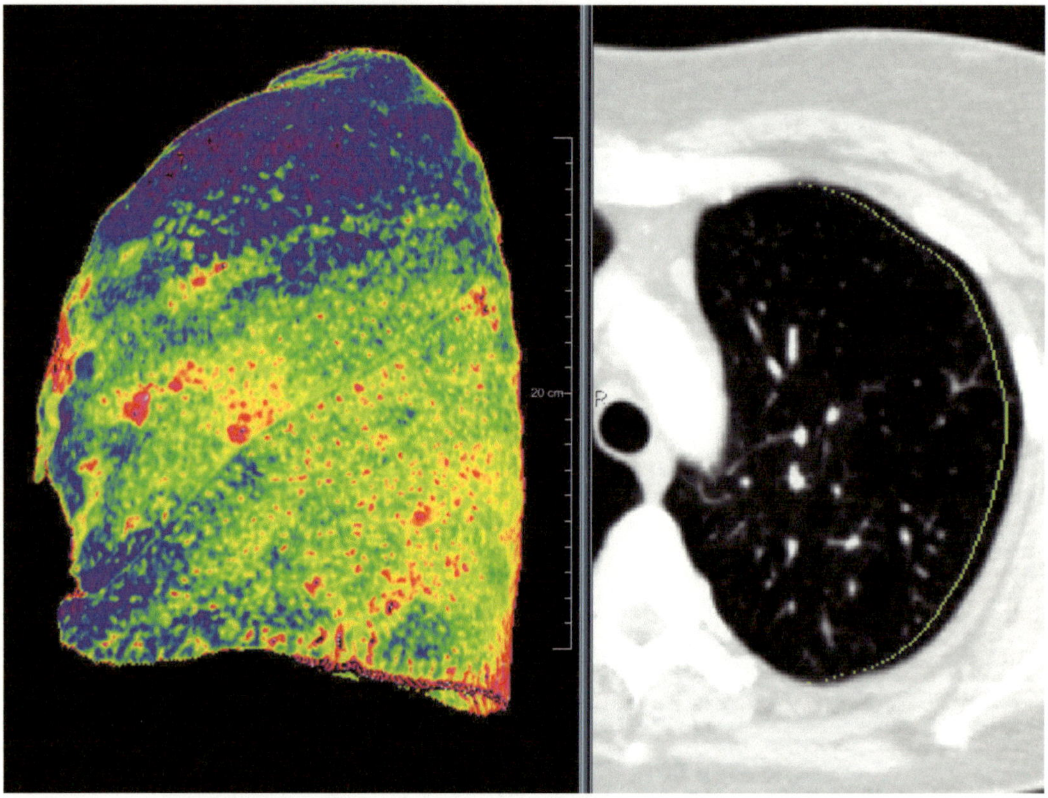

Fig. 3.3 The conventional display of CT data on flat sections provided by the data set is complemented here by the depiction of all image points that, similar to the layers in an onion, are all at a constant distance to the surface of the organ. On the left, you can see a superficial depiction of such a layer, located at approx. 10 mm from the internal thoracic wall. Lung density is colour coded. On the right, you can see the corresponding conventional view.

4. The 3-D reconstruction and visualization techniques

4.1 Lungs, lobes, segments and the bronchial system

The number of publications on the identification of anatomical lung structures rose dramatically after the introduction of MSDCT. Examples of bronchial tree segmentation and analytical methods are found as early on as 1999 in a publication by Preteux and later on in publications by Aykac and Tschirren [Preteux F et al. 1999, Aykac D et al. 2003, Tschirren J et al. 2002]. A variety of algorithms for the automatic segmentation of the lung have been published by Kitasaka, Hu, Leader, Kuhnigk and Sluimer [Kitasaka T et al. 1999, Hu S et al.

2001, Leader JK et al. 2003, Kuhnigk JM et al. 2003, Sluimer I et al. 2005]. A first method on the segmentation of the lobes of the lungs, an algorithm based on fissure detection and knowledge from anatomical atlases, was presented by Zhang [Zhang L et al. 2003]. An alternative method used the Voronoi division of the lung starting at the lobar bronchi for a coarse estimate of the lobes [Zhou et al. 2003]. A method that includes both the areas of vascular and bronchial supply and fissure formations, and thus permits a more rapid interactive refinement of the results, is an integral part of a software solution for parenchyma analysis, developed by Fraunhofer MEVIS [Kuhnigk JM et al. 2005]. Furthermore, also a method for the approximation of lung segments which are not delimited by fissures is available. It was introduced by Krass in 2000 [Krass S et al. 2000] and is based on a similar approach to Zhou's lung lobe segmentation algorithm. The method has currently been further refined which is described in [Welter et al. 2011]. An expanded variant of the lobe segmentation approach developed by Kuhnigk was introduced by Ukill [Ukil S et al. 2005 and 2006]. Methods for the qualitative and quantitative analysis of the lung parenchyma had already been developed in the 1990's by Kalender, Uppaluri and Coxson [Kalender WA et al. 1990, Uppaluri R et al. 1997, Coxson HO et al. 1999] and were further developed over the course of the years [Blechschmidt RA et al. 2001, Hara T et al. 2003, Xu Y et al. 2006]. A first system for quantitative analysis under inclusion of a regional division of the lung, previously achieved through segmentation, was presented by Reinhardt in 2001, whereby Zhou's fissure-based lobe segmentation was used and no further division into subsegments could be undertaken [Reinhardt JM et al. 2001]. There is currently no generally available software for CT-based division of the lung into lobes and segments. There are the following additional challenges when segmenting the supply systems, especially in the case of the lungs: In the segmentation of the bronchial tree, on the one hand, the structures that take a horizontal course in the internal regions are rendered very bright and, on the other hand, the centres of the thinner bronchi that take a diagonal course through the volume are no longer coherent within the meaning of neighbouring relationships in the voxel grid in the discrete reconstruction [Park W et al. 1998, Prêteux F et al. 1999, Ley S et al. 2002]. The focus of current research is the stabilization of automatic segmentation methods that produce a satisfactory segmentation result without interaction from the user [Tschirren J et al. 2005b, Schalthölter T et al. 2002, Hoffmann EA et al. 2003].

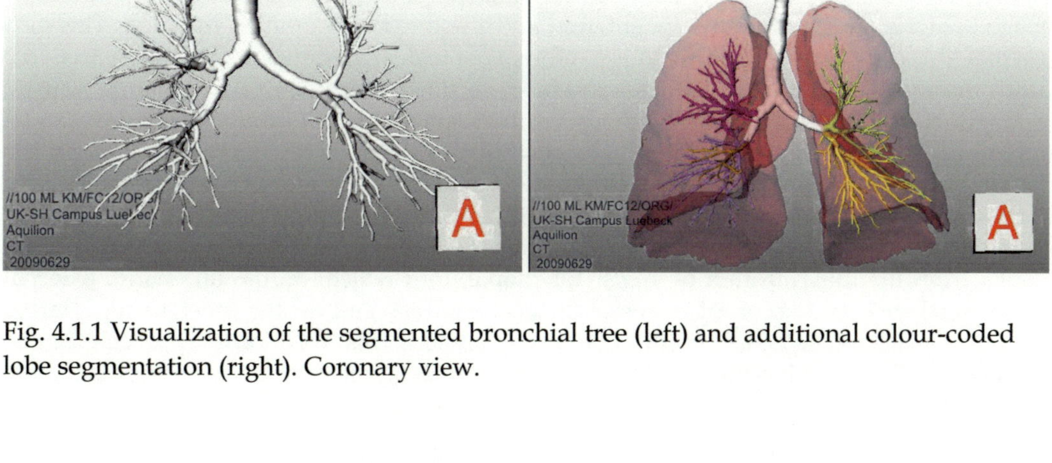

Fig. 4.1.1 Visualization of the segmented bronchial tree (left) and additional colour-coded lobe segmentation (right). Coronary view.

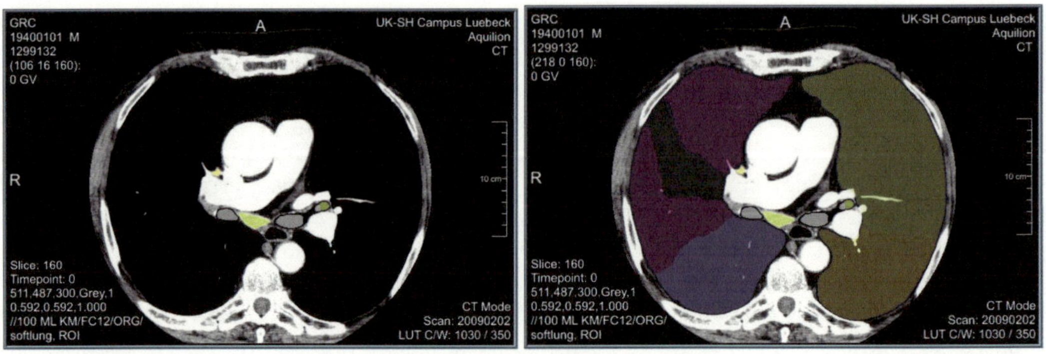

Fig. 4.1.2 Colour-coding of the central vessels and the bronchial system (left). Axial computed tomographic scan of the thorax with colour-coding of the lung lobes. (right)

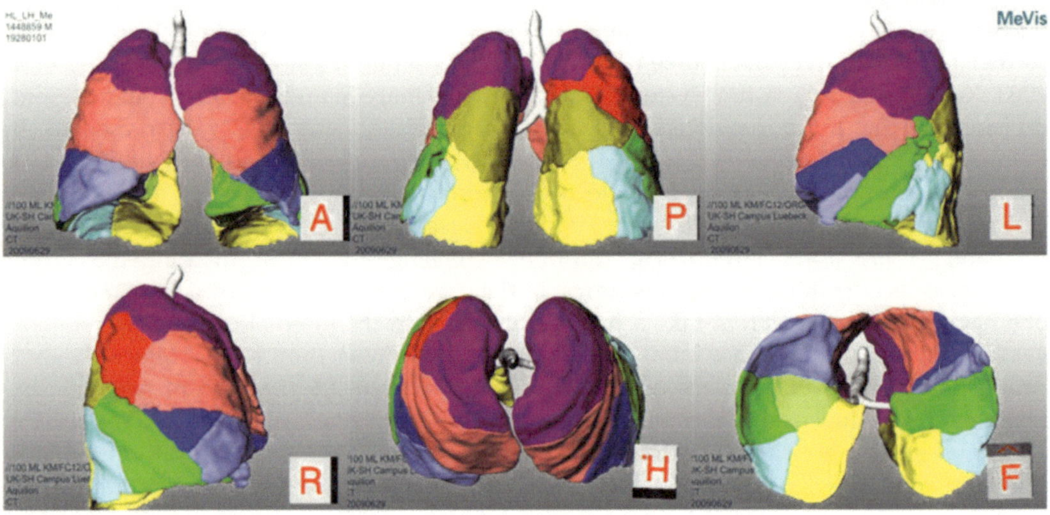

Fig. 4.1.3 3-D visualization of the lungs with colour-coded lung segment analysis.

4.2 Vascular system

The segmentation of pulmonary arteries and veins plays an important role in pre-operative image analysis, in addition to segmentation and the functional units of the lung. This also permits the quantitative determination of morphological parameters for these tree-like supply systems, such as, e.g., diameter and cross-sectional area of vessels, curvature, as well as length or volume of a section. Methods for the segmentation of tubular structures can be broadly divided into two categories. The methods in the first category are based on the determination of the path between two pre-determined end points and subsequently carry out the segmentation on reformatted layers orthogonal to the course of the path [Frangi AF et al. 1999, Hernandez-Hoyos M et al. 2002]. During this process, the calculation of the path results from the minimization of a cost functional, into which, on the one hand, external parameters, such as, e.g. voxel intensity or local contrast, and on the other hand, internal parameters such as, e.g., path length or curvature are fed. This "functional" approach can be efficiently realized and has the advantage that the segmentation of the cross-sections is mainly carried out in 2-D layers. On the other hand, there is no guarantee that the resultant path actually runs parallel to the structure, as length and curvature are taken into consideration in path minimization, which results in non-orthogonal cross-sections in the region of branching and strong curvature, in particular, and thus in erroneous values for diameter and cross-sectional area. Furthermore, these methods are often not suitable for interactive expansions aimed at the improvement or correction of an initial segmentation result.

In contrast, the methods in the second category largely take a 'geometric' approach, i.e., first a 3-D segmentation is carried out on the structure of interest, then its mid-line is determined and, finally, the vessel is measured on reformatted layers that are orthogonal to the mid-line. In this procedure, the mid-line is determined with the aid of skeletonization algorithms that can achieve high levels of accuracy [Lam L et al 1992, Selle D 1999, Borgefors G et al. 2001]. An advantage of this approach is that the user can verify and, if necessary, interactively modify the 3-D segmentation result, prior to calculating the mid-lines. Both approaches can, of course, be combined. For example, it may be meaningful to conduct another, further refined 2-D segmentation of the lumen based on the vascular cross-sections obtained using a geometric approach. During segmentation of the vascular systems, no satisfactory solution has been found to date for the automatic separation of the venous and arterial trees, in particular, which is, however, a prerequisite to producing 3-D depictions that have been coloured in analogous to illustrations in textbooks for each patient for the planning of surgery.

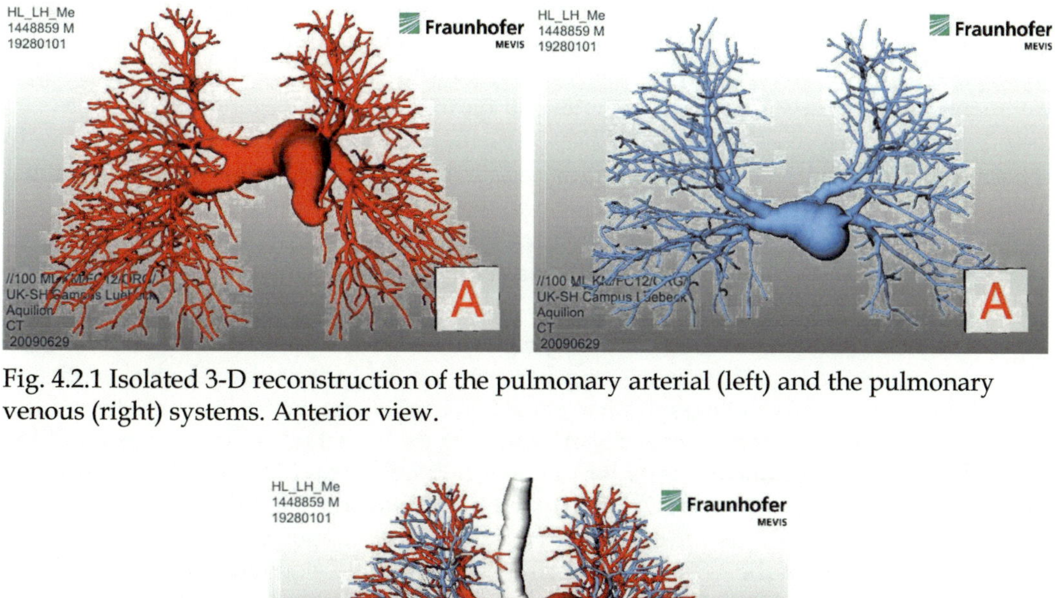

Fig. 4.2.1 Isolated 3-D reconstruction of the pulmonary arterial (left) and the pulmonary venous (right) systems. Anterior view.

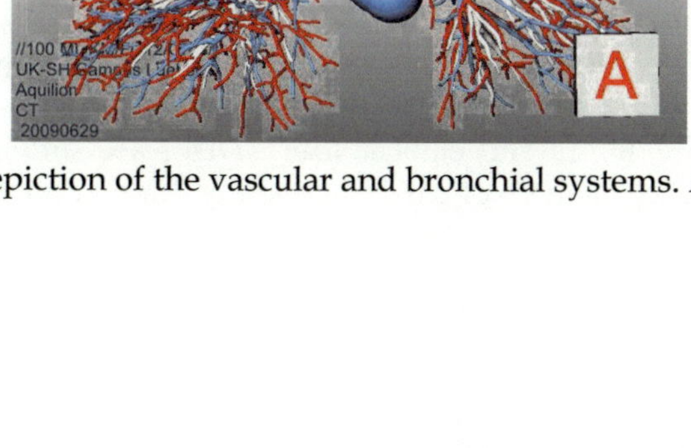

Fig. 4.2.2 Combined depiction of the vascular and bronchial systems. Anterior view.

4.3 Lung tumors and mediastinal lymph nodes

The assessment of the size, shape, location and number of lung tumours plays a substantial role in radiological diagnostics and in the planning of surgical interventions. The locational relationship to structures in lung, in particular, can provide important information on whether a tumorous process is locally restricted to an individual lobe or segment of the lung or whether it extends across multiple lobes or segments, which has a decisive effect on the extent of the resection. In this case, the most important tasks to be fulfilled by the algorithm are the segmentation and the quantification of such masses in the lungs. Research into the segmentation and volumetry of round lung lesions in CT data has, to date, been mainly motivated by CT screening studies for the early recognition of lung cancer. A corresponding emphasis has been placed on the reproducibility of the quantification of small round lesions in the algorithms developed to date. In many cases, these have an almost spherical shape and are generally only in slight contact with the pleura or the vessels. In the approach taken by Kostis [Kostis et al. 2003], a semi-automatic classification into one of very few round lesion models (isolated, close to pleura, with connection to vessels) is made prior to segmentation. After the subsequent initial segmentation with fixed threshold values, the connected, highly dense structures are severed by morphological operations. In 2005, Okada introduced an automated method for the approximation of so-called 'ground glass opacities' (GGO) to ellipsoids [Okada K et al. 2005]. Fetita also used an approach involving an initial segmentation with fixed threshold values and the subsequent application of morphological procedures [Fetita et al. 2003]. However, in this case, global information was also used, while the other methods only based their calculations on a section of the data set. The first commercial software packages that are intended for lung-screening examinations have been introduced on to the market since 2002 (R2, Siemens, GE, Philips). What these tools have in common is that the segmentation of larger and/or more complex tumors with substantial contact to the pleura or vessels is inadequate in many cases and there are often no options available to the user for making corrections, or these options are difficult to operate, as all methods to date for segmentation have been primarily developed for small round lesions.

4.4 Quantitative analysis of lung parenchyma

The standard method for functional lung parenchyma analysis is the selective perfusion scintigraphy. Computed tomography has gained in importance in emphysema diagnostics due to the low sensitivity of conventional x-rays for the detection of emphysema and the low sensitivity of lung function tests for the detection and quantification of early forms of emphysema, in particular [Grosse C and Bankier A 2007]. In addition to the quantification of emphysematous changes in lung parenchyma, computer tomographic scans (CT) also permit determination of the severity of the disease. Recognized standard parameters are the mean lung density (MLD) and the pixel index (PI) or - a synonym - also the emphysema index (EI). The EI can be determined globally or regionally [Blechschmidt, Achenbach]. Thin layer images (1 - 2 mm layer thickness) and the use of a high-resolution algorithm are prerequisites to optimum radiological evaluation. However, constantly improving technologies (4-, 16-, 64-slice CT) also require a large number of images. A data set comprising 300 - 600 images is usually produced, depending on the size of the patient's thorax, which corresponds to 150 - 300 MB storage capacity. However, this quantity of data is of limited practicality to routine clinical use. There are different research software application for quantitative analysis of parenchyma, e. g. MeVisPulmo3D [Kuhnigk JM et al.

2005, Heußel CP et al. 2006], that allows the depiction of emphysematous pulmonary areas, separated into lung, lobe or segment regions. Absolute and relative volumes, MLD and EI can be calculated and quantified selectively. The time-consuming part of the calculation is outsourced to a fully automated pre-processing procedure. The text report that is generated is complemented by two- or three-dimensional results.

Pre-operative 3-D visualization in combination with quantitative analysis of the parenchyma is greatly superior to a conventional CT analysis with a lung function test, especially in the case of extensive pulmonary emphysema (Fig. 4.4.1).

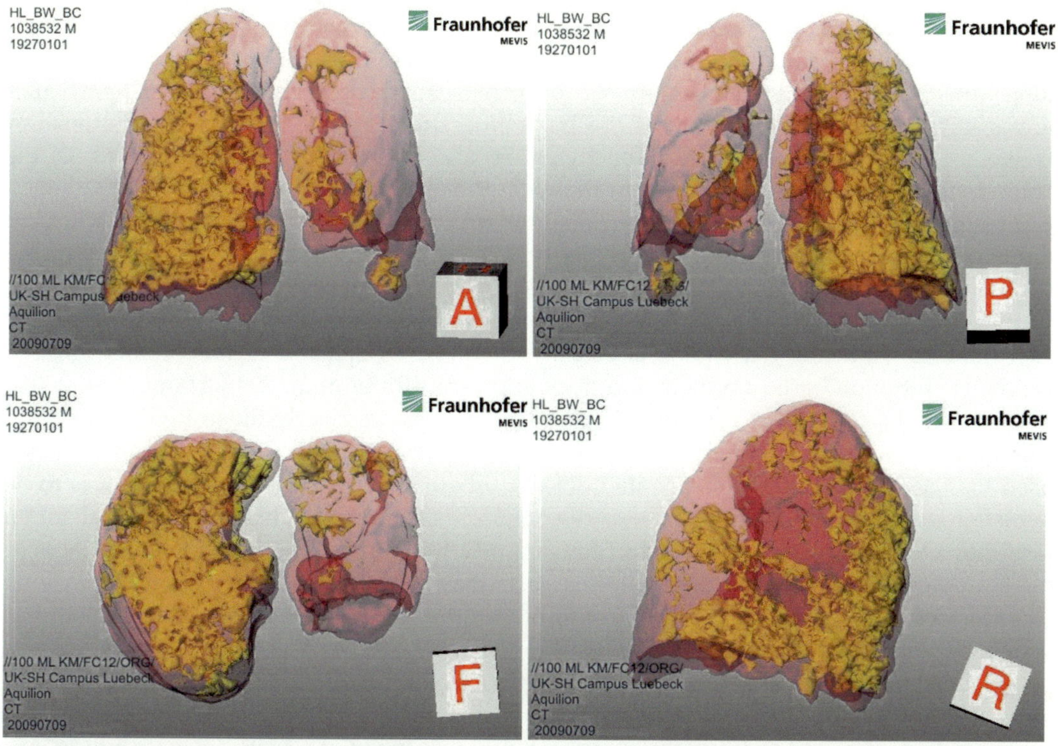

Fig. 4.4.1 Pre-operative 3-D visualization of a patient with extensive lung emphysema in addition to lung cancer of the left lower lobe. View from anterior (A), posterior (P), feet (F) and right side (R).

4.5 Visualization

The visualization of complex medical structures is a current challenge in the field of computer graphics. While algorithms for rapid volume rendering are now part of the functional scope of modern radiological units, to date, special methods for the accentuation of relevant information in the image data generally only exist in the context of prototypic research applications. The depiction of spatially complex anatomical situations that include a variety of diagnostic parameters and can be evaluated intuitively by the surgeon using it must be realized if a precise reproduction of the acquired image data is to be central to the purpose of radiological diagnostics. In the case of spatial visualizations, in particular, the targeted exploration of individual structures, i.e., the furtherance of visibility and

recognition of individual partial objects in a complex spatial scene, generally requires the use of special image-enhancement techniques. Above all, the development of non-photorealistic enhancement techniques that support an intuitive assessment of complex spatial scenes, has a high potential for the efficient implementation of such visualization tasks [Strothotte T et al. 2002, Ibanez L et al. 2005]. For example, the targeted use of contour lines, transparency and shadow projections can substantially improve the visibility of the enhanced objects and the recognition of the shape of the object [Preim B et al. 2002]. The targeted use, focused on specific tasks, of such enhancement techniques for the visualization of medical data is a topic in current research [Ibanez L et al. 2005].
The analysis and visualization of CT data and the production of dynamic image sequences was carried out by Fraunhofer MEVIS, Bremen. In connection with the tasks of planning a lung intervention, the visualization of bronchial and vascular trees is of particular importance. A correct illustration of the branching structure and the spatial relationships between vessels and supplied parenchyma is also important in this case, as is the accentuation of the decrease in vascular diameter towards the periphery.
Conventional visualization techniques, such as volume or surface rendering, reach their limits of applicability in this case, partially due to the fact that the resolution of the image data is too low and partially because of interference from artefacts due to noise and other distortions. Specially developed software permits a rapid and robust visualization of the vascular and bronchial trees. This is based on a surface depiction of the vessels through geometric filtration based on their mid-lines and radii [Ritter et al. 2006, Hahn et al. 2001]. The bronchial tree and the pulmonary vascular trees can be clearly illustrated with a very smooth and natural appearance using these methods. Triangulated surface models are often used for the visualization of segmented objects, where the surface of an object that is to be depicted is approximated using a network composed of triangles. This type of visualization provides a diversity of options, such as, for example, the transparent depiction of surfaces or the simultaneous illustration of multiple objects that penetrate each other, and has a long tradition of use in the field of 3-D computer graphics. For the purposes of surface visualization, Fraunhofer MEVIS has developed a flexible and modular library for the production, modification and visualization of surface models based on so-called winged edge meshes (WEM), that is characterized by a high efficiency and quality and is particularly well suited to interactive applications. The speed at which a surface model can be depicted is essentially determined by the number of triangles used. Although the quality of the visualization increases with the number of triangles, it can become so slow that smooth interactions are no longer possible. The number of triangles can be drastically reduced using a special, locally adapted filtering algorithm, without the quality deteriorating to any great extent. It is even possible to obtain a faster and also more precise visualization by simultaneously increasing the sampling rate.
Besides isosurface representation methods, also (direct) volume rendering is used for 3-D visualization. Volume rendering is the visualization of a three-dimensional data set through the projection of the individual voxels on to an image plane. In this process, the transparency and coloration of the voxels is determined by the grey values and a transfer function. Volume rendering is a reliable and established technique for the depiction of radiological images as this type of visualization does not require segmentation. An illumination model and a multi-dimensional transfer function are often used in modern volume rendering, which include additional attributes for the depiction of the voxel grey

values on to colours and transparencies and thus make special effects possible. For example, vessels or tumours can be highlighted using this technique, with the surrounding areas of the image being illustrated as a transparent silhouette.

5. 3-D reconstruction for the planning of interventions on central tumours

To evaluate the potential of the CT based segmentation and 3-D reconstructions of morphological structures of the lung for thoracic surgery planning 40 cases were analysed. The surgical approach was decided on by the thoracic surgeon undertaking the treatment, while the pre-operative tumour classification was mainly carried out by colleagues in radiology. All 40 CT examinations were initially evaluated without knowledge of the 3-D reconstruction analysis, which is the common procedure in clinical routine. The optimal, oncologically correct surgical intervention was planned. The peri-operative risk assessment with reference to the selected intervention was carried out, also taking into consideration the patient's pulmonary reserve and the general condition. Finally, the oncological approach to resection and the extent of resection were determined individually for each patient. 17 patients were staged as inoperable and not scheduled for surgery. The scheduled surgical strategy which was based on 2-D slices only was documented. In a second step, the 3-D reconstruction analysis was taken into consideration as an additional information and assessment device. In some cases the knowledge of the 3-D analysis lead to a change of the planned surgical procedure. The planned surgical procedure based on the 3-D reconstruction as an additional planning device was documented. The scheduled procedures were then compared to the actually carried out surgical intervention respectively. The assumption of a primary inoperable situation (n = 17 patients) based on the 2-D slices was confirmed by the 3-D reconstruction analysis only in 10 of 17 cases. Finally, 30 patients were scheduled for surgery.

The surgical approach in the 30 patients with operative treatment, selected based on the 2-D slices, corresponded to the therapy that was ultimately carried out in 14 patients (46.7 %, Table 5.1). Ultimately, the final surgical approach was only predicted in just under half of the patients based on the usual 2-D analysis. The risk analysis after the 3-D reconstruction had been viewed revealed a correct predictive outlook in 25 cases (83.3 %) (Table 5.2).

We were not able to classify the operability in 3 patients neither in the 2D nor in the 3D analysis, so we decided to perform a surgical exploration. 4 of the 17 patients - not resectable after 2D analysis - were predicted to be resectable in a curative intention after using the 3D based analysis. In 3 of these 4 patients a curative resection could be performed, the 4th patient turned out to be not resectable despite the 3D analysis.

After neo-adjuvant therapy (stage IIIB), 3 patients became operable (stage IIIA). This stage improvement with a corresponding surgical approach was correctly predicted both based on the 2-D and on the 3-D analysis. No advantage of the 3-D reconstruction was determined in patients after neo-adjuvant therapy with reference to the risk analysis.

		Frequency	Percentage
Valid	Incorrect	16	53.3
	Correct	**14**	**46.7**
	Total	30	100.0

Table 5.1 **Decision based on** 2-D CT slices only (all cases operated on)

		Frequency	Percentage
Valid	Incorrect	5	16.7
	Correct	**25**	**83.3**
	Total	30	100.0

Tab. 5.2 **Decision with** 3-D analysis (all cases operated on)

A comparison of the 2-D and 3-D proposals for surgery reveals 25 congruent and 15 divergent results for all cases (n = 40) and 15 congruent and 15 divergent cases, respectively, for those patients operated on. The analysis of the divergent results (n = 15) revealed the following constellation: out of 15 divergent results, 13 (87 %) had been properly corrected by the 3-D analysis, i.e., the initially incorrect prediction was improved to a correct prediction through the pre-operative use of the 3-D depiction in 13/15 cases. In only 2 cases was the 2-D analysis found to be correct, compared with a subsequent incorrect 3-D analysis. In these cases, the correct 2-D analysis was erroneously changed by the 3-D reconstruction. Patient 1 exhibited status post atypical resection of the left upper lobe with pulmonary metastasis. Given a metastatic relapse in the left lower lobe, the probable operation was regarded as pneumonectomy of the residual lung based on 2-D CT slices. The 3-D representation favoured a lower lobe resection under retention of the partially remaining upper lobe. Pneumonectomy of the residual lung had to be carried out intra-operatively, such that the initial 2-D assessment was confirmed. Patient 2 exhibited a left-central, small-cell bronchial carcinoma with broad-based contact to the aortic arch. While the 2-D analysis indicated inoperability due to a suspected infiltration of the aortic arch, based on the 3-D analysis, the observers thought it would be possible to conduct a resection just within healthy tissue. However, intra-operatively, the tumour infiltration was revealed as even more extensive than on the pre-operative images. The intervention had to be abandoned as an exploration.

In 3 patients, neither the 2-D, nor the 3-D analysis produced a correct analysis of the final surgical strategy. The extent of the resection was underestimated in 2 patients, while it was possible to spare more parenchyma during surgery in 1 patient, when compared with what had been planned based on the analyses.

6. Outlook: Fusion of different modalities

In this outlook we discuss the potential of combining CT information with modalities from nuclear medicine. This discussion is kind of a roadmap of upcoming research in the area of image based preoperative risk assessment and planning of surgical interventions in the lung.

6.1 Functional imaging (SPECT) and data fusion SPECT/3-D

In addition to the depiction of the morphology, the functionality of the original and remaining residual lung tissue is of central interest for a large thoracic resective intervention. The functionality of the lung parenchyma can be assessed with lung function or exercise tests (spirometry, spiroergometry or body plethysmography). At the university hospital Lübeck, selective digital perfusion scintigraphy SPECT (Fig. 6.1.3) is used as the functional imaging method. The examination technique permits a graphic illustration of functional aspects in individual organs. Based on the principle of scintigraphy, a radiotracer is administered intravenously to the patient. The tracer used in lunge perfusion exams is constructed to be fixed in the lung capillaries during first pass. The radionuclides - (Tc99m) -

that are used emit gamma radiation that can be detected and measured with using gamma cameras. One or more gamma cameras rotate around the body and detect the emitted radiation from different directions in space. The distribution of the radiotracer in the lung depends on the amount of blood passing thought the different parts of the lungs. It can be deduced from these planar projections using inverse radon transformation and the distribution can then be depicted in the form of computed tomographic sections through the body. This allows the production of a three-dimensional image of lung function. The substance, Tc-99m-labeled macroaggregated albumin, that is used for perfusion scans has no medicinal effects or side effects as it is used in tiny quantities that produce only small doses of gamma radiation. After about 36 h, 99 % of the material has decayed or been excreted. The levels of radiation exposure are substantially smaller than for an x-ray examination. Beside perfusion scans ventilation scans could be performed using radioisotops of noble gases. As handling of radioactive gases is demanding perfusion scans are preferred at many sites.

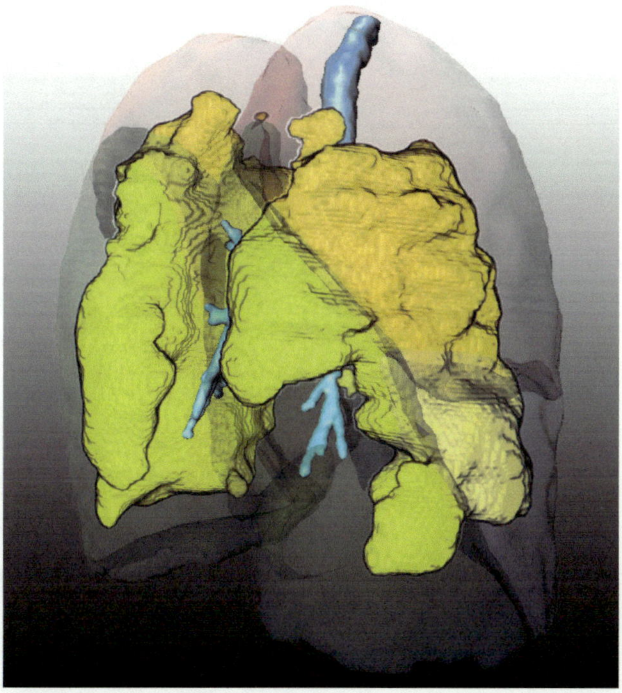

Fig. 6.1.1 Three-dimensional visualization for a patient with severe lung emphysema. Software fusion of SPECT data set with CT data using ManualRegistration in MeVisLab. Ventilated areas are highlighted in colour, non-ventilated areas are depicted semitransparently.

A relatively novel technique is the combination of SPECT and CT to obtain SPECT quantification on a lobar basis. Both scans are therefore used during the examination: CT produces images of the body's morphology, SPECT depicts the perfusion. Superimposed SPECT and CT images then permit a precise local determination of ill perfused areas. As CT data cannot be acquired in the available SPECT scanner we undertook an external fusion of the available image data and subsequent 3-D visualization. In a feasibility experiment, a CT dataset (Clinic for Radiology, University Hospital Schleswig-Holstein (UKSH) , Campus Luebeck) and the tomographic SPECT perfusion data (Clinic for Nuclear Medicine, UKSH, Campus Luebeck) were fused using user guided registration (rigid + scale) (Fig. 6.2) and visualized in 3D externally (Fraunhofer MEVIS / Bremen), and sent back online. Along with the renderings, a quantitative relative and absolute measurement of lung perfusion per lobe and emphysema scores based on the CT data was computed, employing the lung lobe segmentation performed at MEVIS (see Section 5.4). Figure 6.1 shows the corresponding visualization.

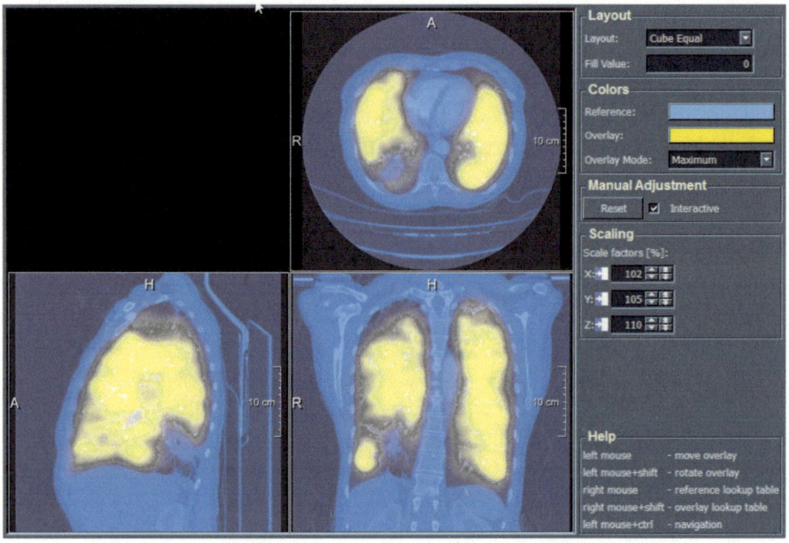

Fig 6.1.2 Reformatted data after fusion with SPECT. Graduated illustration of the ventilation density (dark = reduced ventilation, light = good ventilation).

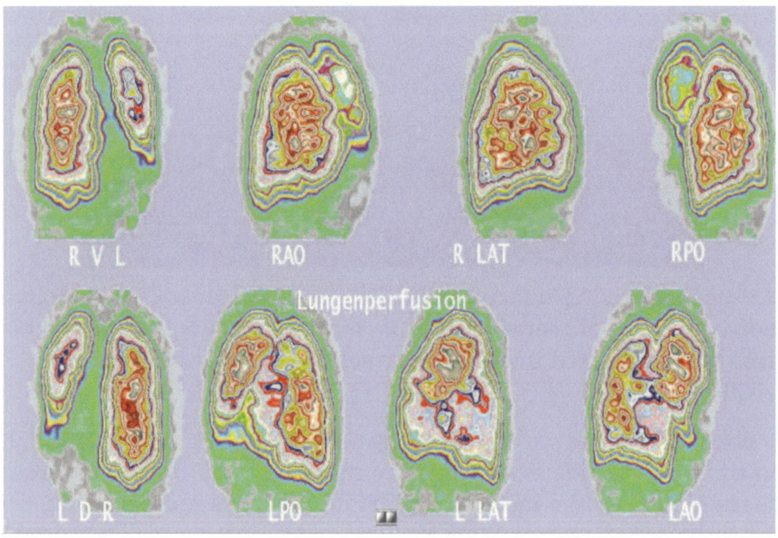

Fig. 6.1.3 Scintigram of the lungs after i.v. administration of a radionuclide (^{99m}Tc). From a higher number of such projection images a 3D-SPECT perfusion image can be reconstructed.

6.2 Fusion of 18-F FDG- PET with 3-D CT

Until recently mostly only anatomy and topography has been illustrated prior to thoracic surgery using MSDCT. In addition to this, the depiction of functional aspects also plays an important role in the planning of surgery. So far scintigraphy of the lungs to illustrate perfusion and, if necessary, ventilation, has been established in clinical routine, as the determination of vessel diameters or the distribution of pulmonary density using CT does not permit secure conclusions with reference to perfusion or ventilation. More recently, positron emission tomography (PET) has become more and more established as an additional diagnostic tool in everyday clinical routine. PET is an imaging method used in nuclear medicine to study the distribution of small doses of radioactively labelled substances in the organism and to thus depict biochemical and physiological functions. In this context, particular interest is in its use in investigating the activity of a suspected tumorous structure, in order to differentiate between scar tissue, artelectasis (non ventilated lung appearing in similar density as the tumor in CT) and tumour tissue in the search for tumour extends, metastases, or within the framework of a staging examination following on from (neo-)adjuvant therapy to assess tumour response to chemotherapy. The fusion of an individual PET finding with 2-dimensional CT images on a light box is difficult and a task that is almost impossible to accomplish for a non-radiologist or nuclear medic, in particular. Therefore most recent PET installations combine a PET an a CT scanner. The CT images from a PET/CT however are commonly not of diagnostic quality. The option of fusing FDG-PET and diagnostic CT images with high 3D resolution was also assessed within the framework of the current study.

For the PET scan a radiopharmaceutical is administered intravenously to the patient at the start of a PET examination. For oncology application mostly 18-FDG is used, a radiolabeled sugar, that has high uptake in tumours and other metabolic highly active areas (e.g. the brain or inflammation areas). In contrast to SPECT, PET uses radionuclides that emit positrons (β^+ rays). The spatial distribution of 18FDG within the body can be deduced from the temporal and spatial distribution of the recorded decay events and a series of cross-sectional images can be calculated. Furthermore, the distribution of the tracer in the volume under investigation can be precisely quantified – which is not as well possible with SPECT - as the absorption of the photons being measured depends only on the thickness of the irradiated tissue and not on the origin of the photons. Oncological PET uses metabolically active glucose as the radionuclide (also called radiopharmaceutical or tracer), in which a hydroxyl group on C6 of the sugar molecule is replaced by the radionuclide F18. FDG-6-phosphate cannot undergo any further metabolism after phosphorylation and accumulates in tissue ('metabolic trapping'). Metabolically active processes taking place in tumours and metastases can thus be depicted and distinguished from non-metabolically active structures like scar tissue. In PET-CT, the patient is passed through the two detector rings for CT and PET, one after the other (in housing for the equipment). The images that are produced are automatically fused in the computer. In contrast to a conventional thoracic CT, a so-called low-dose CT scan is sufficient for a PET-CT. The exposure to radiation for a pure PET examination using F-18 is about 4mSv and is thus in the range of a computed tomography on the thorax. For a feasibility study the digital PET images were fused to the high resolution diagnostic CT data externally (Fraunhofer MEVIS, Bremen) in order to create 3D visualization incorporating the functional PET information. The CT data (Clinic for Radiology, University Hospital Schleswig-Holstein (UKSH) , Campus Lübeck) and digital

PET images (Clinic for Nuclear Medicine, UKSH, Campus Luebeck) were sent separately online, fused with user guidance in dedicated MeVisLab software prototypes (Figs. 6.2.1 and 6.2.2) and rendered in 3D externally (Fraunhofer MeVis, Bremen), the data structures allowing interactive 3D visualizations were then sent back to Lübeck online. The advantages of a high-dose CT became clear: only with high resolution CT data an acceptable image quality will be feasible for 3D visualizations. They provide a greatly improved fused image quality when compared with a low-dose CT image. However, as PET-CT is a rather expensive imaging method, it is not currently available across the board in Germany.

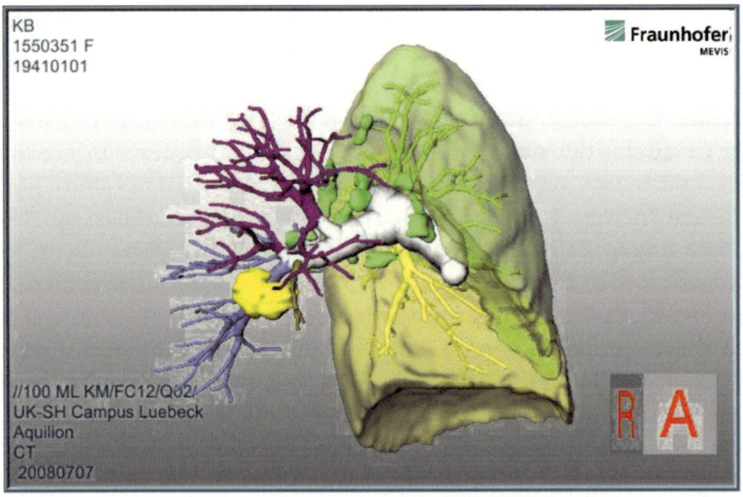

Fig. 6.2.1 67-year-old patient with a suspected local relapse of an adenocarcinoma in the right lower lobe. Status post primary transthoracic radiation therapy with initial functional inoperability (tumor highlighted in yellow).

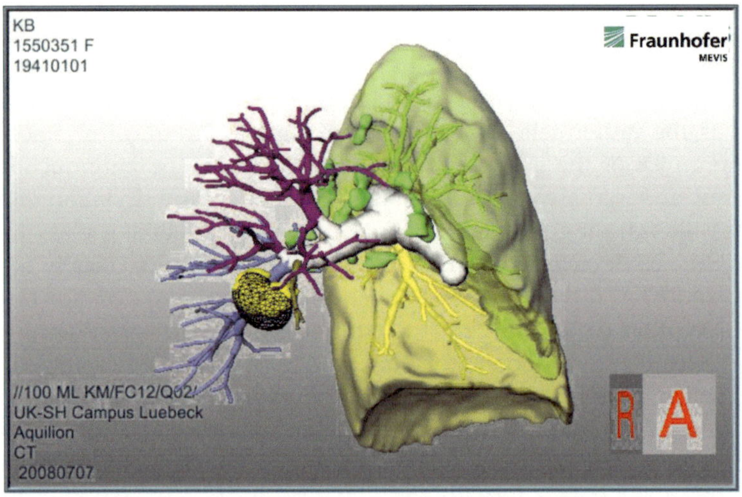

Fig. 6.2.2 PET-CT image fusion. Clear superimposition of metabolically active areas on the F18-PET (black grid lines) with the tumor (yellow).

7. Limits of 3-D reconstruction

The basic prerequisite for a subsequent optimal and meaningful 3-D reconstruction is the initial CT. Standard CT quality (5mm sections) does not permit adequate 3-D reconstruction. Distances between layers that are too great or CT layers that are too thick result in 3D-images of poor quality containing little information and possibly in inaccurate results of software based segmentations. In turn, if no, or too little, contrast agent is administered, this results in a deficient depiction of the intra-thoracic vascular supply. The initial CT must therefore fulfil the following requirements: }{Hochauflösendes Computertomogramm (mindestens 4-Zeiler), maximale Schichtdicke 2 mm, maximaler Schichtabstand 1,5mm undKontrastmittelgabe zur Gefäßdarstellung. | high-resolution computed tomography scan (minimum 4-slice), maximum layer thickness 2 mm, maximum distance between layers 1.5 mm and administration of contrast agent for vascular depiction.}
The thresholds for 3-D imaging are identical to those for an axial 2-D CT: The differentiation between a solid tumour and a post-stenotic atelectasis is just as impossible as the secure delimitation of a point of contact between a tumour and a potential infiltration of a vascular wall or solid mediastinal organs.
Even so, the image analysis and 3-D reconstruction constitutes an enormous gain in quantitative and qualitative information for the surgeon. In addition to the quantitative depiction and calculation of tumour size and tumour volume, the lobe volumes and calculations of distances, it is mainly the qualitative advance that is of importance when compared with an axial 2-D CT. The possibility of segmentation permits the selective observation of tumour, vascular system or bronchial tree and is vastly superior to the visual depiction in 2 planes. The method of anatomical 3-D reformatting currently provides the best possible imaging for pre-operative risk analysis in complex thoracic interventions.
In the medium term, computer analysis should also be used for intra-operative detection of lung tumours and for navigation during VATS. However, prior to this, the problem that is specific to the lungs, e.g. changes in locational anatomy due to the peri-operative atelectasis, must be clarified and a full understanding must be gained.

8. Summary

The segmentation and 3-dimenstional visualization of thoracic morphology based on CT is a novel and highly promising method for pre-operative imaging and risk analysis for central lung tumours. This allows a visualization of the tumour in combination with colour-coded lobe and segment association and the anatomical relationship to neighbouring structures. Furthermore, the depiction and calculation of lung volumes and emphysematous portions permits estimates of the expected residual functionality of the lung. The 3-dimensional image that can be moved in all planes, in combination with the possibility of anatomical segmentation, is easier and more simple for the observer to understand than the 2-D scans used to date with/without the associated radiological information.

9. Acknowledgments

This work has been financially supported by grant DFG PE 199/20-1 of the german society for research. The referred software is based on contributions of many current and former researchers at Fraunhofer MEVIS. It is also a result of a lot of fruitful discussions with a variety of thoracic surgeons throughout Germany within and beyond the frame of the ongoing project.

10. References

Alexander E (2001) 3rd. Optimizing brain tumor resection. Midfield interventional MR imaging. Neuroimaging Clin N Am.11(4):659-72.

Aykac D, Hoffman EA, McLennan G, Reinhardt JM (2003) Segmentation and analysis of the human airway tree from three-dimensional X-ray CT images. IEEE Trans Med Imaging. 22(8):940-50.

Blechschmidt RA, Werthschuetzky R, Loercher U (2001) Automated CT image evaluation of the lung: a morphology-based concept. IEEE Trans Med Imaging 20(5):434-42.

Borgefors G, Ramella G, Sanniti di Baja G (2001) Hierarchical Decomposition of Multiscale Skeletons. IEEE Trans Pattern Anal Mach Intell. 23:1296-1312.

Bornik A, Beichel R, Reitinger B, Gotschuli G, Sorantin E, Leberl F, Sonka M (2003) Computer aided liver surgery planning: An augmented reality approach. In: Medical Imaging 2003: Visualization, Image-Guided Procedures and Display. Vol. 5029: 395-406.

Centers for Disease Control and Prevention: http://www.cdc.gov/niosh/topics/cancer/

Coxson HO, Rogers RM, Whittall KP, D'yachkova Y, Paré PD, Sciurba FC, Hogg JC (1999) A quantification of the lung surface area in emphysema using computed tomography. Am J Respir Crit Care Med. 159(3):851-6.

Dicken V, Kuhnigk JM, Bornemann L, Zidowitz S, Krass S, Peitgen HO (2005) Novel CT data analysis and visualization techniques for risk assessment and planning of thoracic surgery in oncology patients. In: Lemke HU, Inamura K, Doi K, Vannier MW, Farman AG, editors (eds). Computer Assisted Radiology and Surgery. Amsterdam: Elsevier: 783-787.

Dicken V, Wein B, Schubert H, Kuhnigk JM, Krass S, Peitgen HO (2003) Novel Projection Views for Simplified Reading of Thorax CT Scans with Multiple Pulmonary Nodules. In: Lemke H-U, Vannier MW, Inamura K, Farman AG, Doi K, Reiber JHC, editors (eds). Computer Assisted Radiology and Surgery. Amsterdam:Elsevier: 59-64.

Frangi AF, Niessen WJ, Hoogeveen RM, van Walsum T, Viergever MA (1999) Model-based quantitation of 3-D magnetic resonance angiographic images. IEEE Trans Med Imaging. 18(10):946-56.

[FUSION] http://www.somit-fusion.de/SF/index.php

Hahn, H.K.; Preim, B.; Selle, D.; Peitgen, H.-O.; , "Visualization and interaction techniques for the exploration of vascular structures," Visualization, 2001. VIS '01. Proceedings , vol., no., pp.395-578, 21-26 Oct. 2001

Grenacher L, Thorn M, Knaebel HP, Vetter M, Hassenpflug P, Kraus T, Meinzer HP, Buechler MW, Kauffmann GW, Richter GM (2005) The role of 3-D imaging and computer-based postprocessing for surgery of the liver and pancreas. Rofo 177(9):1219-1226.

Grosse C, Bankier A (2007) Bildgebung des Lungenemphysems. Radiologe 47(5):401-6.

Hara T, Yamamoto A, Zhou X, Iwano S, Itou S, Fujita H, Ishagaki T (2003) Automated volume measurements of pulmonary emphysema on 3-D chest CT images. In: Lemke HU, Vannier MW, Inamura K, Farman AG, Doi K, Reiber JHC editors (eds.). Computer Aided Radiology and Surgery. Berlin: Springer. pp:1043-1048.

Heussel CP, Achenbach T, Buschsieweke C, Kuhnigk J, Weinheimer O, Hammer G, DFüber C, Kauczor HU (2006) Quantifizierung des Lungenemphysems in der Mehrschicht-CT mittels verschiedener Softwareverfahren. RöFo 178(10):987-998.

Hernández-Hoyos M, Orkisz M, Puech P, Mansard-Desbleds C, Douek P, Magnin IE (2002) Computer-assisted analysis of three-dimensional MR angiograms. Radiographics. 22(2):421-36.

Hildebrand P, Kleemann M, Schlichting S, Martens V, Besirevic A, Roblick U, Bruch HP, Bürk C (2009) Prototype of an online navigation system for laparoscopic radiofrequency ablation. Hepatogastroenterology 56(96):1710-3.

Hildebrand P, Martens V, Schweikard A, Schlichting S, Besirevic A, Kleemann M, Roblick U, Mirow L, Bürk C, Bruch HP (2007) Evaluation of an online navigation system for laparoscopic interventions in a perfused ex vivo artificial tumor model of the liver. HPB(Oxford) 9(3):190-4.

Hoffmann EA, Reinhardt JM, Sonka M, Simon BA, Guo J, Saba O, Chon D, Samrah S, Shikata H, Tschirren J, Palagyi K, Beck KC, McLennan G (2003) Chracterizytion of the intestitial lung diseases via density-based and texture-based analysis of computed tomography images of lung structure and function. Acad Radiol. 10(10):1104-1118.

Hu S, Hoffman EA, Reinhardt JM (2001) Automatic lung segmentation for accurate quantitation of volumetric X-ray CT images. IEEE Trans Med Imaging. 20(6):490-8.

Hünerbein M, Gretschel S, Rau B, Schlag PM (2003) Reducing trauma with minimally invasive surgery. Evidence and new strategies. Chirurg 74:282-289.

Ibanez L, Aylward SR, Kindlmann G (2005) Hot Topics in 3D Medical Visualization. SIGGRAPH 2005 Tutorial.

Jolesz FA (2005) Future perspectives for intraoperative MRI. Neurosurg Clin N Am. 16(1):201-13.

Kalender WA, Rienmüller R, Seissler W, Behr J, Welke M, Fichte H (1990) Measurement of pulmonary parenchymal attenuation: use of spirometric gating with quantitative CT. Radiology. 175(1):265-8.

Kitasaka T, Mori K, Hasegawa J, Toriwaki J (1999) Automated extraction of the lung area from 3-D chest X-ray CT images based upon the 3-D shape model deformation. In: Lemke HU, Vannier MW, Inamura K, Farman AG, Doi K, editors (eds.). Computer Assisted Radiology and Surgery. Amsterdam: Elsevier. pp.194-198.

Kostis WJ, Reeves AP, Yankelevitz DF, Henschke CI (2003) Three-dimensional segmentation and growth-rate estimation of small pulmonary nodules in helical CT images. IEEE Trans Med Imaging 22(10):1259-1274.

Kuhnigk JM, Hahn H, Hindennach M, Dicken V, Krass S, Peitgen HO (2003) Lung lobe segmentation by anatomy-guided 3D watershed transform. In Sonka M, Fitzpatrick JM, editors (eds.). Medical Imaging 2003: Image Processing. Bellingham: SPIE. pp:1482-1490.

Kuhnigk JM, Dicken V, Zidowitz S, Bornemann L, Kuemmerlen B, Krass S, Peitgen HO, Yuval S, Fend HH, Rau WS, Achenbach T (2005) New Tools for Computer Assistance in Thoracic CT. Part 1. Functional Analysis of Lungs, Lung Lobes, and Bronchopulmonary Segments. RadioGraphics 25:525-536.

Krass S, Selle D, Boehm D, Jend HH, Kriete A, Rau WS, Peitgen HO (2000) Determination of bronchopulmonary segments based on HRCT data. In: Lemke HU, Vannier MW, Inamura K, Farman AG, Doi K editors (eds). Computer Assisted Radiology and Surgery. Amsterdam: Elsevier. pp:584-589.

Krebsatlas der Bundesrepublik Deutschland: http://www.krebsatlas.de

Lam L, Lee SW, Suen CY (1992) Thinning Methodologies - A Comprehensive Survey. IEEE Trans Patt Anal Mach Intell. 14:869-885.

Lang H, Radtke A, Hindennach M, Schroeder T, Fruehauf NR, Malagó M, Bourquain H, Peitgen HO, Oldhafer KJ, Broelsch CE (2005) Impact of virtual tumor resection and computer-assisted risk analysis on operation planning and intraoperative strategy in major hepatic resection. Arch Surg 140(7):629-38; discussion 638.

Leader JK, Zheng B, Rogers RM, Sciurba FC, Perez A, Chapman BE, Patel S, Fuhrman CR, Gur D (2003) Automated lung segmentation in X-ray computed tomography: development and evaluation of a heuristic threshold-based scheme. Acad Radiol.10(11):1224-36.

Ley S, Mayer D, Brook BS, van Beek EJ, Heussel CP, Rinck D, Hose R, Markstaller K, Kauczor HU (2002) Radiological imaging as the basis for a simulation software of ventilation in the tracheo-bronchial tree. Eur Radiol. 12(9):2218-28.

Limmer S, Dicken V, Kujath P, Krass S, Stoecker C, Wendt N, Unger L, Hoffmann M, Vogt FM, Kleemann M, Bruch HP, Peitgen HO (2010) Dreidimensionalen Rekonstruktion von zentralen Lungentumoren basierend auf CT-Daten : Erste klinische Erfahrungen. Der Chirurg 81(9):833–840.

Okada K, Comaniciu D, Krishnan A. Robust (2005) Anisotropic Gaussian Fitting for Volumetric Characterization of Pulmonary Nodules in Multislice CT. IEEE Trans Med Imaging. 24(3):409-423.

Oldhafer KJ, Hoegemann D, Stamm G, Raab R, Peitgen HO, Galanski M (1999) 3-dimensional (3-D) visualization of the liver for planning extensive liver resections. Chirurg 70(3):233-8.

Park W, Hoffmann EA, Sonka M (1998) Segmentation of intrathoracic airway trees: a fuzzy logic approach. IEEE Trans Med Imaging. 17(4):489-497

Preim B, Ritter F. Techniken zur Hervorhebung von Objekten in medizinischen 3d-Visualisierungen. In: Simulation und Visualisierung. Ghent: SCS. pp:187-200

Prêteux F, Fetita C, Capderou A, Grenier P (1999) Modeling, segmentation, and caliber estimation of bronchi in high resolution computerized tomography. J. Electron. Imaging 8(1):36-45

Reinhardt JM, Guo J, Zhang L, Bilgen D, Hu S, Uppaluri R, Long RM, Saba OI, McLennan G, Sonka M, Hoffmann EA (2001) Integrated system for objective assessment of global and regional lung structure. In: Niessen WJ, Viergever MA editors (eds.). Lecture Notes in Computer Science 2208. Berlin: Springer. pp:1384-1385

Ritter, F.; Hansen, C.; Dicken, V.; Konrad, O.; Preim, B.; Peitgen, H.-O.; , "Real-Time Illustration of Vascular Structures," Visualization and Computer Graphics, IEEE Transactions on , vol.12, no.5, pp.877-884, Sept.-Oct. 2006

Schalthölter T, Lorenz C, Carlsen IC, Renisch S, Deschamps T (2002) Simultaneous segmentation and tree reconstruction of the airways for virtual bronchoscopy. In: Sonka M, Fitzpatrick JM editors (eds.). Proceedings of SPIE Vol. 4684 Medical Imaging: Image Processing: Bellingham

Selle D (1999) Analyse von Gefäßstrukturen in medizinischen Schichtdatensätzen für die computergestützte Operationsplanung. Aachen: Shaker Verlag.

Sluimer I, Prokop M, van Ginneken B (2005) Toward automated segmentation of the pathological lung in CT. IEEE Trans Med Imaging. 24(8):1025-38.

Stoecker C, Dicken V, Krass S, Kuhnigk JM, Peitgen HO, et al. (2009) CT-based patient individual anatomical modeling of the lung and its impact on thoracic surgery. In O. Dössel, & W. C. Schlegel (Eds.), World Congress on Medical Physics and Biomedical Engineering (pp. 1592–1595). IFMBE Proceedings, 25(4). München: Springer-Verlag.

Strothotte T, Schlechtweg S (2002) Non-Photorealistic Computer Graphics: Modeling, Rendering and Animation. San Francisco: Morgan Kaufmann Publischers.

Tormenti MJ, Kostov DB, Gardner PA, Kanter AS, Spiro RM, Okonkwo DO (2010) Intraoperative computed tomography image-guided navigation for posterior thoracolumbar spinal instrumentation in spinal deformity surgery. Neurosurg Focus 28(3):E11.

Tschirren J, McLennan G, Palagyi K, Hoffmann EA, Sonka M (2005a) Matching and anatomical labeling of human airway tree. IEEE Trans Med Imaging. 24(12):1540-7.

Tschirren J, Hoffman EA, McLennan G, Sonka M (2005b) Intrathoracic airway trees: segmentation and airway morphology analysis from low-dose CT scans. IEEE Trans Med Imaging. 24(12):1529-39.

Ukil S, Hoffman EA, Reinhardt JM (2005) Automatic lung lobe segmentation in x-ray CT images by 3D watershed transform using anatomic information from the segmented airway tree. In SPIE Conf. Medical Imaging 2005: Image Processing. pp.556-567

Ukil S, Sonka M, Reinhardt JM (2006) Automatic segmentation of pulmonary fissures in x-ray CT images using anatomic guidance (Proceedings Paper) Medical Imaging 2006: Image Processing. 61440N

Uppaluri R, Mitsa T, Sonka M, Hoffman EA, McLennan G (1997) Quantification of pulmonary emphysema from lung computed tomography images. Am J Respir Crit Care Med. 156(1):248-54.

Welter S, Stoecker C, Dicken V, Kuehl H, Krass S, Stamatis G (2011) Lung segment geometry study: Simulation of largest possible tumours that fit into bronchopulmonary segments. The Thoracic and Cardiovascular Surgeon (accepted).

Xu Y, Sonka M, McLennan G, Guo J, Hoffmann EA (2006) MDCT-based 3-D texture classification of emphysema and early smoking related lung pathologies. IEEE Trans Medical Imaging. 25(4):464-475.

Zhou X, Kobayashi S, Hayashi T, Murata N, Hara T, Fujita H, Yokoyama R, Kiryu T, Hoshi H, Sato M (2003) Lung structure recognition: a further study of thoracic organ recognitions based on CT images. In: Lemke HU, Vannier MW, Inamura K, Farman AG, Doi K, Reiber JHC, editors (eds.). Computer Aided Radiology and Surgery. Berlin:Springer. pp:1025-1030.

13

CT Scanning and Dental Implant

Yeon-Jo Choi[1], Sang-Ho Jun[2], Young-Dae Song[3],
Myoung-Woo Chang[4] and Jong-Jin Kwon[5]
[1,2,3,5]Department of Dentistry Korea University Medical Center
[4]Restorative Dentistry and Biomaterials Sciences
Harvard School of Dental Medicine
[1,2,3,5]Korea
[4]U.S.A.

1. Introduction

1.1 Osseointegration and bone density

Osseointegrated screw-shaped titanium implants that support dental prosthesis have been used to restore function and esthetics of missing teeth with favorable clinical results. Restoration using dental implants is now the most popular treatment in the field of dentistry. Since Brånemark P-I reported the treatment using titanium-made dental implants for the edentulous patient in 1977, there has been enormous advancement in the field of implant dentistry.

Successful osseointegration, which is an utmost determining factor for the success of implant treatments, has been viewed as the direct, structural, and functional connection existing between ordered, living bone and the surface of a functionally loaded implant (Fig. 1 a to d). Many clinical studies and investigations were performed to propose success criteria for dental implants. Albrektsson et al. report in 1986 was specific for implants with rigid fixation and is widely used today (Table 1).

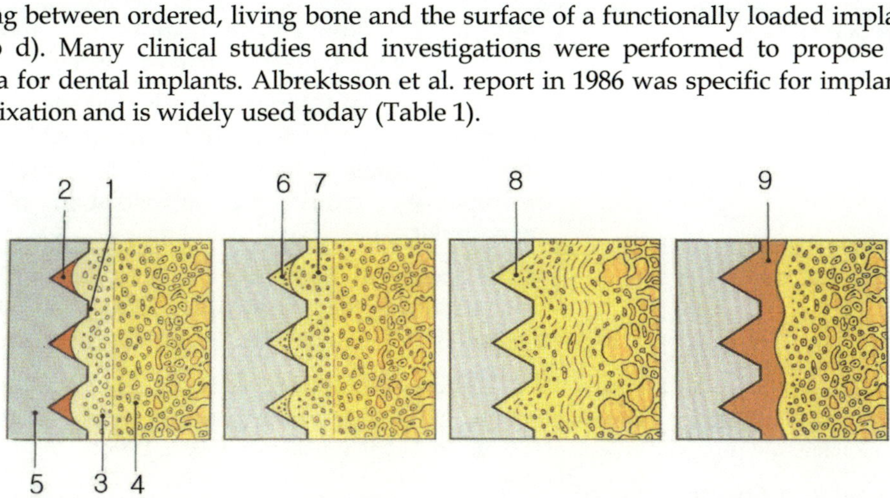

From Brånemark P, Zarb G, Albrektsson T. Introduction to osseointegration. In: Brånemark PI, ZarbGA, Albrektsson T (eds). Tissue-integrated Prostheses: Osseointegration in clinical Dentistry. Chicago: Quintessence, 1985:12.

Fig. 1. Diagrammatic representation of biology of osseointegration

Fig. 1a The threaded bone site cannot be made perfectly congruent to the implant. Object of making a threaded socket in bone is to provide immobilization immediately after installation and during the initial healing period. The diagram is based on relative dimensions of fixture and fixture site. 1 = contact between fixture and bone (immobilization); 2= hematoma in closed cavity. Bordered by fixture and bone; 3= bone that was damaged by unavoidable thermal and mechanical trauma; 4= original undamaged bone; and 5 = fixture.
Fig. 1b During the unloaded healing period, the hematoma becomes transformed into new bone through callus formation (6). Damaged bone, which also heals, undergoes revascularization, and demineralization and remineralization (7).
Fig. 1c After the initial healing period, vital bone tissue is in close contact with fixture surface, without any other intermediate tissue. Border zone bone (8) remodels in response to the masticatory load applied.
Fig. 1d In unsuccessful cases nonmineralized connective tissue (9), constituting a kind of pseudoarthrosis, forms in the border zone at the implant. This development can be initiated by excessive preparation trauma, infection, loading too early in the healing period before adequate mineralization and organization of hard tissue has taken place, or supraliminal loading at any time, even many years after integration has been established. Once lost, osseointegration cannot be reconstituted. Connective tissue can become organized to a certain degree, but is not a proper anchoring tissue because of its inadequate mechanical and biologic capacities, resulting in creation of a locus minorisresistentiae.

Immobility	An individual, unattached implant is immobile when tested clinically
No periimplantradioducency	A radiograph does not demonstrate any evidence of periimplant radiolucency
Vertical bone loss	Vertical bone loss is less than 0.2mm annually following the implant's first year of service
No symptoms	Individual implant performance is characterized by an absence of persistent and/or irreversible signs and symptoms such as pain, infections, neuropathies, paresthesia, of violation of the mandibular canal
Long term survival rate	In the context of the above, a success rate of 85% at the end of a 5-year observation period and 80% at the end of a 10-year period are minimum criteria for success

From Albrektsson T, ZarbGA, Worthington P et al: The long-term efficacy of currently used dental implants: a review and proposed criteria of success, Int J Oral MaxillofacImplants 1986;1:1.

Table 1. Criteria for Implant Success

Implant stability, an indirect indication of osseointegration, is a measure of the clinical mobility of an implant and plays an essential role in the long-term success of dental implants. It is classified into two; 1) primary and 2) secondary. Primary stability mostly comes from mechanical engagement of cortical bone, and it is a function of local bone quality and quantity, the geometry of an implant (i.e. length, diameter, and type), and the placement technique used. Primary stability occurs at the time of implant placement and is related to the level of primary bone contact and to the biomechanical properties of the surrounding bone. Secondary stability offers biological stability through remodeling and regeneration of surrounding bone, and results after the formation of secondary bone contact of woven and lamellar bone. During the early phase of healing process after implant placement osseointegration of the implant relies on primary or mechanical stability, and secondary or biological stability plays a major role for osseointegration with the decrease of primary stability over time (Fig. 2).

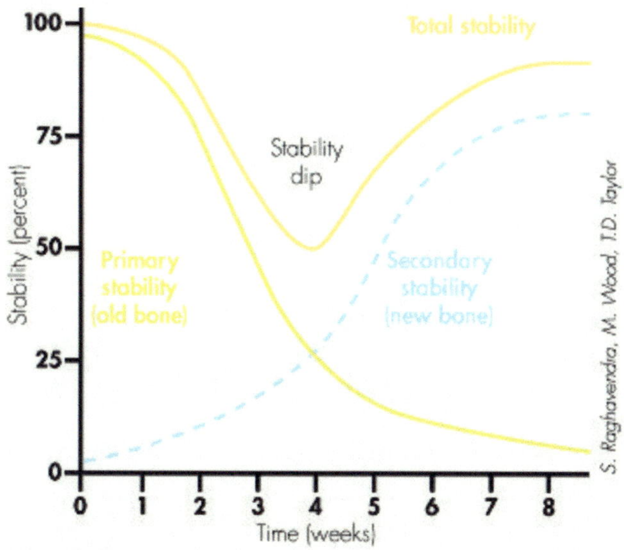

Fig. 2. Implant Stability Dip

Primary stability is a requirement of successful secondary stability. The latter, however, dictates the time of functional loading. Secondary stability has been shown to begin to increase at 4 weeks after implant placement.

Osseointegration and implant stability is affected by various factors during healing process (Table 2).

Factors affecting primary stability
Bone quality and quantity
Surgical technique, including the skill of the surgeon
Implant; geometry, length, diameter, surface characteristics
Factors affecting secondary stability
Primary stability
Bone regeneration and remodeling
Implant surface conditions

Table 2. Factors affecting implant stability

Available bone is particularly important in implant dentistry and describes the external architecture or volume of the edentulous area considered for implants. In addition, bone has an internal structure described in terms of density or quality, which reflects the strength of the bone. The density of available bone in an edentulous site is a determining factor in treatment planning, implant design, surgical approach, healing time, and initial progressive bone loading during prosthetic reconstruction.

The classification of bone density and its relation to dental implant treatments have been evaluated in the last three decades. Linkow in 1970, classified bone density into three categories:

Class I bone structure: This ideal bone type consists of evenly spaced trabeculae with small cancellated spaces.

Class II bone structure: The bone has slightly larger cancellated spaces with less uniformity of the osseous pattern.

Class III bone structure: large marrow-filled spaces exist between bone trabeculae.

Linkow stated that Class III bone results in a loose-fitting implant; Class II bone was satisfactory for implants; and Class I bone was a very satisfactory for implant restoration.

In 1985, Lekholm and Zarb listed four bone qualities based on both the radiographic assessment, and the sensation of resistance experienced by the surgeon when preparing the implant placement (Table 3; Fig. 3).

Quality 1: Entirely homogeneous compact bone

Quality 2: A thick layer of compact bone surrounding a core of dense trabecular bone

Quality 3: A thin layer of cortical bone surrounding dense trabecular boneof favorable strength

Quality 4: A thin layer of cortical bone surrounding a core of low-density trabecular bone

Bone type	Grade 1	Grade 2	Grade 3, 4
Cortical bone	Thick	Moderate	(very)Thin
Trabecular bone	Dense	Moderate	(very)Poor

Table 3. Tactile evaluation of the cortical and trabecular bone during surgery

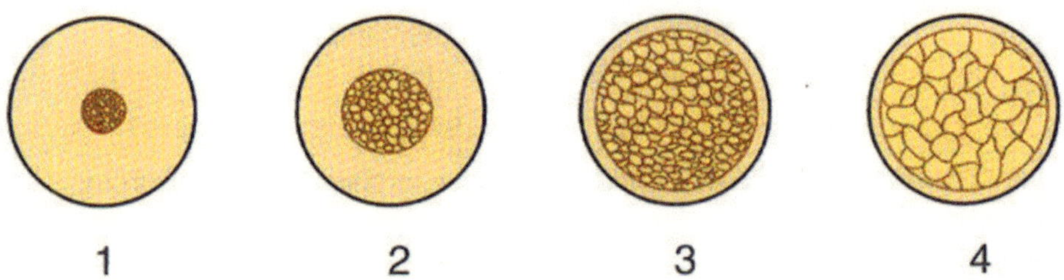

Fig. 3. Grading system for bone quality assessment (Lekholm & Zarb 1985).

In 1988, Misch defined four bone density groups based on macroscopic cortical and trabecular bone characteristics (Table 4). Based on Misch classification of bone density, human jaw bone is divided into the four regions and listed in Table 5.

Bone	Density
D1	Dense cortical bone
D2	Thick dense to porous cortical bone on crest and coarse trabecular bone within
D3	Thin porous cortical bone on crest and fine trabecular bone within
D4	Fine trabecular bone

Table 4. Misch Bone Density Classification

Bone	Anterior maxilla	Posterior maxilla	Anterior mandible	Posterior mandible
D1	0	0	6	3
D2	25	10	66	50
D3	65	50	25	46
D4	10	40	3	1

Table 5. Usual Anatomic Location of Bone Density Types (% Occurrence)

Osseointegrated implants have created a revolution in functional and esthetic rehabilitation in clinical dental practice. The surgical protocol proposed by Brånemark in 1969 included a 2-stage surgical technique: The implant was placed in bone and completely covered by oral mucosa, so that functional loading was avoided during the initial healing period of the bone tissue. The recommended healing period before functional loading was 6-month for maxilla and 4-month for mandible (Fig. 4).

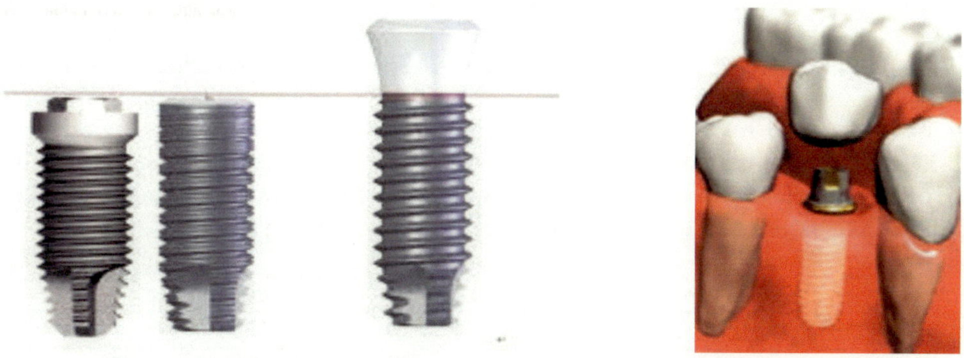

A B C

Fig. 4. Three Different Surgical approaches: (A) 2-stage (healing submerged, then uncovery surgery), (B) 1-stage (implant with permucosal healing, no uncovery surgery), and (C) immediate restoration (restoration placed at the time of the surgical placement).

However, the requirement of a healing period under submerged and stress-free conditions has been questioned. Research into immediate loading protocols has shown encouraging results since the 1980s. Several studies involving immediate loading of implants placed using a 1-step surgical protocol have been published in an attempt to improve the esthetic results, reduce the treatment period, and simplify the treatment process. In immediate loading protocols, an implant is placed in bone and loaded at once or within 48 hours of surgery. Immediate loading of dental implants has recently gained popularity due to such advantages from both clinicians and patients.

A fundamental prerequisite for the success of immediate loading of dental implants is bone density and primary stability at the time of insertion and following functional loading of the implant. If strong mechanical retention resulting from primary stability is not gained at the time of implant placement, there is a high risk of implant failure due to immediate functional or occlusal loading applied onto the implant. A poor bone density has been indicated as the main risk factors of implant failure as it may be associated with excessive bone resorption and impairment in the healing process compared with higher density bone. Therefore, the bone density of recipient sites of implants has to be precisely analyzed before, during, and after implant placement for the long-term success.

The three fore-mentioned classifications of bone density heavily rely on the clinician's tactile sensation of drilling into jaw bone during implant placement and the subjective radiographic evaluation of the clinician. Presently, more objective diagnostic analyses have been suggested to evaluate bone density at various time points and to estimate a long term prognosis based upon measured implant stability: 1) Housefield units (Hu) scale of computed tomography (CT), 2) Insertion torque value, 3) Removal torque.

2. Computed tomography

CT was invented by Housefield and was announced to the imaging world in 1972, but it had its origins in mathematics(1917) and astrophysics(1956). The first CT scanners appeared in medical imaging departments during the mid-1970s and were so successful that they largely replaced complex tomography by the early 1980s.

The power and usefulness of CT for maxillofacial imaging and diagnosis were apparent as soon as high resolution CT was introduced in early 1980s. CT was used for imaging the temporomandibular joint, evaluating dental-bone lesion, assessing maxillofacial deformities, and preoperative and postoperative evaluation of the maxillofacial region. CT provides a unique means of postimaging analysis of proposed surgery or implant sites by reformatting the image data to creat tangential and cross-sectional tomographic images of the implant site. The density of structures within the image is absolute and quantitative and can be used to differentiate tissues in the region and characterize bone quality(Table 6).

Density	Hounsfield Units
D1	1250
D2	850-1250
D3	350-850
D4	150-350
D5	<150

Table 6. Bone quality

CT enables the evaluation of proposed implant sites and provides diagnostic information that other imaging or combinations of imaging techniques cannot provide. The utility of CT for dental implant treatment planning was evident, but the access to these imaging techniques was limited. And even though advances enhanced diagnostic skills, there were inherent shortcomings to medical scanners used for dental purposes. Because medical scanners were not developed for dental reformatting, there existed inherent errors such as distortion, magnification, and positioning problems that led to inaccuracies when reformatted(Table 7).

advantages	Negligible magnification
	Relatively high-contrast image
	Various views
	Three-demensional bone models
	Interactive treatment planning
	Cross-referencing
limitations	Cost
	Technique sensitive
indications	Interactive treatment planning
	Determination of bone density
	Vital structure location
	Subperiosteal implant fabrication
	Determination of pathology
	Preplanning for bone augmentation

Table 7. Computed Tomography

This was overcome with the advent of sophisticated scanning appliances, stereolithographic resin bone models, interactive software, computer-generated surgical guides, and CT-based image-guided navigation system, which allowed for ideal placement and prosthetic outcome to be established.

Although the clinical problems of medical scanners have been remedied, there still existed numerous disadvantages-radiation exposure and availability. The amount of radiation exposure of medical scans has been shown to be excessive and unnecessary. It has been postulated that radiation exposure for a scan involving the maxilla and mandible is equivalent to approximately 20 panoramic radiographs.

3. Cone beam CT

3.1 A new type of CT

To overcome some of the disadvantages of conventional medical CT scanners, a new type of CT specific for dental applications has recently been developed. The x-ray dose absorbed by the patient during CT scanning may limit the use of this modality for routine diagnosis or repeated surveys. However, a new type of CT-CBCT(Cone Beam Computed Tomography) machine for the purpose of dental and maxillofacial imaging has been introduced (NewTom, Model QR-DVT 9000; QR, Verona, Italy) (Fig. 5) that lessens the patient's radiation exposure. The average absorbed radiation dose from a CBCT scanner (NewTom 3G) is approximately 12.0 mSv. This dose is equivalent to five D-speed dental x-rays or 25% of the radiation from a typical panoramic radiograph. Medical scanners acquire images that use radiation doses of 40 to 60 times that of CBCT doses.

The CBCT technique was employed previously in radiotherapy using fluoroscopic systems or modified simulators to obtain cross-sections of the patient in the same geometric conditions as the treatment. It was also used in vascular imaging and in microtomography of small specimens for biomedical and industrial applications. Nowadays, radiotherapy has become another relevant field for this machine.

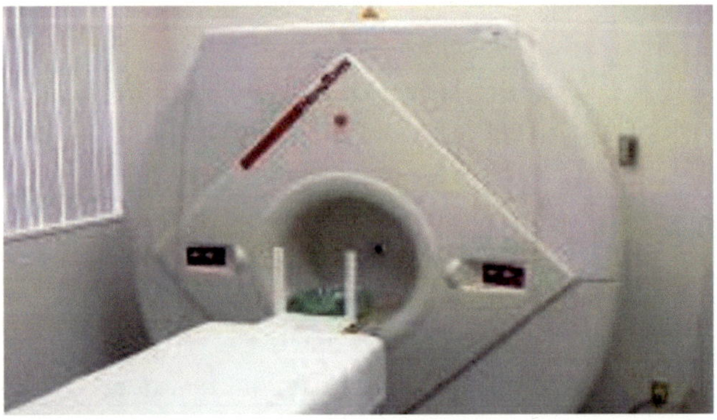

Fig. 5. Cone-beam computerized tomography (CBCT) device (NewTom)

In May 2001, CBCT imaging for dentistry was introduced to the United States by QR srl of Verona, Italy, the manufacturer of the New-Tom. This same company has recently developed a new model named NewTom 3G. Besides the latter, we can presently find four other models: I-CAT (Imaging Sciences International, Hatfield, USA), 3D Panoramic X-ray CT scanner PSR 9000N (Asahi Roentgen, Kyoto, Japan), CB MercuRay (Hitachi Medico Technology Corporation, Kashiwa, Chiba, Japan), and 3D Accuitomo (J. Morita, Kyoto, Japan). Specifications of these cone beam devices devoted to dentistry are shown in Table. 8.

Cone beam CT devices	Company	Size of Reconstructed Image(diameter x height)	X-ray source voltage (kV)	X-ray source current (xtime) mA(s)	Scanning time (s)	Voxel size (xy)	Min reconstr uct. Inc. or cubic
3D Accuitomo	J.Morita, Kyoto, Japan	4x3,4x4,6x6	60-80 (step 1kV)	1-10 mA (step 0.1mA)	18	0.125	0.125
NewTom 9000	Quantitative Radiology, Verona, Italy	13x13	110	15 mA	72	0.29	0.2
NewTom 3G		8x8,10x10,13x13,15x15, 18x18,22,22	110	15 mA	36	0.16-0.42	0.16
I-CAT	Imaging Sciences, Hatfield, Pennsylvania, USA	16x21,16x13,16x8,16x8	120	12.48 mAs, 23.87 mAs, 46.72 mAs	10,20,40	0.2-0.4	0.2
CB MercuRay	Hitachi, Medical, Kyoto, Japan	5.12x5.12,10.2x10.2, 15x15, 19x19	60-120 (step 20kV)	10 or 15 mA	10	0.1-0.4	0.1
3D Panoramic X-ray CT scanner PSR 9000N	Asahi Roentgen, Kyoto, Japan	3.6x4, 4.1x4	60-100 (step 1kV)	2-12 mA (step 2mA)	20,30	0.1-0.15	0.1-0.15

Table 8. Company, X-ray source voltage, X-ray source current (x time), scanning time, in plane voxel size and reconstruction increment for each cone beam CT device

This technique uses a cone-shaped x-ray beam centered on an x-ray area detector and is termed cone-beam CT (CBCT). As in conventional CT imaging, quantitative bone density measurements expressed in HU can be retrieved (quantitative CBCT [QCBCT]).Volume data can be acquired in a single rotation of the beam and detector (Fig. 6)

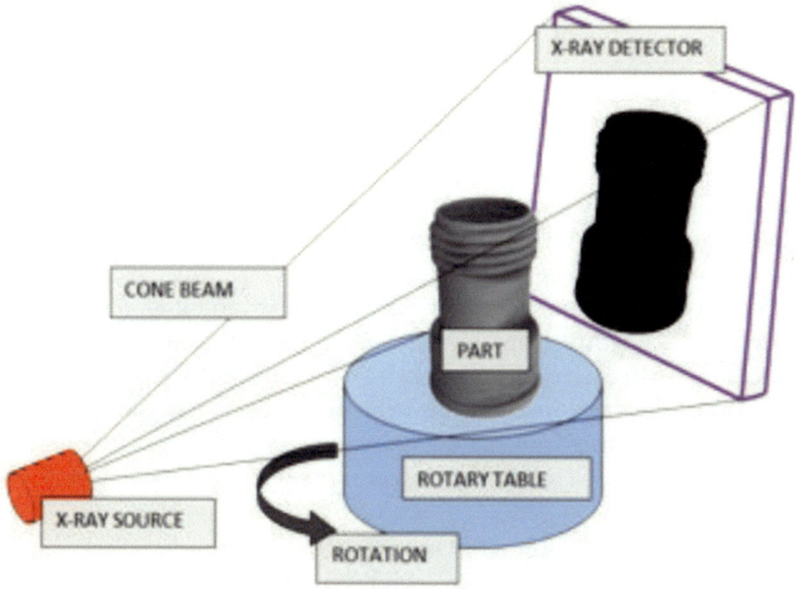

Fig. 6. Cone-shaped x-ray beam centered on an x-ray area detector

The amount of radiation absorbed by the patient for each scan is reportedly 0.62 mGy.Utilization of CBCT clearly illustrates the true 3-D shape and size of all anatomical structures. By combining CBCT and 3-D treatment planning, implants are being placed with ideal prosthetic results.

3.2 Image quality

Image quality on cone beam computed tomography was established that the generation of the CT hardware, data acquisition, and parameters such as slice thickness and interval of the reconstruction can determine the imaging resolution. Schulze et al. demonstrated high-contrast structures with the CBCT device. In addition, several authors revealed excellent image acquisition for different structures such as morphology of the mandible, location of the inferior alveolar canal, and even for the relationship of radioopaque templates to the bone. The error factor in CBCT is determined by the size of the voxel (Fig. 7).

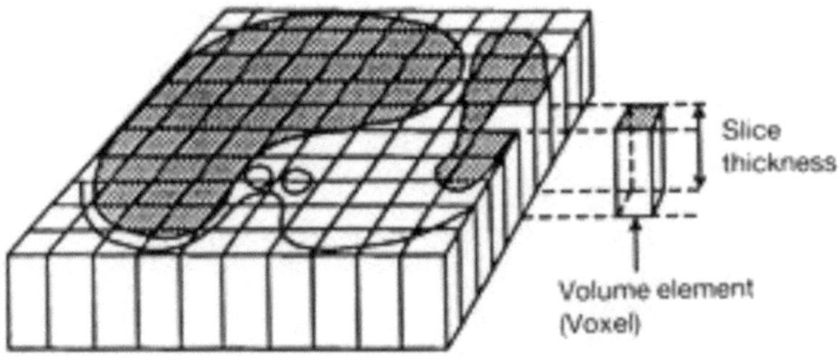

Fig. 7. Voxel Voxel, short for volume pixel, is the smallest distinguishable box-shaped part of a three-dimensional image. Voxelization is the process of adding depth to an image using a set of cross-sectional images known as a volumetric dataset. The dataset is processed when slices are stacked in computer memory based on inter-pixel and inter-slice distances to accurately reflect the real world sampled volume. Now that the data set exists as a solid block of data, the pixels in each slice have taken on volume and are now voxels. For a true 3-D image, voxels must undergo opacity transformation. Opacity transformation gives voxels different opacity values. This is important when it is crucial to expose interior details of an image that otherwise would be hidden by darker more opaque outside-layer voxels.

3.3 CBCT Imaging for implant installation

Implant Installation through the use of CBCT has dramatically helped to improve the placement of implants. Several imaging modalities have been used for the pre-surgical evaluation of implant sites. The panoramic, periapical and cephalometric images contain superimpositions, have large information voids related to depth and are affected by projection geometry so that measurements are not reliable. Only tomography, conventional CT scans and cone beam CT scans provide the information desired about each implant site. When the imaging goals are extended to occlusion, maxillomandibular spatial relationships and the temporomandibular joint then cone beam CT scans stands alone as the best value. Cone beam CT creates the opportunity to extend the information yield beyond the conventional imaging methods and is an ideal modality for implant planning. CBCT produces accurate 3 dimensional image data (Fig. 8). The field of view is scalable and one scan can include the entire maxillofacial region including the maxilla, mandible, base of skull and TMJs. The small voxel size would allow feature detection size and dimensional accuracy in the range of 0.2-0.8 mm. A single cone beam CT scan contains enough information to satisfy the imaging objectives stated above including maxillomandibular spatial relationships. The software used to create the images utilizes tools that accurately mark the delineation of the nerve and provide 1:1 images, allowing for accurate measurements. Software is used to display and visualize the anatomy in a way that is clinically meaningful. The software allows for multiplanar reformation and display.

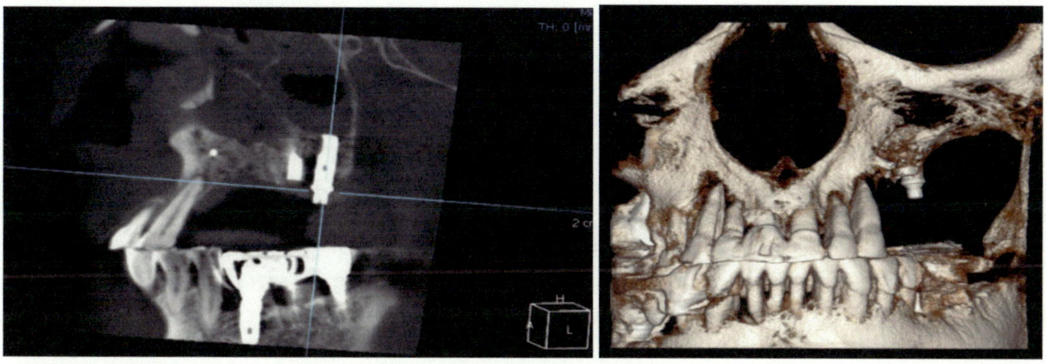

Fig. 8. Accurate 3 dimensional image data of Cone Beam CT (AZ-3000 CT, ASAHI)

But, many surgeons require additional information. They desire the ability to integrate the CBCT data into implant surgery. Using CBCT without any type of radiographic markers or a 3-D program that places implants into the study can be as analogous to arriving at a fork in the road with no directional signs leaving the surgeon unable to understand the true treatment plan (Fig. 9).

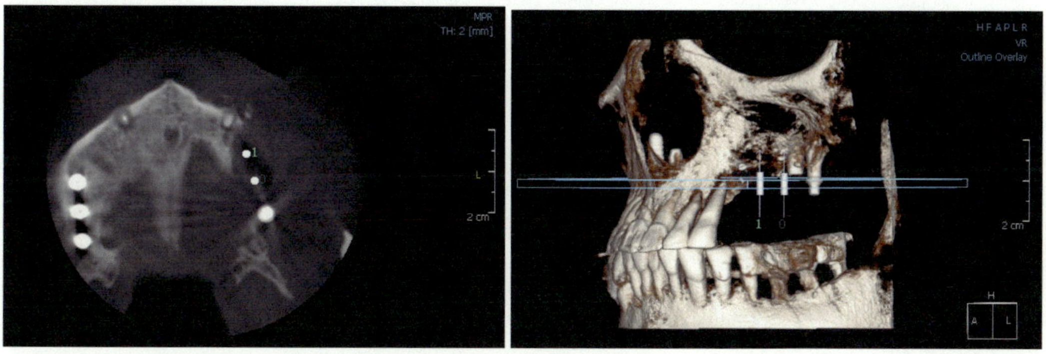

Fig. 9. Virtual Imaging of Implant Installation (AZ-3000 CT, ASAHI)

4. Insertion torque value

The cutting resistance refers to the energy required in cutting of a unit volume of bone (Friberg*et al.*, 1995) while the insertional torque occurs during the fixture tightening procedure (Ueda *et al.*, 1991). Both of these measurements consider the lateral compression force and friction at the interface during implant insertion and are mainly influenced by the tolerance of the fixture thread design (O'Sullivan *et al.*, 2000). Many researchers also used the peak insertional torque value, which is generated during the last fixture tightening step, as an indicator of primary implant stability.

A non-destructive quantitative method is necessary to measure the implant stability (Rasmusson et al.1998). A precise and scientifically established method for the evaluation of the bone quality/primary stability is the measure of the insertion torque (Al-Nawas et al. 2006; Rabel et al. 2007). The cutting resistance, during implant insertion, has been recommended in the evaluation of bone quality (Johansson et al. 2004). A high IT value probably indicates that the implant is stable from a mechanical point of view (Ito et al. 2008).

In cutting resistance analysis (CRA), originally developed by Johansson and Strid and later improved by Friberg et al in in vitro and in vivo human models, the energy (J/mm3) required for a currentfed electric motor in cutting off a unit volume of bone during implant surgery is measured. This energy was shown to be significantly correlated with bone density, which has been suggested as one of factors that significantly influences implant stability. To minimize the interoperator variation, hand pressure during drilling was controlled. CRA can be used to identify any area of low-density bone (or poor-quality bone) and to quantify bone hardness during the low-speed threading of implant osteotomy sites. A torque gauge incorporated within the drilling unit (eg, Osseocare; Nobel Biocare, Göteborg, Sweden) can be used to measure implant insertion torque in Ncm to indirectly represent J/mm3. Insertion torque values have been used to measure bone quality in various parts of the jaw during implant placement.

CRA gives a far more objective assessment of bone density than clinician-dependent evaluation of bone quality based on Lekholm and Zarb classification. Clinical relevance was demonstrated by studies that showed the highest frequency of implant failures in jaws with advanced resorption and poor bone quality, often seen in maxilla. Therefore, cutting resistance value may provide useful information in determining an optimal healing period in a given arch location with a certain bone quality.

The major limitation of CRA is that it does not give any information on bone quality until the osteotomy site is prepared. CRA also cannot identify the lower "critical" limit of cutting torque value (ie, the value at which and implant would be at risk). Furthermore, longitudinal data cannot be collected to assess bone quality changes after implant placement. Its primary use, therefore, lies in estimating the primary stability of an implant. For instance, in Misch's 6 time-dependent stages of implant failure-(1)surgical, (2)osseous healing, (3) early loading, (4) intermediate, (5)late, and (6) long-term- CRA can only provide information on the first 2 stages. Estimation of implant primary stability alone from CRA is still of value, as high implant failure rates are observed in the first 3 phases. Nonetheless, long-term evaluation of implant stability after implant placement, phases 3 to 7, is desired and should not be overlooked. This Limitation has led to development of other diagnostic tests. Table 9 summarizes CRA.

advantages	Detect bone density
	High correlation between cutting resistance and bone quality
	Reliable method to assess bone quality
	Identify bone density during surgery
	Can be used in daily practice
disadvantages	Can only be used during surgery

Table 9. Advantages and disadvantages of CRA

5. Removal torque value

The removal torque refers to the torsional force necessary for unscrewing the fixture and was first investigated by Johansson and coworkers (Johansson *et al.*, 1998). The removal torque value was recorded using a torque manometer calibrated in Newton-centimeters (Ncm).

Unlike CRA, which measures the bone density and the resistance to cutting torque, the reverse torque test (RTT), proposed by Roberts et al. and developed by Johansson and Albrektsson, measures the "critical" torque threshold where bone-implant contact (BIC) was destroyed. This indirectly provides information on the degree of BIC in a given implant. In the study conducted by Johansson and Albrektsson, a reverse torque was applied to remove implants placed in the tibiae of rabbits 1, 3, 6, and 12 months postsurgery. Reverse torque value and histologic evaluation showed that greater BIC could be achieved with a longer healing time. Similar observations at the histologic level have been made in other animal studies. Removal torque value (RTV) as an indirect measurement of BIC or clinical osseointegration was later reported to range from 45 to 48 Ncm in 404 clinically osseointegrated implants in humans. Sullivan et al further speculated that any RTV greater than 20Ncm may be acceptable as a criterion for a successful osseointegration, since none of the implants in their study could be removed during abutment connection at 20Ncm. It was further suggested that RTT is, therefore, a reliable diagnostic method for verification of osseointegration.

However, this method has been criticized as being destructive. Brånemark et al cautioned about the risk of irreversible plastic deformation within peri-implant bone and of implant failure if unnecessary load was applied to an implant that was still undergoing osseointegration. Furthermore, a 20Ncm threshold RTV for successful osseointegration has not yet been supported by scientific data. The threshold limit varies among patients depending on the implant material and the bone quality and quantity. A threshold RTV may be lower in type 4bone than in denser bone, for instance. Hence, subjecting implants placed in this bone type to RTV may result in a shearing of BIC interface and cause implant failure. Furthermore, RTV can only provide information as to "all or none" outcome (osseointegrated or failed); it cannot quantify degree of osseointegration. Hence, RTT is only used in experiments and has no clinical meaning.

6. Periotest

Periotest (Siemens AG, Benshein, Germany) uses an electromagnetically driven and electronically controlled tapping metallic rod in a handpiece (Fig. 10).

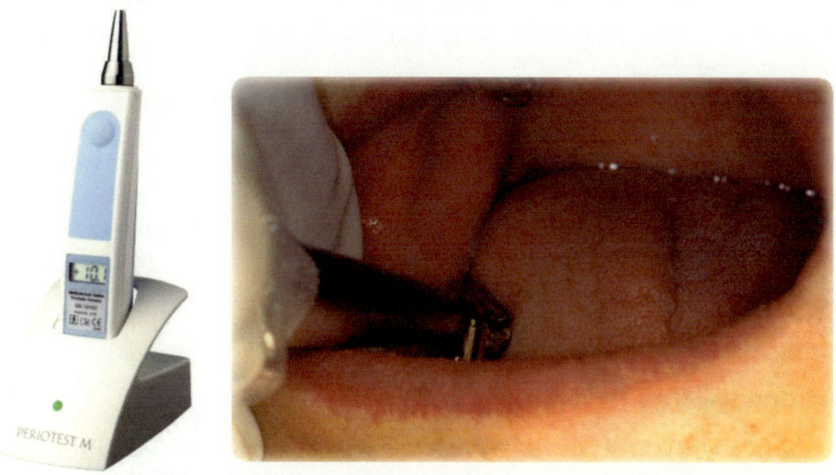

Fig. 10. Periotest (Siemens AG, Benshein, Germany)

Response to a striking or "barking" is measured by a small accelerometer incorporated into the head. Contact time between the test object and tapping rod is measured on the time axis as a signal for analysis. The signals are then converted to a unique value called the Periotest value (PTV), which depends on the damping characteristics of tissues surrounding teeth or implants. In the case of a natural tooth, the buffering capacity of the PDL poses a problem in analyzing the distribution of impact force exerted on a tooth. When dynamic characteristics are analyzed based upon an assumption that the whole periodontal structure functions as a mechanical unit, it is difficult to model the attenuation from the PDL. The soft tissue, including the periosteum, is considered a viscoelastic medium; thus, Hooke's law does not apply to the behavior of the PDL under and applied load. Thus, viscoelasticity of the PDL has always posed a difficulty in analysis of the physical characteristics of periodontal tissue. By contrast, bone-implant interface with no PDL is believed to be similar to the serial spring model which follows Hooke's law, and mobility measurement is considered easier.

Most reports of the use of a natural tooth mobility detector such as Periotest to measure implant mobility have pointed out a lack of sensitivity in these devices. Such devices permit a very wide dynamic range (in case of Periotest, PTV is -8 to +50) to permit the measurement of a wide variety of natural tooth mobility. However, the dynamic range used for measuring implant mobility is very limited. Thus, the sensitivity of these devices is insufficient to measure implant mobility.

In the use of mobility measurement to assess implant stability, the presence or absence of a PDL makes a crucial difference. Similar to impact/vibration testing, values measured with Periotest are significantly influenced by excitation conditions, such as position and direction. The Periotest user's manual contains clear instructions about striking point position and angle:"The Periotest measurement must be made In a midbuccal direction" and "During measurement the Periotest handpiece must always be held perpendicular to the tooth axes."

Even if it could be assumed that PTV precisely reflects the condition of BIC(bone implant contact) as reported by previous studies, an average PTV has no importance. Despite a wide variation in host factors such as bone density, normal PTV of an osseointegrated implant falls in a relatively narrow zone (-5 to +5) within a wide scale (-8 to +50). Therefore, the measured PTV may falsely be interpreted as having a small standard deviation and therefore viewed as having a good accuracy. PTV cannot be used to identify a "borderline implant" or "implant in the process of osseointegration" which may or may not continue to a successful osseointegration.

It has been suggested that these limitations of Periotest measurement have been suggested to be strongly related to the orientation of excitation source or striking point. In vitro and in vivo experiments demonstrated that the influence of striking point on PTV is much greater than the effects from increased implant length due to marginal bone resorption or other excitation conditions such as the angle of the handpiece or repercussion of a rod. Unfortunately, controlling these influential factors is extremely difficult. Despite some positive claims for Periotest, the prognostic accuracy of PTV for implant stability has been criticized for a lack of resolution, poor sensitivity, and susceptibility to operator variables.

7. RFA (resonance frequency analysis)

The resonance frequency analysis (RFA) method was presented by Meredith et al in 1996. RFA is a noninvasive diagnostic method that measures implant stability and bone density at various time points using vibration and a principle of structural analysis (Fig. 11).

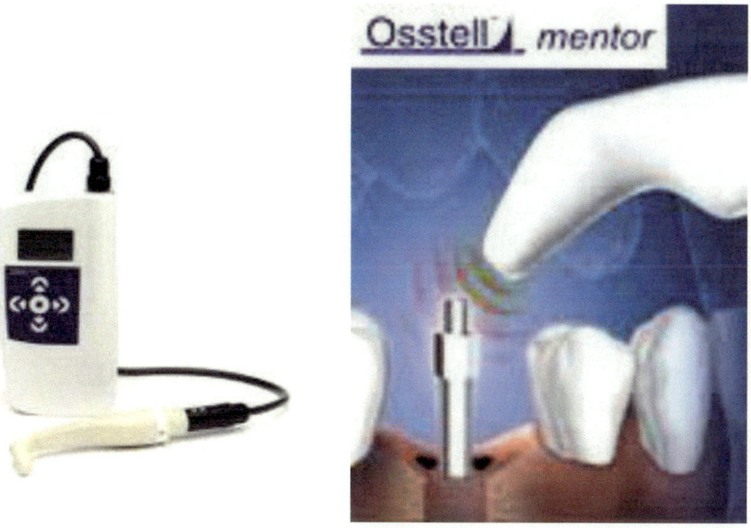

Fig. 11. RFA (Osstell AB, Göteborg, Sweden)

This method uses a small L-shaped transducer that is fastened by a screw to the implant or to the mucosa-penetrating abutment. Two piezoceramic elements are attached to the vertical beam. Using a personal computer, a frequency response analyzer, and dedicated software, the vertical beam of the transducer is vibrated over a range of frequencies, typically 5 kHz to 15 kHz, through one of the piezoceramic elements. The other serves as a receptor for the signal. Resonance peaks from the received signal indicate the first flexural resonance frequency of the measured object. In vitro and in vivo studies have suggested that this resonance peak may be used to assess implant stability in a quantitative manner.

It is assumed that an implant and the surrounding bone function as a single unit; thus, a change in stiffness is considered to represent the change of osseointegration of an implant. A steady-state sinusoidal force in a form of sine wave is applied to the implant-bone unit to measure the implant stability via resonance. Frequency and amplitude are then picked up as a response. Higher frequency and sharp peak indicate more stable implant, whereas a wider and lower peak and lower frequency indicate implant failure. In brief, RFA may be a useful method in predicting the prognosis of the implant after surgery.

8. Dominant frequency sound analyzer

This device (Fig.12) is still under the state of prototype, and it's mechanism of striking a target object is quite similar to that of periotest. Periotest measures the contact time of striking rod onto implant surface, and implant stability can be predicted by utilizing the contact time. Sound analyzer evaluates stability of the implant in a different way of analyzing specific striking sound of the implant compared with periotest. The sound of multiple strikes of an object is collected, graphically analyzed (Fig.13), and numerically displayed in average. Depending on the degree of osseointegration and implant stability different sound is produced from the same implant. Further investigations are still necessary to demonstrate versatile application of this device into the field of dentistry based on clinical evidences.

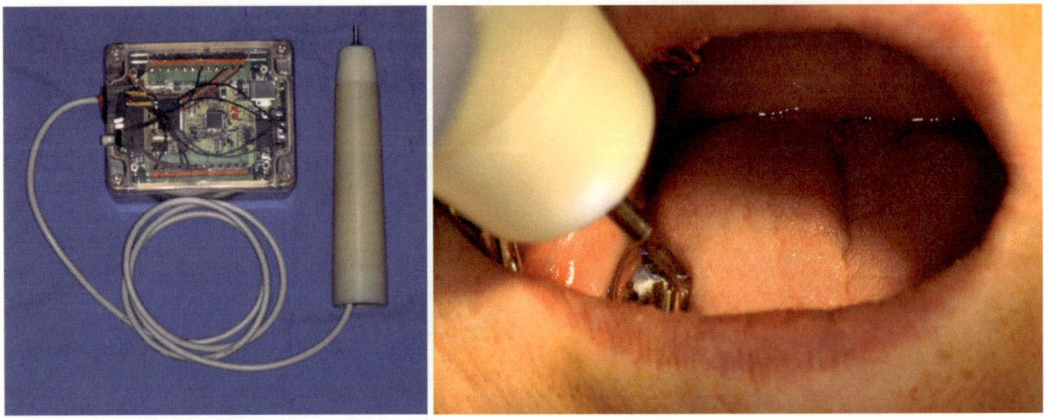

Fig. 12. Dominant Frequency Sound Analyzer

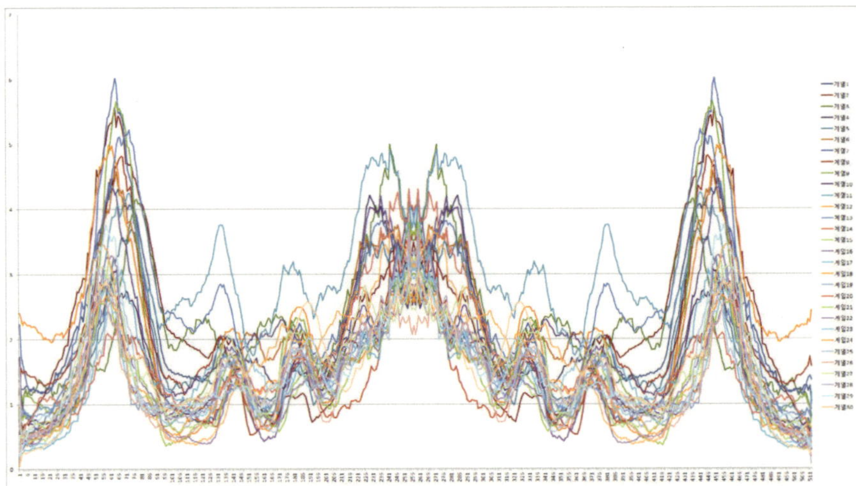

Fig. 13. Graphical analysis of sound analyzer

9. Clinical implications

Currently the use of osseointegrated implants to treat partially or completely the edentulous arch is considered reliable and predictable, with a success rate of 98% or higher. Among the factors affecting implant success, Bone density and implant stability are key factors to take into account and important for implant osseointegration, which has been widely demonstrated by several authors. Clinical studies show greater implant survival in the mandible than in the maxilla, due to the area's characteristics of bone density; more type I, II, or III bones are observed in the mandible than in the maxilla. New 3-D cone beam CT (CBCT) analyzes and classifies implant placement sites based on the bone density in Housefield units (Hu) with high reliability. With the aid of this high technology equipment it is possible to make an accurate treatment plan for the number, size, and location of implants along with the bone density at the implant placement sites and predict prognosis of the treatment before surgery. Periapical or panoramic radiographs are not very beneficial to determine bone density because the lateral cortical plates often obscure the trabecular bone density. In addition, classification of bone density on periapical or panoramic radiographs depends on clinician's subjective evaluation. The values of Housefield units are numerically displayed on CBCT, and bone density of the installation site is objectively classified by the numbers. Also, 3-D image of the operation sites allows to view precise vital structure locations and reduce the risk of damage to the structures during surgery. Now, measurements of periotest, insertion torque, or resonance frequency are widely used for the evaluation of implant stability before and after surgery. Many studies evaluated correlations between bone density measured by CBCT and implant stability by periotest, insertion torque, and resonance frequency analysis. It was reported that implant stability measured by RFA is most likely to have a positive relation with bone density measured by CBCT. However, there is no definite correlation between these three methods reported up to now. Along with the advancement of technology, it will be possible in near future to match the data obtained from CBCT to that of periotest, insertion torque, or RFA and predict long-term implant stability by utilizing CBCT.

10. References

Adell R, Ericksson B, Lekholm U, Branemark PI, Jemt T. A long-term follow-up study of osseointegrated implants in the treatment of totally edentulous jaws. Int J Oral Maxillofac Implants 1990;5:347-59.

Aparicio C. The use of the Periotest value as the initial success criteria of an implant:8-year report. Int J Periodontics Restorative Dent 1997;17:150-161.

Albrektsson T, Hansson T, Lekholm T. Osseointegrated dental implants. Dent Clin North Am 1986;30:151-174.

Albrektsson T, Zarb GA, Worthington P et al:The long-term efficacy of currently used dental implants: a review and proposed criteria of success, Int J Oral MaxillofacImpl 1:1-25, 1986.

Albrektsson T. A multicenter report on osseointegrated oral implants. J Prosthet Dent 1988;60:75-84.

Andersson J-E, Svartz K: CT scanning in the preoperative planning of ossointegrated implants in the maxilla, Int J Oral MaxillofacSurg 17:33-35, 1988.

Aral Y, Tammiasalo E, Iwai K: Development of a compact computed tomographic apparatus for dental use, Dentomaxillofac Radial 28A:245-248, 1999.

Arvidson K, Bystedt H, F4rykholm A, von Konow L, Lothigius E, A 3-year clinical study of Astra dental implants in the treatment of edentulous mandibles. Int J Oral Maxillofac Implants 1992;7:321-9.

Branemark P-I, Hansson BO, Adell T, et al. Osseointegrated implants in the treatment of the edentulous jaw. Experience from a 10-year period. Scand J PlastReconstrSurg 1977: 11 (Suppl.16): 39-94.

Branemark P-I, Zarb GA, Albrektsson T. Introduction to Osseointegration. In: Branemark P-I, Zarb GA, Albrektsson T (eds). Tissue-Integrated Prostheses Osseointegration in Clinical Dentistry. Chicago: Quintessence, 1985:11-76.

Brooks RA: comparative evaluation of CT scanner technology. In Fullerton GD, Zagzebski JA, editor: Medical physics monograph no. 6. Medical physics of CT and ultrasound: tissue imaging and characterization, New York, 1980, American Institute of physics.

Brunski JB. Biomechanical factores affecting the bone-dental implant interface. Clin Mater 1992;10:153-201.

Buser D, Mericske-Stern R, Bernard JP, et al. Long-term evaluation of non-submerged ITI implants. Part1: 8-year life table analysis of a prospective multi-center study with 2359 implants. Clin Oral Implants Res 1997;8:161-172

Buser D, Nydegger T, Hirt Hp, Cochran DL, Nolte LP. Removal torque values of titanium implants in the maxilla of miniature pigs. Int J Oral Maxillofac Implants 1988;13:611-619

Cann CE: Quantitative CT for for determination of bone mineral density: a review, Radiology 141:718-724, 1982.

Clark DE, Danforth RA, barnes RW et al: Radiation absorbed from dental implant radiography: a comparison of liner tomography, CT scan, and paroramic and intraoral techniques, J Oral Implants 3:156-164, 1990.

Cochran KL, Schenk RK, Lussi A, Higginbottom FL, Buser D. Bone response to unloaded and loaded titanium implants with a sandblasted and acid-etched surface: A histometric study in the canine mandible. J Biomed Mater Res 1998;40:1-11.

Cranin AN, Silverbrand H, Sher J et al: The requirements and clinical performance of dental implants. In Smith DC, Williams DF, editors: Biocompatibility of dental materials, vol4, p198, Boca Raton, Fla, 1982, CRC Press.

Dae-Hyun Lee, Young Ku, In-Chul Rhyu, Jeong-Ug Hong, Cheol-Woo Lee, Min-Suk Heo, Kyung-Hoe Huh.A clinical study of alveolar bone quality using the fractal dimension and the implant stability quotient. J Periodontal Implant Sci. 2010 February; 40(1): 19–24.

Dental implants:benefit and risk, A National Institutes of Health-Harvard consensus development conference, Publication 81:1531,Washington DC, 1980, U.S.Dept of Health and Human Services.

Derhami K, Wolfaardt JF, Faulkner G, Grace M. Assessment of the Periotest device in baseline mobility measurements of craniofacial implants. Int J Oral Maxillofac Implants 2995;10:221-229.

Engquist B, Bergendal T, Kallus T, Linden U. A retrospective multicenter evaluation of osseointegrated implants supporting overdentures. Int J Oral Maxillofac Implants 1988;3:129-134

Engstrom H, Svendsen P: Computed tomography of the maxilla in edentulous patients, Oral Surg Oral Med Oral Pathol 52:557-560, 1981.

Fjellstrom C-A, Strom C: CT of the edentulous maxilla intended for osseo-integrated implants, J CraniomaxillofacSurg 15:45-46, 1987.

Friberg B, Jemt T, Lekholm U. Early failures in 4,641 consecutively placed Branemark dental implants: A study from stage 1 surgery to the connection of completed prostheses. Int J Oral Maxillofac Implants 1991;6:142-146

Friberg B, Sennerby L, Grondahl K, Bergstorm C, Back T, Lekholm U. On cutting torque measurements during implant placement: A 3-year clinical prospective study. Clin Implant Dent Relat Res 1999;1:75-83

Friberg B, Sennerby L, Merredith N, Lekholm U. A comparison between cutting torque and resonance frequency measurements of maxillary implants. A 20-month clinical study. Int J Oral Maxillofac Surg 1999;28:297-303.

Friberg B, Sennerby L, Roos J, Johansson P, Strid CG, Lekholm U. Evaluation of bone density using cutting resistance measurements and microradiography: An in vitro study in pig ribs. Clin oral Implants Res 1995;6:164-171.

Friberg B, Sennerby L, Roos J, Lekholm U. Identification of bone quality in conjunction with insertion of titanium implants. A pilot study in jaw autopsy specimems. Clin Oral Implants Res 1995;6:213-219

Gapski R, Wang HL, Mascarenhas P, Lang NP. Critical review of immediate implant loading. Clin Oral Implants Res 2003;14:515-517.

Genant HK: Quantitative computed tomography: update, Calcif Tissue Int 41:179-186,1987.

Helms C, Morrish R, Kirocos LT: Computed tomography of the TMJ: preliminary considerations, Radiology 141:718-724, 1982.

Hendee WR: the physical principles of computed tomography, Boston, 1983, Little, brown.

Herrmann I, Lekholm U, Holm S, Kultje C. Evaluation ofpatient and implant characteristics as potential prognosticfactors for oral implant failures. Int JOralMaxillofacImplants 2005;20:220–30.

Hounsfield GN: Computerized transverse axial scanning (tomography), Br J Radial 46:1016-1022, 1973.

Ito K, Gomi Y, Sato S, Arai Y, Shinoda K (2001) Clinical application of a new compact CT system to assess 3-D images for the preoperative treatment planning of implants in the posterior mandible. A case report. Clin Oral Implants Res12:539–542

Ito K,Yoshinuma N,Goke E, Arai Y, Shinoda K. Clinical application of a new compact computed tomography system for evaluating the outcome of regenerative therapy: A case report. J Periodontol 2001;72: 696–702.

Jemt T, Lekholm U, Adell R. Osseointegrated implants in the treatment of partially edentulous patients: A preliminary study on 876 consecutively placed fixtures. Int J Oral Maxillofac Implants 1989;4:211-217

Jensen O, The Carter hypothesis. In: Buser K, Kahlin C, Schenk RK (eds). Guided Bone Regeneration in Implant Dentistry. Hong Kong: Quintessence, 1994:238-239.

Joe Merheb, Nele Van Assche, Wim Coucke, Reinhilde Jacobs, Ignace Naert, Marc Quirynen. Relationship between cortical bone thickness or computerized tomography-derived bone density values and implant stability. Clinical oral implants research.21, 2010;612-617.

Johansson C, Albrektsson T. Integration of screw implants in the rabbit: A 1-year follow-up of removal torque of titanium implants. Int J Oral Maxillofac Implants 1987;2:69-75

Johansson CB, Albrektsson T. A removal torque and histomorphometric study of commercially pure niobium and titanium implants in rabbit bone. Clin Oral Implants Res 1991;2:24-29

Johansson CB, Sennerby L. Albrektsson T. A removal torque and histomorphometric study of bone tissue reactions to commercially pure titanium and vitallium implants. Int J Oral Maxillofac Implants 1991;6:437-441

Johansson P, Strid K. Assessment of bone quality from cutting resistance during implant surgery. Int J Oral Maxillofac Implants 1994;9:279-288

Jun SH, Chang BM, Weber HP, Kwon JJ. Comparison of initial stability parameters and histomorphometric analysis of implants inserted into extraction sockets: human fresh cadaver study. Int J Oral Maxillofac Implants. 2010 Sep-Oct;25(5):985-90.

Jurzeler MB, Quinones CR, Schupbach P, Vlassis JM, Strub JR, Caffesse RG. Influence of the suprastructure on the perio-implant tissues in eagle dongs. Clin Oral Implants Res 1995;6:139-148

Kim KD, Jeong HG, Choi SH et al: Effect of mandibular positioning on pre-implant site measurement of the mandible in reformatted CT, Int J PeriodontRset Dent 23:177-183, 2003.

Kircos LT: Quantitative implant imaging with a focus on interactive computed tomography: successful implant cases. Are they possible? For how long?Lecture, March 13-14, 1994, Loma Linda University.

Lekholm U. Zarb Ga, Albrektsson T (eds). Tissue-integrated Prostheses: Osseointegration in Clinical Dentistry. Chicago:Quintessence, 1985;199-209

Lindh T, Gunne J, Tillberg A, Molin M. A meta-analysis of implants in partial edentulism. Clin Oral Implants Res 1998;9:80-90

Linkow LI, Chercheve R: Theories and techniques of oral implantology, vol. I, St Louis, 1970, Mosby.

MaGivney GP, Haughton V, Strandt IE et al: A comparison of computer-assisted tomography and data-gathering modalities in prosthodontics, Int J Oral Maxillofac Implants 1:55-58, 1986.

McKinney RV, Koth DC, Steflik DE:Clinical standards for dental implants. In Clark JW, editor: Clinical dentistry, p198, Harperstown, PA, 1984, Harper & Row.

Meredith N. Assessment of implant stability as a prognostic determinant. Int J Prosthodont 1998;11:491-501

Meredith N. Shagaldi F, Alleyne D, Sennerby L, Cawley P. The application of resonance frequency measurements to study the stability of titanium implants during healing in the rabbit tibia. Clin Oral Implants Res 1997;8:234-243.

Mihoko Atsumi, Sang-hoon Park, Hom-Lay Wang. Methods used to Assess Implant Stability: Current Status, Quintessence2007 Vol 22, number 5, 743-754

Misch C, Meffert RM. Implant quality of health scale: A clinical assessment of the health disease continuum In: Mish C(ed). Dental Implant Prosthetics. St Louis: Elsevier Mosby, 2005;596-603

Misch CE: Bone character: second vital implant criterion. Dent Today 39-40, June/July 1988.

Misch CE: Density of bone: Effect on treatment plans, surgical approach, healing, and progressive loading, Int J Oral Implant 6:23-31, 1990.

Morris HE, Ochi S, Crum P, Orenstein I, Plezia R. Bone density: Its influence on implant stability after uncovering. J Oral Implantol 2003;29:263-269

Mozzo P, Procacci C, Tacconi A, Martini PT, Andreis IA (1998) A new volumetric CT machine for dental imaging based on the cone-beam technique: preliminary results. Eur Radiol 8:1558–1564

Mozzo P, Procacci C, Tacconi A: A new volumetric CT machine for dental imaging based on the cone-beam technique, Eur Radial 8:1558-1564,1988.

Mozzo P, Procacci C,Tacconi A,Martini PT,Andreis IA.A new volumetric CT machine for dental imaging based on the cone-beam technique: Preliminary results. Eur Radiol 1998;8: 1558–1564.

Naert IE, Rosenberg D, van Steenberghe D, Tricio JA, Nys M. The influence of splinting procedures on the periodontal and peri-implant tissue damping characteristics. A longitudinal study with the Periotest device. J Clin Periodontal 1995;22:703-708

Nakagawa Y, Kobayashi K, Mishima, Ishii H, Asada K, Ishibashi K (2002) Preoperative application of limited cone beam computerized tomography as an assessment toll before minor oral surgery. Int J Oral Maxillofac Surg 31:322–327

Norton MR, Gamble C: Bone classification: an objective scale of bone density using the computerized tomography scan, Clin Oral Implants Res 12:79-84,2001.

O'Sullivan D, Sennerby L, Jagger D, Meredith N. A comparison of two methods of enhancing implant primary stability. Clin Implant Dent Relat Res 2004;6:48-57

Olive J, Aparicio C. Periotest method as a measure of osseointegrated oral implant stability. Int J Oral Maxillofac Implants 2990;5:390-400

Rasmusson L, Meredith N, Kahnberg KE, Sennergy L. Stability assessments and histology of titanium implants placed simultaneously with autogenousonlay bone in the rabbit tibia. Int J Oral MaxillofacSurg 1998;27:229-235.

Roberts WE, Helm FR, Marshall KJ, Gongloff RK, Rigid endosseous implants for orthodontic and orthopedic anchorage. Angle Ortho 1989;59:247-256

Roberts WE, Smith RK, Zilberman Y, Mozsary PG, Smith RS. Osseous adaptation to continuous loading of rigid endosseous implants. Am J Orthod 1984;86:95-111

Romanos GE, Toh CG, Siar CH, Wicht H, Yacoob H, NentwigGH. Bone–implant interface around titanium implantsunder different loading conditions: a histomorphometricalanalysis in the Macacafascicularis monkey. Journal ofPeriodontology 2003;74:1483–90.

Sarment D, Sukovic P, Clinthorne N: Accuracy of implant placement with a stereolithogrphic surgical guide, Int J Oral maxillofacImpl 18:571-577, 2003.

Schnitman PA, Shulman LB: Recommendations of the consensus development conference on dental implants,J Am Dent Assoc 98:373-377,1979.

Schulze D, Heiland M, Schmelzle R, Rother UJ (2004) Diagnostic possibilities of cone-beam computed tomography in the facial skeleton. Int Congr Ser 1268:1179–1183

Sennerby L, Roos J. Surgical determinants of clinical success of osseointegrated oral implants: A review of the literature. Int J Prosthodont 1998;11:408-420.

Song YD, Jun SH, Kwon JJ. Correlation between bone quality evaluated by cone-beam computerized tomography and implant primary stability. Int J Oral Maxillofac Implants. 2009 Jan-Feb;24(1):59-64.

Shahlaie M, Gantes B, Schulz E et al: Bone density assessments of dental implant sites: quantitative computed tomography, Int J Oral Maxillifac Implants 18:224-231, 2003.

Sullivan DY, Sherwood RL, Collins TA, Krogh PH. The reverse torque test: A clinical report. Int J Oral Maxillofac Implants 1996;11:179-185

Swartz MS, Rothman SLG, Rhodes ML et al: Computed tomography. 1. Preoperative assessments of the mandible for edentulous implants surgery, Int J Oral Maxillofac Implants 2: 137-141, 1987

Teerlinck J, Quirynen M, Darius P, van Steenberghe D. Periotest: An objective clinical diagnosis of bone apposition toward implants. Int J Oral Maxillofac Implants 1991;6:55-61.

Tjellstrom A, Jacobsson M, Albrektsson T. Removal torque of osseointegrated craniofacial implants: A clinical study. Int J Oral Maxillofac Implants 1988;3:287-289

Van Steenberghe D, Lekholm U, Bolender Ch, et al. The applicability of osseointegrated oral implants in the rehabilitation of partial edentulism: a prospective multicenter study on 558 fixtures. Int J Oral Maxillofac Implants 1990;5:275-81.

Vannier MW: Craniofacial computed tomography scanning: technology, application, and future trends, Orthod Craniofacial Res 6(suppl 1):23-30, 2003.

14

Three-Dimensional CT Analysis of Congenital Scoliosis and Kyphosis: A New Classification

Shiro Imagama[1], Noriaki Kawakami[2] and Naoki Ishiguro[1]
[1]*Department of Orthopaedic Surgery, Nagoya University Graduate School of Medicine*
[2]*Department of Orthopaedic Surgery, Meijo Hospital*
Japan

1. Introduction

With advances in spine surgery, congenital spine deformity can now be treated with corrective fusion and osteotomy, even in young children. In these patients, the spine has various complications of vertebral anomalies and congenital fusion. A successful and safe outcome of corrective surgery requires evaluation by imaging preoperatively. Congenital spinal anomaly has conventionally been evaluated on plain radiographs using the classification described by Winter et al. in 1973 (Winter et al. 1973) as formation failure, segmentation failure, and mixed type (Table 1).

1. Failure of formation	Complete failure of formation (hemivertebra, butterfly vertebra)
	Partial failure of formation (wedged vertebra)
2. Failure of segmentation	Unilateral failure of segmentation (unilateral unsegmented bar)
	bilateral failure of segmentation (block vertebra)
3. Miscellaneous	Mixed type

Table 1. Winter's classification of congenital scoliosis on plain radiographs, as first described by Winter et al. in 1973 (partially modified for simplicity)

It is now clear that the complicated anomalies and the relationship between anterior and posterior components cannot be fully evaluated on plain radiographs only. We often encounter intraoperative findings that differ from preoperative findings on plain radiographs. Therefore, improved imaging evaluation of congenital anomalies is important to avoid difficulties during surgery. Preoperative 3-dimensional CT evaluation (3DCT) is very useful in this respect (Newton et al. 2002, Nakajima et al. 2007) since it allows clearer observation of morphology and fusion compared to plain radiographs (Fig. 1). Based on evaluation of many cases with 3DCT, we have established a new classification of congenital spine anomaly (Kawakami et al. 2009). In this chapter, we introduce the utility of 3DCT and describe variations of congenital deformity detected by 3DCT, based on Winter's classification of deformity.

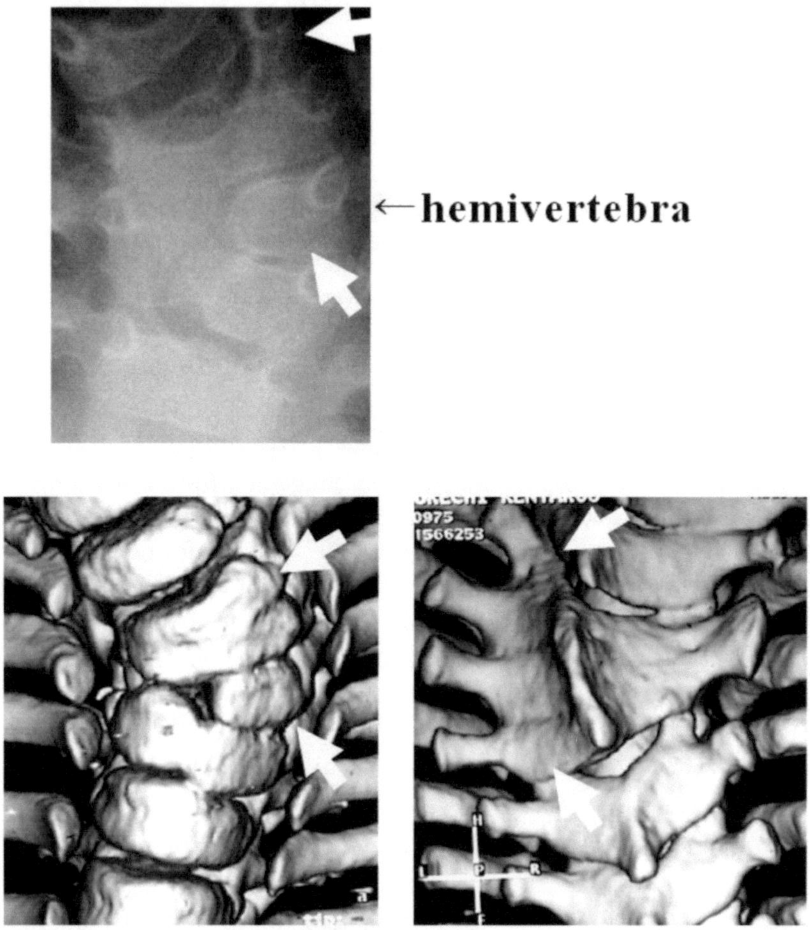

Fig. 1. **Congenital scoliosis of a hemivertebra with posterior fusion.** A hemivertebra (arrow) on the upper side may be missed and without 3DCT it can be difficult to evaluate the relationships of morphologic changes with anterior and posterior bony fusion.

2. Three-dimensional analysis of congenital anomaly

2.1 Formation failure

2.1.1 3DCT evaluation of morphology

Formation failures in Winter's classification are defined by morphology, and include a hemivertebra with one lateral pedicle, a butterfly vertebra, and a wedge vertebra with a bipedicle. However, evaluation of the morphology of the anterior component can be difficult and evaluation of posterior components is often particularly difficult on plain radiographs. In contrast, 3DCT effectively reveals the morphology of the anterior and posterior components of the spine, and these images show that there are various patterns of posterior components.

First, we show a fully segmented hemivertebra and fully segmented hemilamina (Fig. 2). A plain radiograph shows the morphological change of the vertebra and suspected hemivertebra because of scoliosis, but does not reveal the details, whereas these are shown clearly on 3DCT. This type is a half structure of normal anterior and posterior components, which may be understood easily.

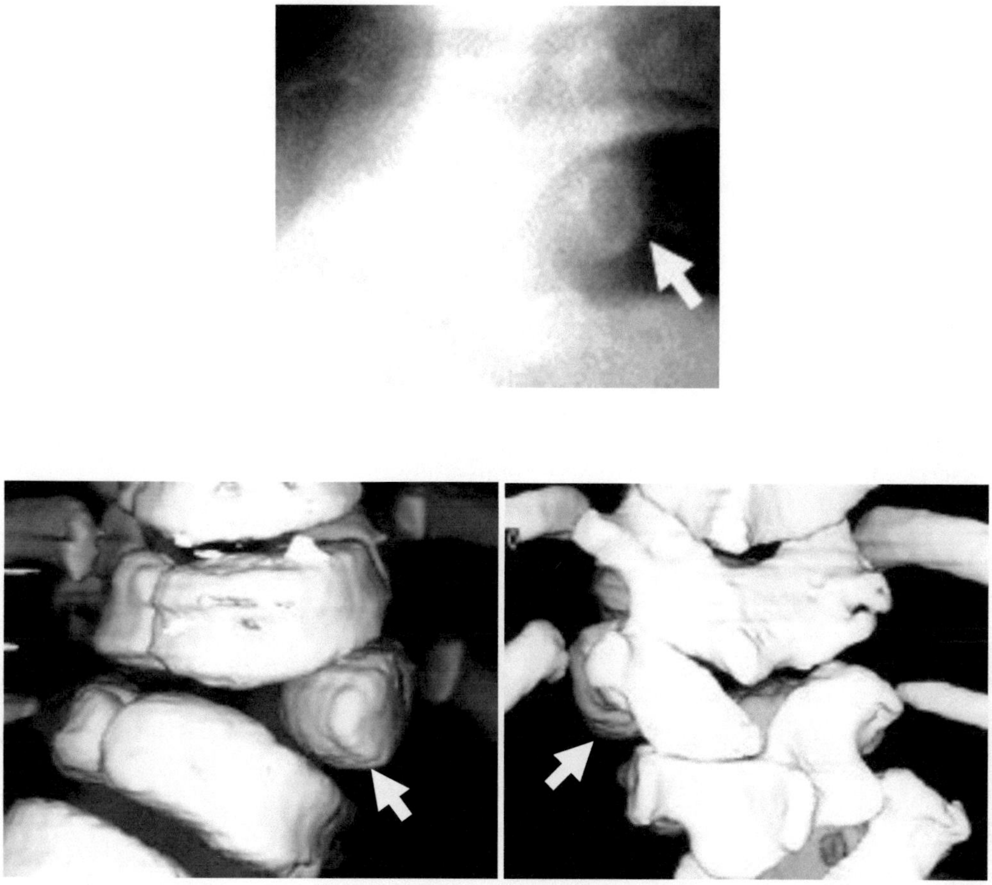

Fig. 2. **Fully-segmented hemivertebra with hemilamina.** The 3DCT images show a combination of a hemivertebra (anterior) and hemilamina (posterior) without bony fusion (arrow). In contrast, the plain radiograph shows no details of the morphology of the anterior and posterior components.

There are also other types of posterior components with a hemivertebra, including fully segmented bilamina (Fig. 3) and spina bifida (Fig. 4).

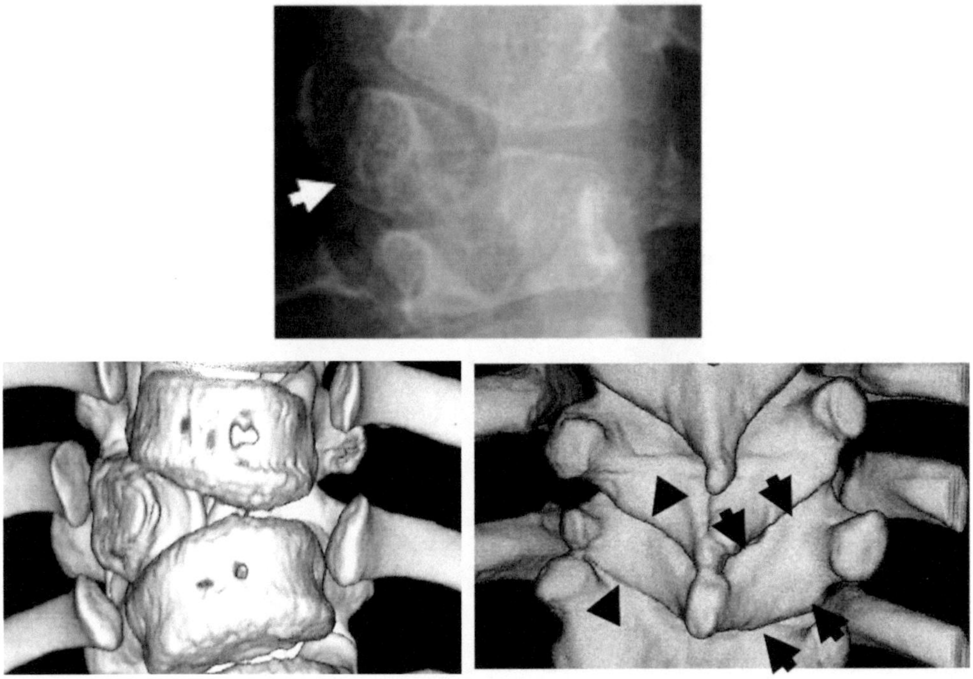

Fig. 3. **Fully-segmented hemivertebra and fully segmented bilamina.** A plain radiograph shows a hemivertebra (white arrow), but does not show the posterior components. 3DCT clearly showed bilamina that differed from the case in Fig. 2 (black arrow: same side of hemivertebra, arrowhead: opposite side of hemivertebra).

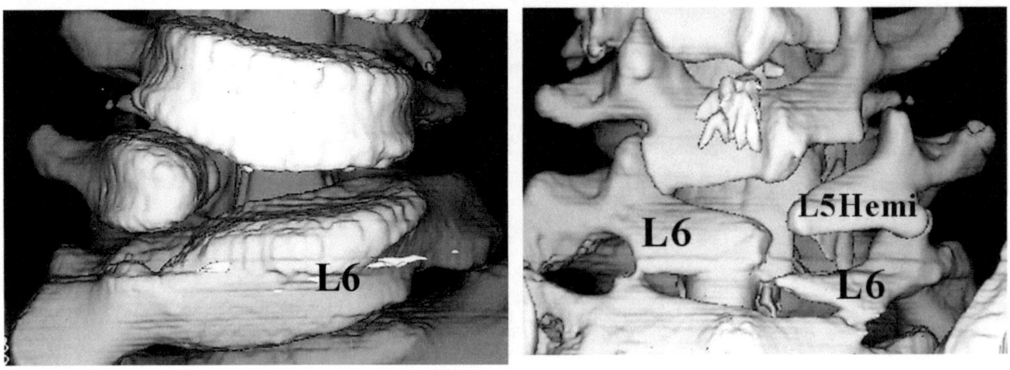

Fig. 4. **Fully-segmented hemivertebra and spina bifida.** The spina bifida type has a characteristic morphology of the posterior component. This type is located around the sacrum in most cases.

We show a summary of the combination of morphology of anterior and posterior components in formation failure in Table 2. For butterfly vertebra and lateral wedged vertebra, it is also likely that the morphology of the posterior component may vary, as for hemivertebra. There are many possible combinations of formation failures in both anterior and posterior components based on evaluation by 3DCT (Fig. 5).

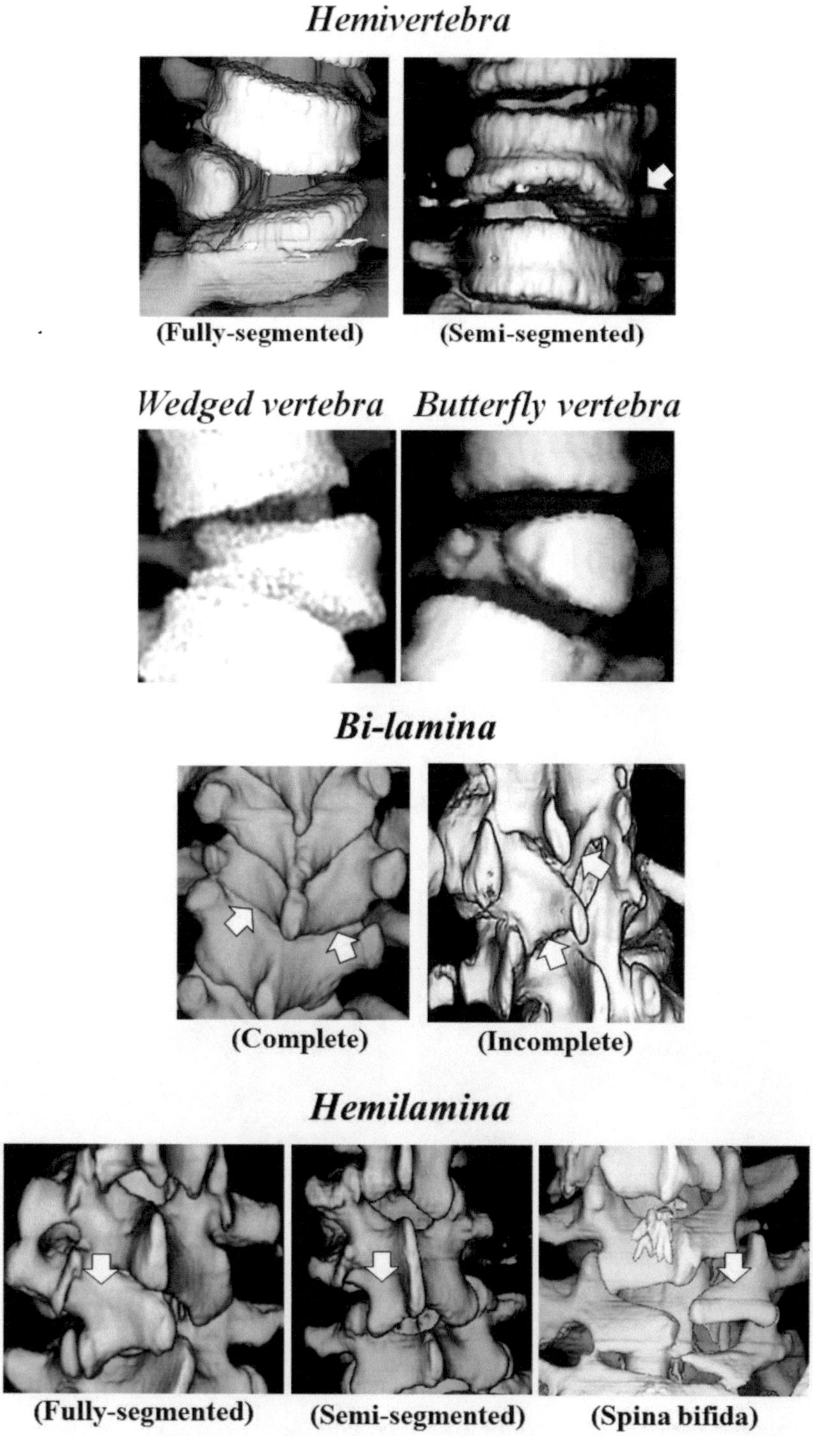

Fig. 5. Typical variation of type of formation failure in anterior and posterior components based on 3DCT. Arrows indicate formation failures.

Anterior component	Posterior component
Hemivertebra (hemi-pedicle)	Fully segmented hemilamina
	Semisegmented hemilamina
	Spina bifida
	Bilamina (complete or incomplete)
Butterfly vertebra (bipedicle)	Wedged lamina
	Spina bifida
Lateral wedged vertebra (bipedicle)	Wedged lamina

Table 2. Combination of morphology of anterior and posterior components in formation failure.

Segmentation failure may also occur in anterior and/or posterior components (semisegmented hemivertebra, semisegmented hemilamina) (Fig. 5) and solitary malformation and multiple anomalies must also be taken into account (Kawakami et al. 2009).

2.1.2 Anteroposterior (AP) unison anomaly and discordant anomaly

Malformed vertebrae in the solitary group and the simple type in the multiple malformation group may be explained by formation failure of vertebral components one by one. The usual pattern can be referred to as "an anteroposterior unison anomaly" (Nakajima et al. 2007). However, 3DCT findings indicate that posterior components are sometimes mismatched with anterior components. This malformation pattern can be referred to as "anteroposterior discordant anomaly"(Fig. 6). It also appears that this type is due to formation failure, segmentation failure, and mixed type (described below).

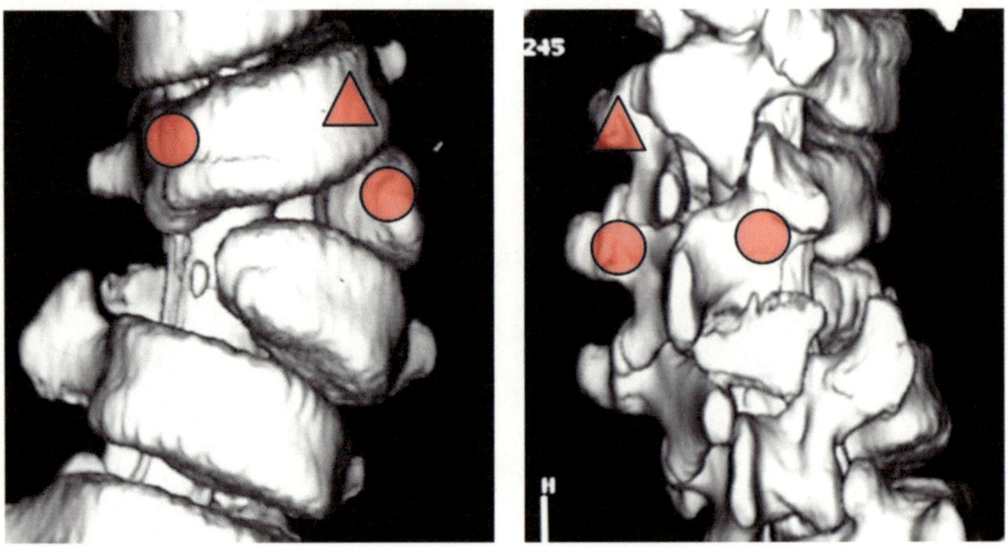

Fig. 6. **Anteroposterior (AP) discordant anomaly.** Left hemivertebra composed of the same lamina with the right upper segment at posterior. The anterior component is not matched to a posterior component (AP discordant anomaly).

2.2 Segmentation failure

Bony fusion (segmentation failure) and formation failure are often seen in 3DCT, with more cases than expected having a mixed type in Winter's classification (Fig. 7). The semisegmented hemivertebra and semisegmented hemilamina shown in Fig. 5 can be evaluated based on unsegmented morphological changes. However, other types of bony fusion (i.e. segmentation failure) can be identified by 3DCT evaluation. Therefore, we introduce segmentation failure in this chapter. Since evaluation of all cases of segmentation failure as one group is complicated, we examined these cases in categories of segmentation failure alone (without formation failure) (Imagama et al. 2004) and formation failure with segmentation failure (mixed type in Winter's classification) (Imagama et al. 2005).

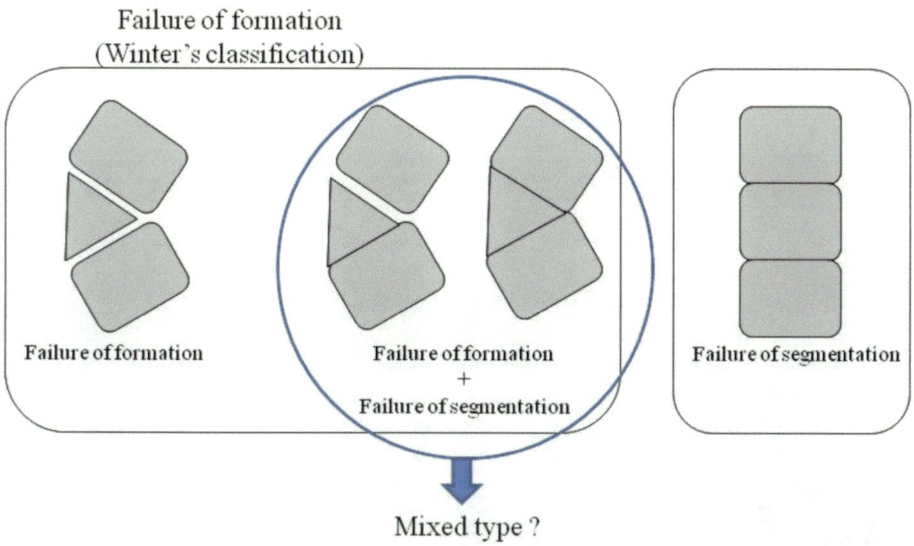

Fig. 7.**Ambiguous border of segmentation failure.** Failure of formation in Winter's classification includes fully segmented, semisegmented, and nonsegmented hemivertebrae. However, semisegmented and nonsegmented vertebrae have the same characteristics of segmentation failure as a block vertebra with segmentation failure (Kawakami et al. 2009). Therefore, failure of formation in Winter's classification also includes mixed type.

2.2.1 Segmentation failure (without formation failure)

3D-CT images for 25 patients with congenital scoliosis (failure of segmentation) were examined to determine the fusion abnormalities of the vertebral bodies and those of the laminae, pedicles, ribs and transverse processes. The vertebral body was defined as the anterior component, the pedicle, transverse process and rib as the lateral components, and the lamina and spinous process as the posterior components. We classified the 25 cases into three groups and investigated the posterior features in each group. One group had anterior fusion only (group A: 8 cases), the second had anterolateral fusion (group AL: 14 cases), and the third had posterior fusion only (group P: 3 cases) on 3DCT. In this series, we did not find any cases of lateral fusion only. In group A, all vertebral bodies had a posterior component with which they originally belonged (i.e. unison) (Fig. 8). All cases had normal posterior structures that were fully segmented.

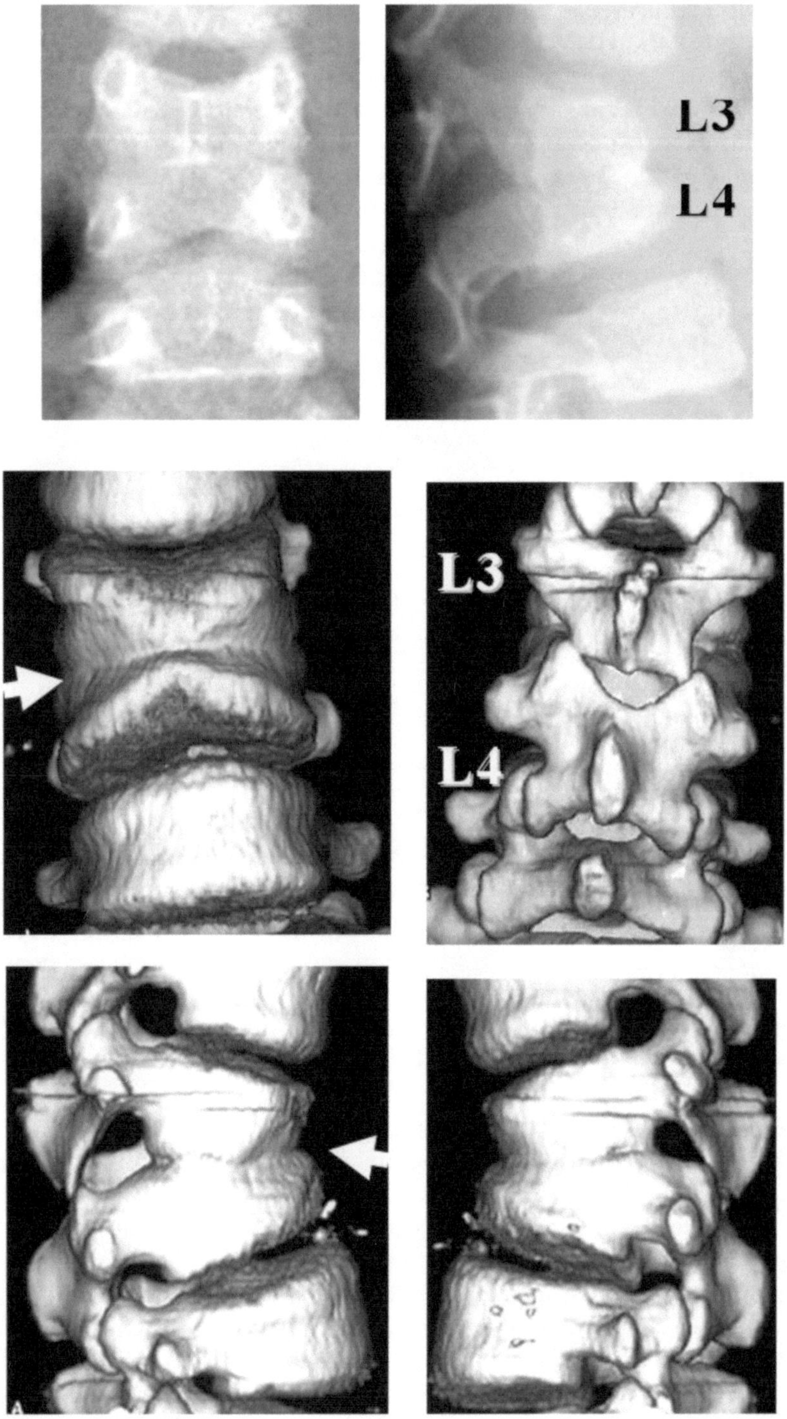

Fig. 8. **Segmentation failure only (group A).** These cases had anterior fusion (arrow) with normal posterior components.

In group AL, all cases had congenital fusion posterior components. In all cases in group AL, the vertebral bodies paired with posterior components with which they originally belonged (i.e. unison) (Fig. 9).

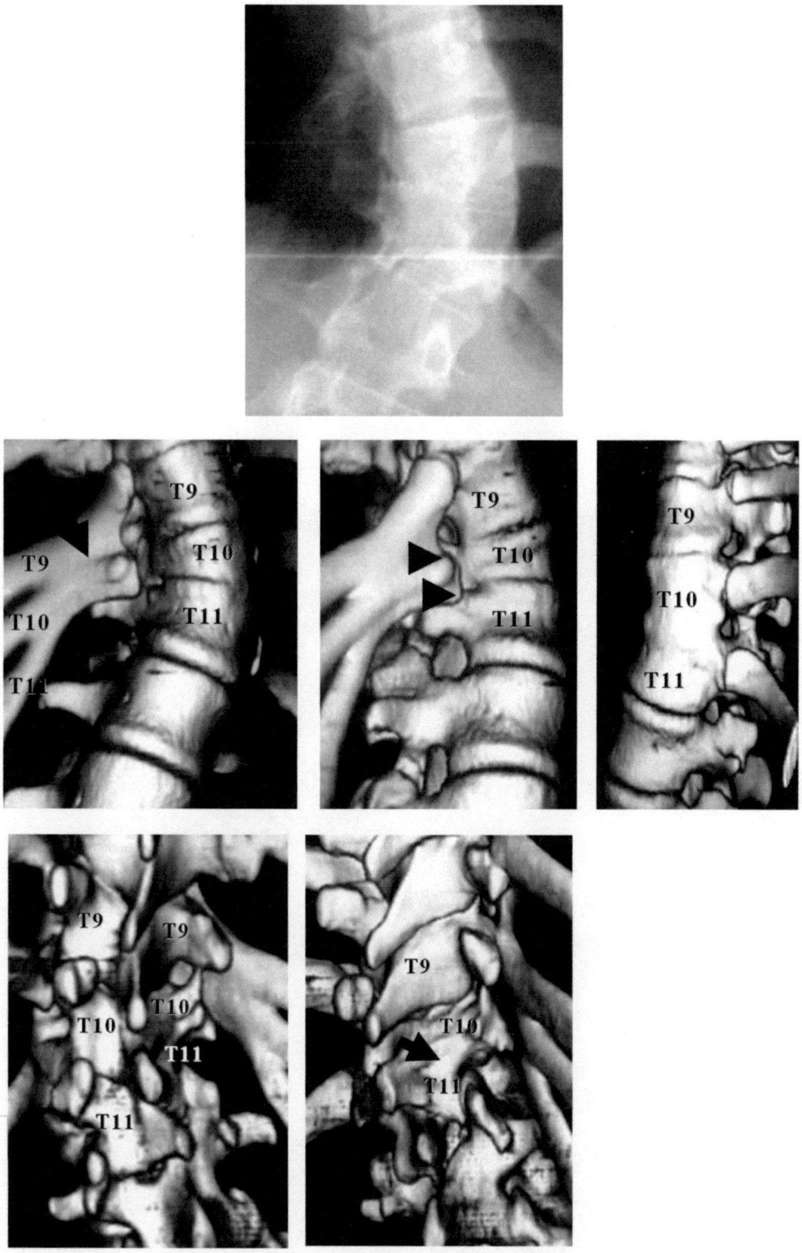

Fig. 9. **Segmentation failure only (group AL).** In this case, anterior, lateral (pedicle, transverse process and ribs) (arrowhead) and posterior (arrow) components were fused only on the left side, with no fusion on the right side.

In group P, posterior components (lamina and spinous process) were fused. Two cases showed unison anomalies (Fig. 10) and one had a discordant anomaly in which the vertebral bodies made another pair with posterior components with which they did not originally belong (Fig. 11). We also accidentally noticed that there may be a type of hemilamina only without another anomaly, as shown in Fig. 11.

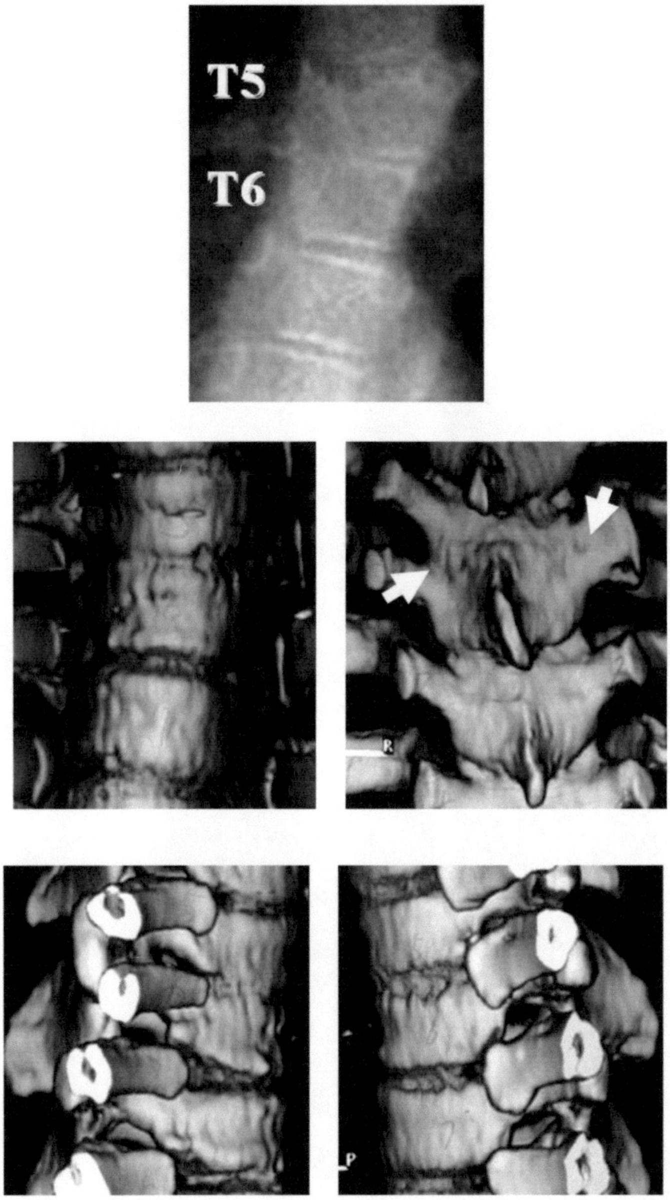

Fig. 10. **Posterior segmentation failure (group P: AP unison type).** This case showed no anterior and lateral fusion, but laminas and spinous processes at T5 and T6 were fused (arrow) with the corresponding anterior components.

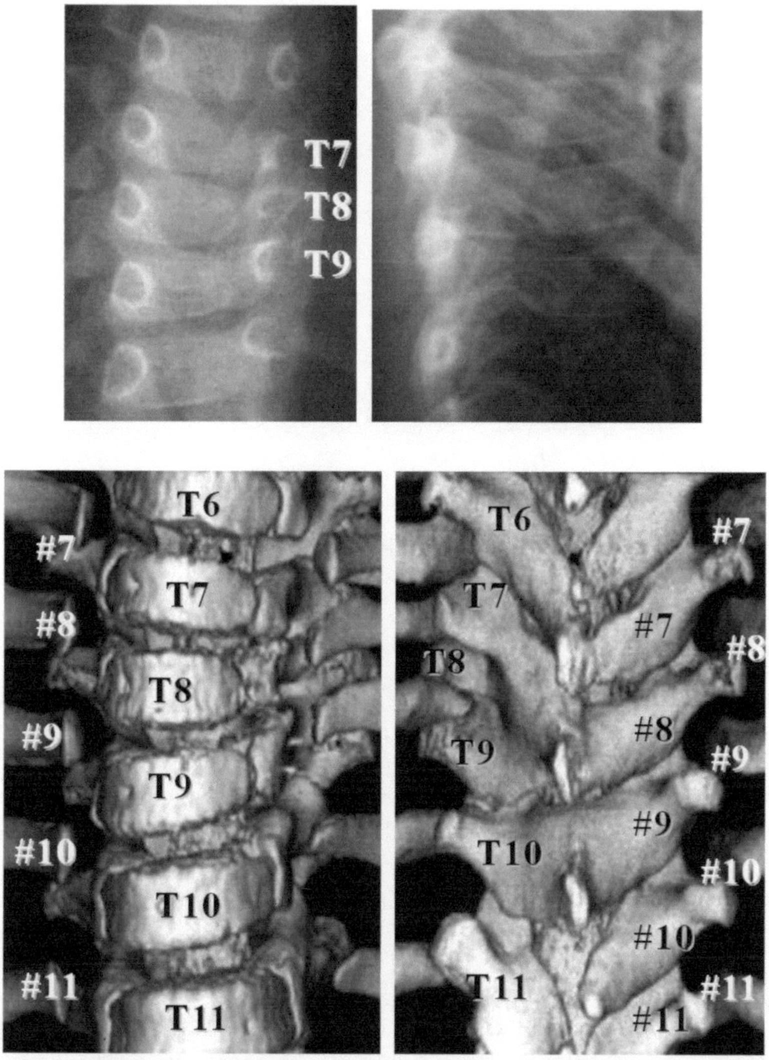

Fig. 11. **Posterior segmentation failure (group P: AP discordant type).** This case showed no anterior and lateral fusion, but laminas and spinous processes at T7 to T9 were fused. The posterior structure on the right side did not correspond to the components on the left side, which can be viewed as anterior components.

In evaluation of segmentation failure alone on 3DCT, the fusion type was divided into three categories: fused anterior only (group A), fused anterior, lateral and posterior components on the same side (group AL), and posterior fusion only (group P). All cases in group AL had posterior segmentation failure, and thus may be an ALP group, with group AL requiring further division. We speculated that the lateral component (the pedicle) may be the key to extending the fusion to the anterior and posterior parts in categories of segmentation failure alone (Fig.12). However, we do not have sufficient cases to draw this conclusion and further studies are needed. We also note that discordant anomalies were seen only in group P in this series of segmentation failure alone without vertebral formation failure.

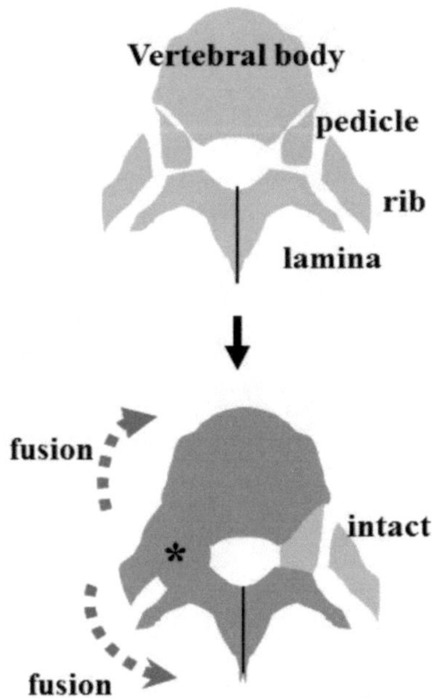

Fig. 12. **Proposed process of segmentation failure.** There were no cases of anterior and lateral segmentation failure, anterior and posterior segmentation failure, or lateral and posterior segmentation failure at the same side. Conversely, all cases with lateral fusion had anterior, lateral, and posterior fusion at the same side. Therefore, we speculate that the pedicle (asterisk) is the origin of the fusion in the cases of segmentation failure alone.

2.2.2 Formation failure with segmentation failure: Mixed type in Winter's classification

Next, we evaluated the mixed type in Winter's Classification. In this category, the combination of morphological anomalies and fusion varied and were the most complicated. We first divided the cases into hemivertebra or butterfly vertebra, and examined the relationship of fusion between the abnormal vertebral body and upper and lower adjacent segments. Here, we describe the results of this study (Imagama et al. 2005).

We examined 40 patients with congenital scoliosis (failure of formation) by 3D-CT to determine the morphological abnormalities of the vertebral bodies and the laminae, pedicles, ribs, and transverse processes. We excluded cases with segmentation failure only, which has been described above. We investigated the anterior, lateral and posterior features and evaluated the type of vertebral anomaly, incarcerated or nonincarcerated hemivertebra, and AP unison anomaly and AP discordant anomaly.

Twenty-seven of the cases had hemivertebra and 13 had butterfly vertebrae. There were fifteen incarcerated vertebra. As expected, the morphological features of the deformed vertebra and the adjacent vertebra had many variations of fusion. Anterior fusion only was present in 12 cases (group A), anteroposterior fusion was found in 16 cases (group AP), anterior, lateral, and posterior fusion was present in 6 cases (group ALP), and posterior fusion only was found in 6 cases (group P). There were no cases with lateral fusion only (group L in the classification), similarly to the evaluation of segmentation failure only. Many cases showed anterior and posterior components combined and fused with the adjacent components, which differed from the evaluation of segmentation failure alone (Fig. 13, Table 3). Plain radiographs and 3DCT images for each group are shown in Figs. 14-17.

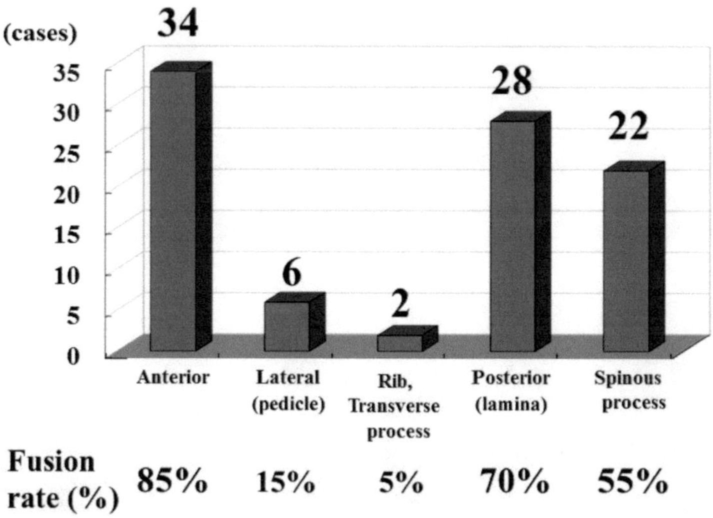

Fig. 13. **Fusion rate for each component in the mixed type.** Among cases with hemivertebra and/or butterfly vertebra, fusion was common for anterior and posterior components and seemed to be less frequent for lateral components.

Vertebral formation failure	n	Segmentation group			
		A (n=12)	AP (n=16)	ALP (n=6)	P (n=6)
Hemivertebra	27	8	13	3	3
Hemivertebra+ Butterfly vertebra	10	2	2	3	3
Butterfly vertebra	3	2	1		

Table 3. Classification of segmentation based on vertebral failure of formation

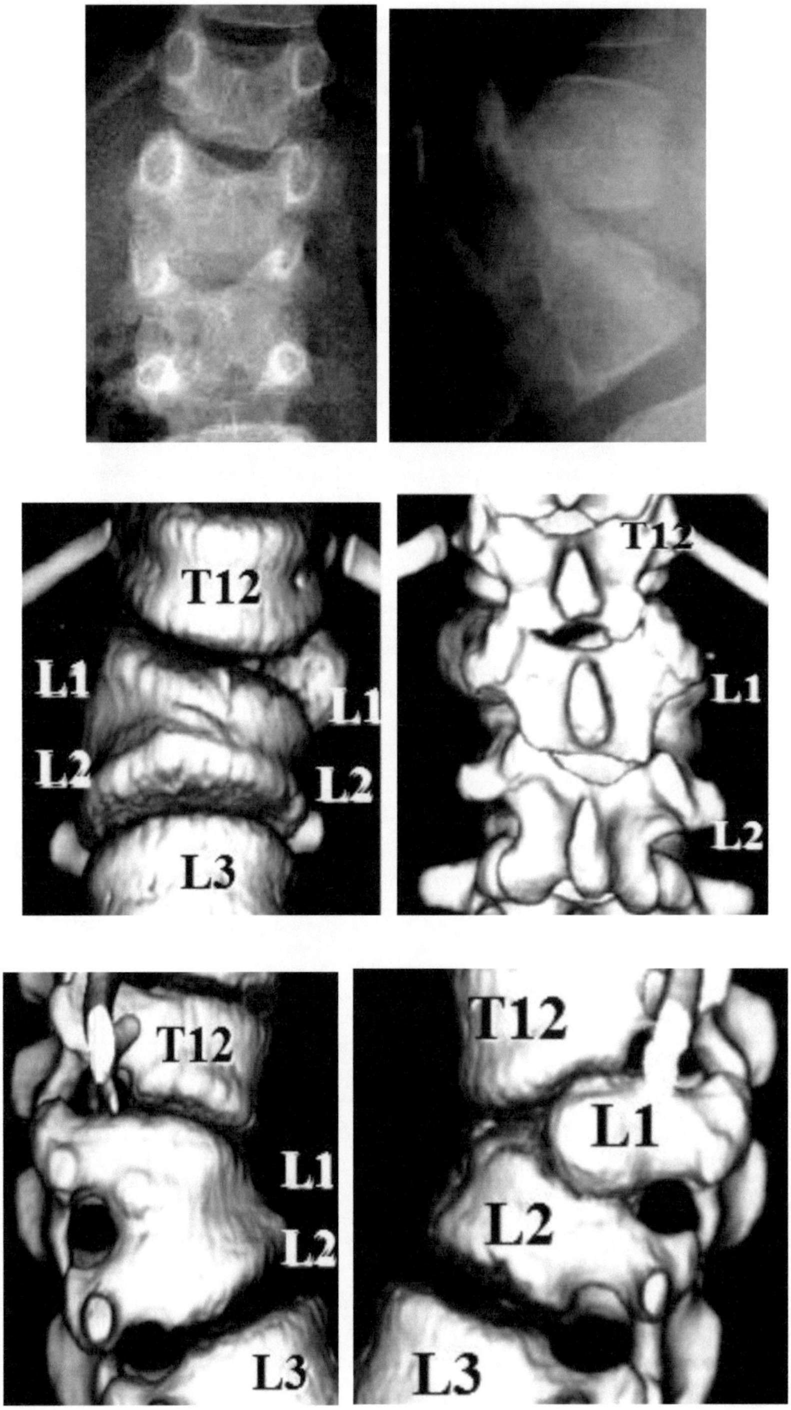

Fig. 14. **Images for group A.** This case has an L1 butterfly vertebra and only the right side of the vertebra was fused.

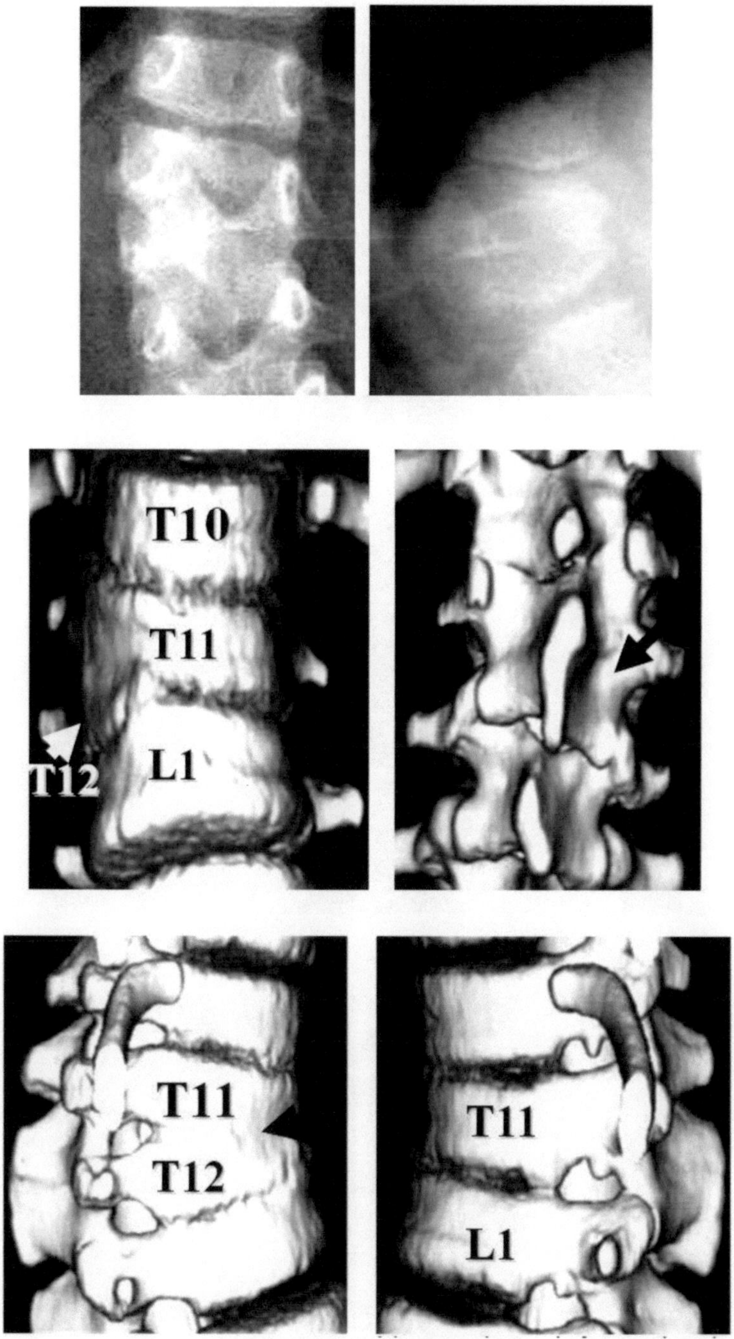

Fig. 15. **Images for group AP.** This case has a left T12 hemivertebra and anterior and posterior components were fused (arrow), with no lateral fusion. There was no incarceration hemivertebra.

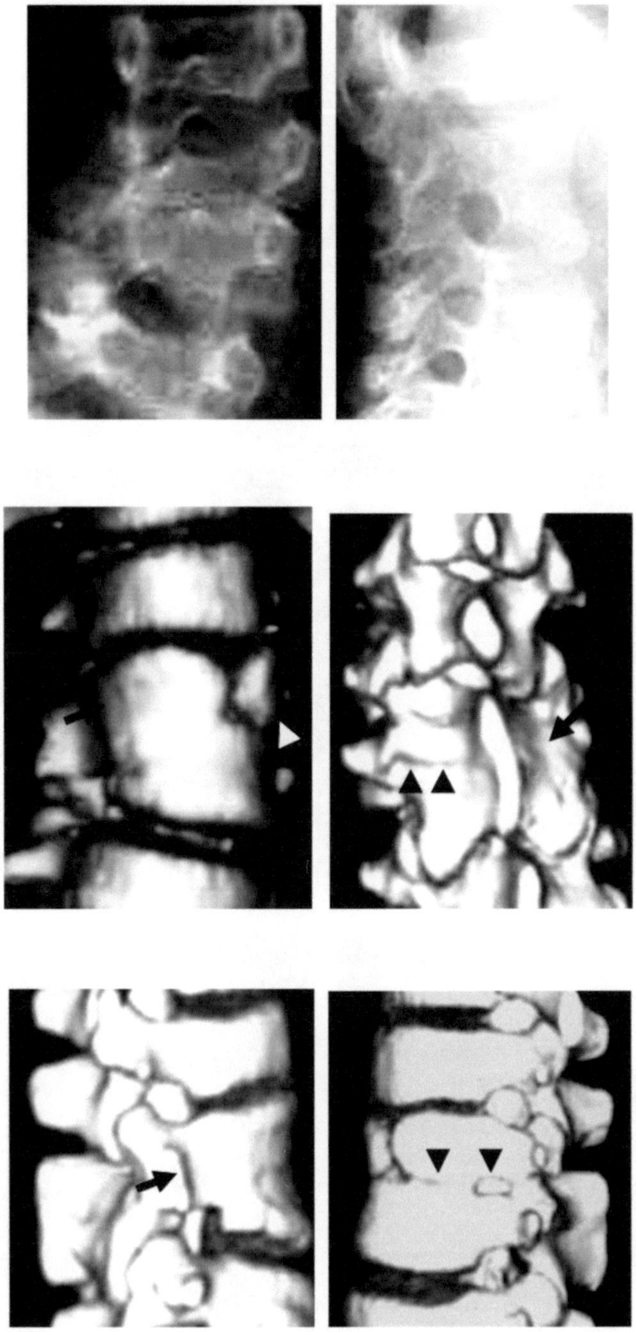

Fig. 16. **Images for group ALP.** This case has an L2 butterfly vertebra and right anterior, lateral and posterior components were fused (arrow). However, there was no complete fusion on the left side (arrowhead).

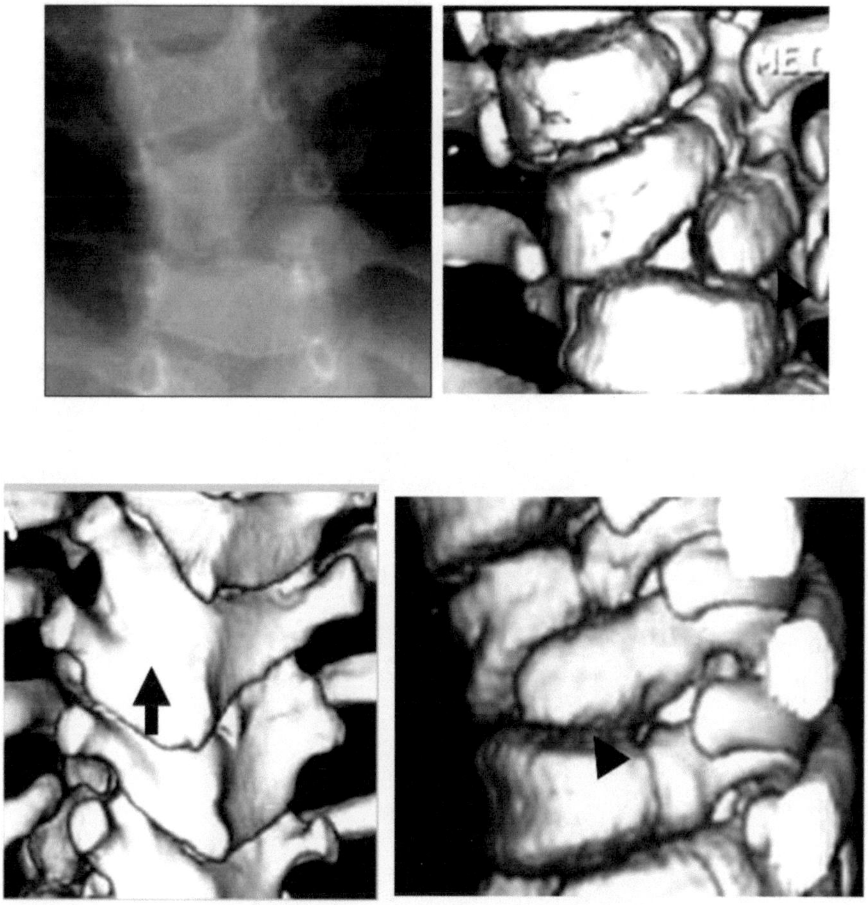

Fig. 17. **Images for group P.** This case has a left T9 hemivertebra and posterior fusion only (arrow), without anterior and lateral fusion (arrowhead). Incarceration was also seen at the T8 vertebra.

The above classification demonstrates the various types of formation failure with segmentation failure. There was no discordant type in the mixed type, but this may be because segmentation failure prevented evaluation of the correspondence between anterior and posterior components. Instead, we found an AP discordant *segmentation* anomaly (Fig. 18). This case had an anterior component fused with the lower site, but the laminae fused with the upper opposite adjacent laminae.

In this evaluation, there was no clear trend for segmentation failure or formation failure, including incarceration. However, various types of formation and segmentation failure were found in the study, and this is useful for performance of further research and for reference in preparing a surgical plan.

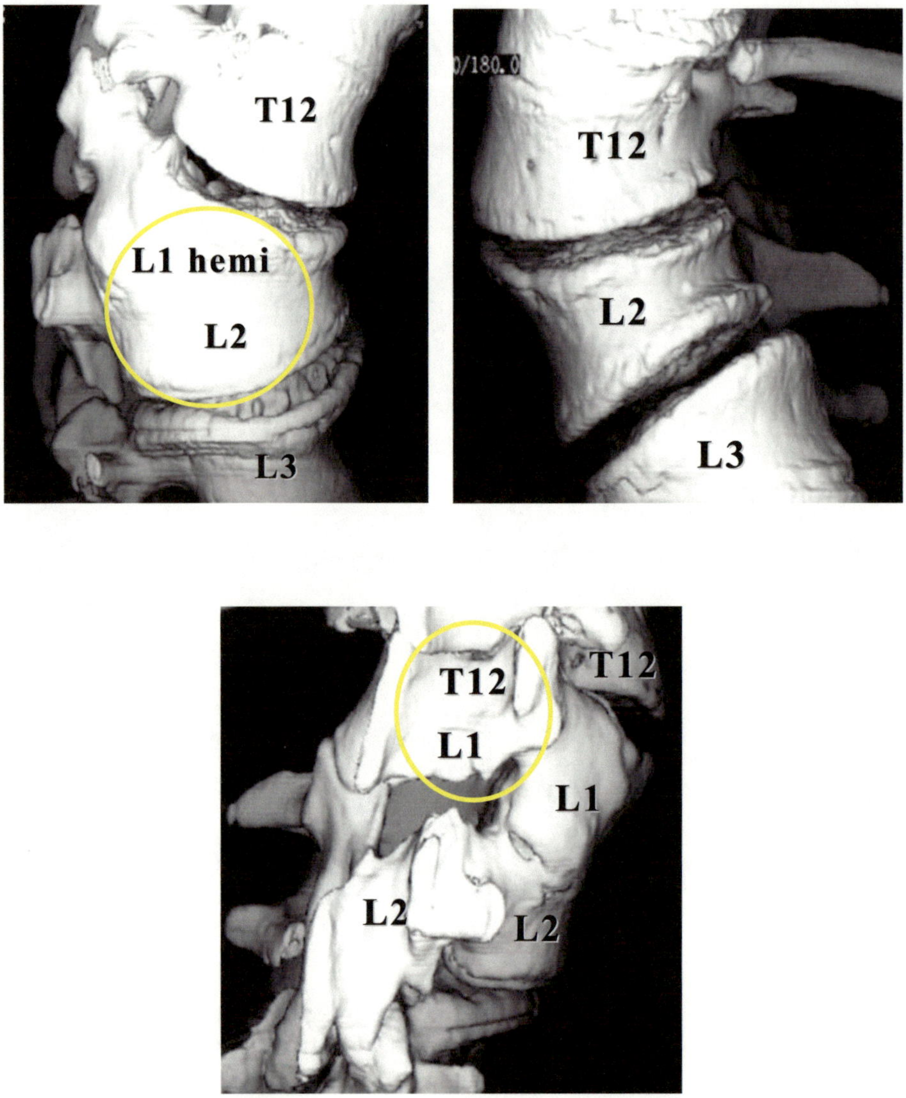

Fig. 18. **AP discordant segmentation anomaly.** This case has a right L1 hemivertebra and anterior fusion with L2. However, on the posterior side the L1 lamina was fused with T12, rather than L2.

2.3 Summary of anteroposterior unison anomaly and discordant anomaly

We first recognized the mismatch of anterior and posterior components and named this "AP discordant anomaly". However, this may be somewhat complicated to understand, and therefore we describe the scheme in detail. There are some variations of discordant anomaly according to the presence and location of formation failure and segmentation failure. The scheme on the left in Fig. 19A is normal. When the anterior component (vertebra) has no anomaly, it is possible for AP discordant anomaly with hemilamina to occur with or without posterior segmentation failure (Figs. 11, 19A right). If anterior formation failure is present, AP discordant anomaly can occur (Figs. 6, 19B). When anterior segmentation failure is present, AP discordant anomaly may occur (Fig. 19C). As an unusual type of AP discordant anomaly, AP discordant *segmentation* anomaly can also be present when the level of segmentation is mismatched between anterior and posterior components (Figs. 18, 19D). It may sometimes be difficult to evaluate AP discordant anomaly, so it may be useful to refer to the anterior and posterior components using the rib and the transverse process. That is, when the same rib is seen in the anterior and posterior views in 3DCT images, it is easier to evaluate the anomaly. AP discordant anomaly at the lumbar spine seems to be easier to evaluate compared to that at the thoracic spine.

There are clearly several types of AP discordant anomaly and the above findings are important for reference during surgery. Osteotomy from a posterior approach is now performed and in this method resection of anterior components from the posterior approach is performed blindly. Therefore, it is important to consider AP discordant anomaly for performing safe and accurate surgical procedures.

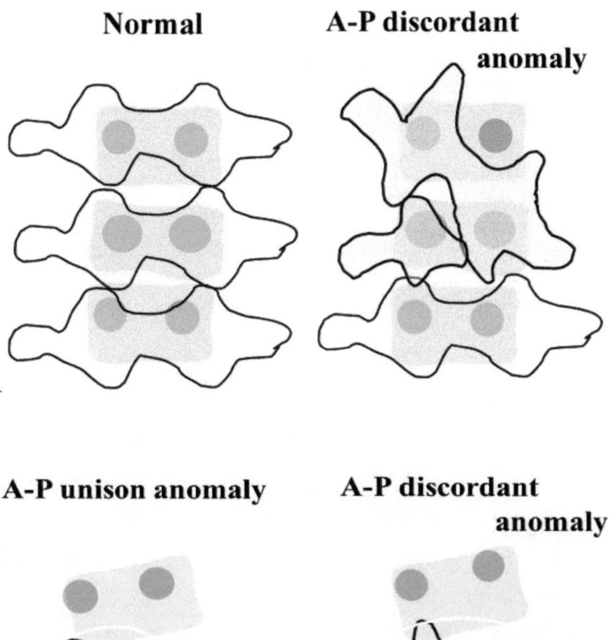

A

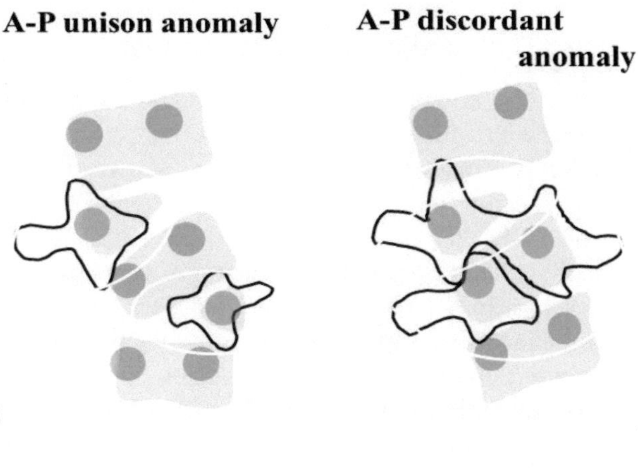

B

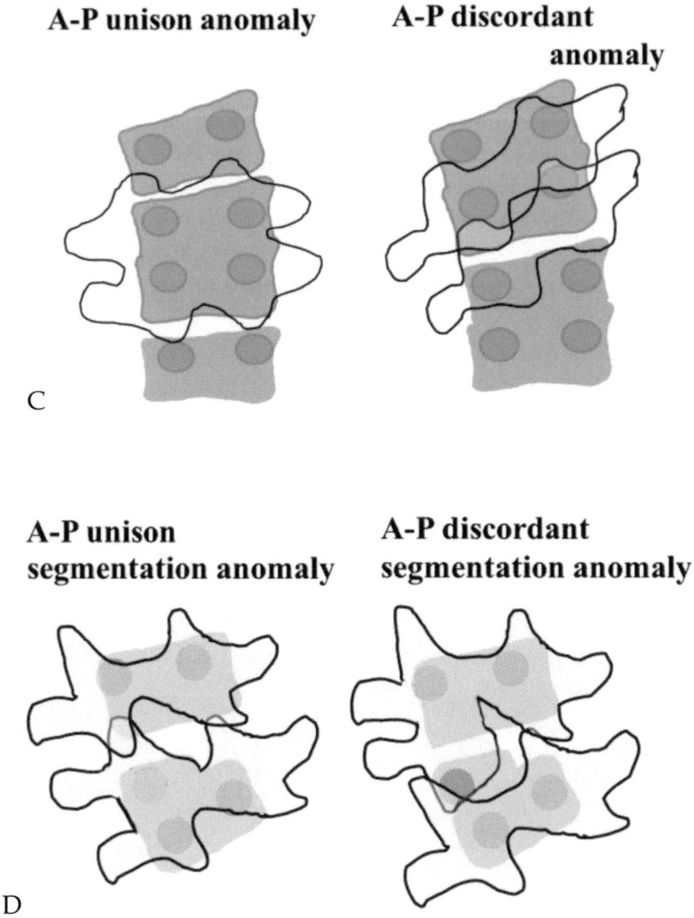

Fig. 19. **Scheme of AP discordant anomaly.** There are several type of AP discordant anomaly based on the location and presentation of formation failure and segmentation failure.

3. Conclusion (A new 3D classification of congenital anomaly)

We have evaluated congenital anomaly with 3DCT images for several years as described above, and developed a new classification of congenital scoliosis and kyphosis(Kawakami et al. 2009). This work clearly illustrated the limitation of two-dimensional classification, showed the clinical significance of 3D analysis of congenital vertebral anomalies, and allowed the proposal of a new 3D classification of these anomalies. The large volume of information obtained by 3DCT, including the various morphologies, patterns of segmentation, solitary or multiple, and unison or discordant, complicates the classification (Fig. 20). However, we believe that this approach provides a closer view of the reality of vertebral abnormalities based on analysis of 3DCT images, compared to past classifications. This new classification of congenital scoliosis based on 3D imaging is needed to understand the etiology and embryology of the disease, as well as to determine an operative strategy.

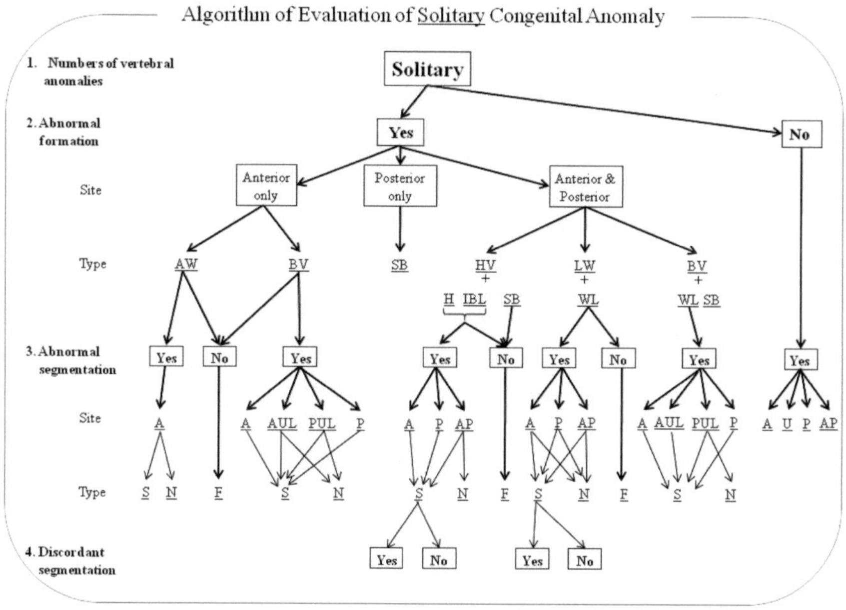

A

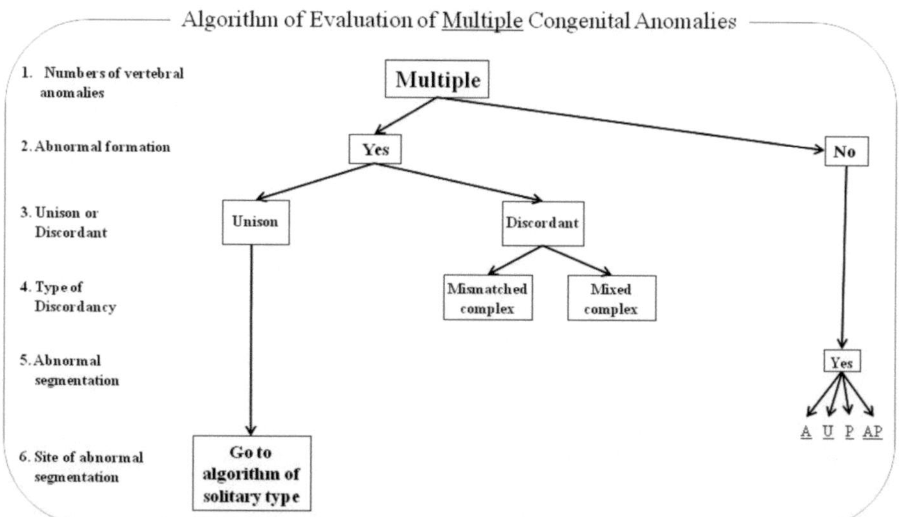

B

Fig. 20. **Algorithm of evaluation of congenital anomalies.** There are algorithms for the solitary type (A) and for the multiple type (B). If more than 2 congenitallyabnormal vertebrae exist in whole spinal column, we should follow the algorithm for the multiple type. This algorithm helps to clarify the characteristics of abnormal vertebra. A indicates anterior; P, posterior; BV, butterfly vertebra; W, wedged vertebra; HV, hemivertebra; SB, spina bifida; AW, anterior wedged vertebra; LW, lateral wedged vertebra; H, hemilamina; IBL, incomplete bilamina; WL, wedged lamina; AUL, anterior unilateral; PUL, posterior unilateral; S, semisegmented; N, nonsegmented; F, fully segmented; U, unilateral; AP, anteroposterior(Kawakami et al. 2009).

4. References

Imagama, S. et al.(2004). The three-dimensional analysis of congenital scoliosis–segmentation failure. *J Jpn Scoliosis Soc*;19:33–7.

Imagama, S. et al.(2005). Spacial relationships between a deformed vertebra and an adjacent vertebra in congenial scoliosis–failure of formation. *J Jpn Scoliosis Soc*;20:20–5.

Kawakami, N. et al.(2009). Classification of Congenital Scoliosis and Kyphosis: A New Approach to the Three-Dimensional Classification for Progressive Vertebral Anomalies Requiring Operative Treatment. *Spine*;34:1756–65

Nakajima, A. et al.(2007). Three-Dimensional analysis of formation failure in congenital scoliosis. *Spine* ;32:562–7.

Newton, PO. et al.(2002). Utility of three dimensional and multiplanar reformatted computed tomography for evaluation of pediatric congenital spine abnormalities. *Spine*;27:844–50.

Winter, RB.; Moe, JH.& Wang, JF.(1973). Congenital Kyphosis—Its natural history and treatment as observed in a study of one hundred thirty patients. *J Bone Joint Surg Am*;55:223–56.

Part 4

Treatment Planning

15

Computed Tomography of Osteolysis Related to Total Ankle Replacement

Ia Kohonen[2], Helka Koivu[1], Kimmo Mattila[2] and Hannu Tiusanen[1]
[1]Department of Internal Medicine, Rheumaorthopaedic Unit,
[2]The Medical Imaging Centre of Southwest Finland,
Turku University Hospital,
[1]Turku
[2]Finland

1. Introduction

Increasing number of patients come to computed tomography (CT) imaging with orthopaedic hardware including total ankle replacement (TAR). These patients have either implant related complaints, or they are imaged due to other medical causes with the prosthesis in the imaged body area. Inventions in CT; first helical computed tomography and later, multidetector computed tomography (MDCT) have made imaging of bones and joints extremely fast and precise, resulting in less motion artifacts and thinner sections (Lee et al., 2007; Ohashi et al., 2005; West et al., 2009). With modern scanners image data is routinely obtained as isotropic or near isotropic voxels. This allows image reconstruction in any arbitrary plane without loosing image quality and also 3D volume rendered images (West et al., 2009).

CT is useful when imaging ankle after TAR especially in the situations when the patient has implant related symptoms or periprosthetic osteolysis is suspected and the radiographs cannot determine the condition. Cahir et al. (2007) and Keogh et al. (2003) have shown the usefulness of CT in imaging painful hip after total hip replacement. Periprosthetic osteolysis and aseptic loosening are common complications after TAR (Berquist, 2006; Besse et al., 2009; Koivu et al., 2009; Kokkonen et al., 2011; Rodriguez et al., 2010). CT reveals osteolytic changes around prosthesis components in ankle better than radiographs (Besse et al., 2009; Hanna et al., 2007; Koivu et al., 2009; Rodriguez et al., 2009). CT may also be useful in other total ankle replacement related conditions, e.g. periprosthetic fracture, subluxation and dislocation of prosthesis components, infection, impingement and heterotopic ossification.

This article is not a comprehensive encyclopedic review of CT scanning of total ankle prostheses. Our aim was to review previous literature of CT in osteolysis related to total ankle prosthesis. This article also contains short description of total ankle replacements.

2. Periprosthetic osteolysis

Periprosthetic osteolysis is a common problem with total joint replacements. The exact pathogenesis of osteolysis still remains unclear, but both biological and mechanical factors likely contribute (Jacobs et al., 2001; Konttinen et al., 2005; Saleh et al., 2004; Purdue et al., 2006). Osteolysis in hip arthroplasty has been widely studied and was originally described as cement disease (Jones & Hungerford 1987). Currently it is commonly regarded as a foreign body reaction due to cement, polyethylene or metallic wear particles (Dumbleton et al., 2002; Harris, 1995; Jacobs et al., 2001; Konttinen et al., 2005; Saleh et al., 2004; Santavirta, 2005; Purdue et al. 2006). Numerous proinflammatory cytokines participate to the process in response to implant-derived wear particles and recent studies have shown that RANK/RANKL/OPG pathway might have a crucial role in osteoclastogenesis and osteolysis (Holt et al., 2007; Purdue et al., 2006; Saleh et al., 2004). Wear particles are considered the single most important factor in development of osteolysis, but the specific nature of this process is likely dependent of numerous parameters, including patterns of wear, type of prosthesis and host factors (Dumbleton et al., 2002; Jacobs et al., 2001; Purdue et al., 2006).

Previous studies on total hip replacement have shown that radiographs underestimate the size of periprosthetic osteolytic lesions (Puri et al., 2002; Walde et al., 2005) and some of the existing lesions may even remain undetected on radiographs (Looney et al., 2002). The hip prosthesis studies have demonstrated mean time-interval from total hip replacement to detectable osteolytic lesions on radiographs to vary between five and ten years (Park et al., 2004; Puri et al., 2002). Looney et al. (2002) found correlation between osteolysis and polyethylene wear. However, in another study (Puri et al., 2002) correlation between volumetric bone loss and linear wear of the polyethylene was not established.

Patients with periprosthetic osteolysis may remain asymptomatic for a long time despite of the lesions around prosthesis components. Because osteolysis is a progressive phenomenon (Purdue et al., 2006) and probably results finally in component failure, it is important to detect these lesions around prosthesis components as early as possible. CT may be useful in monitoring the progress of these lesions around components.

3. Total ankle replacement

Total ankle replacement has emerged since the introduction of the third generation total ankle implants. The first generation total ankle replacements from 1970s and 1980s were non-anatomical and did not respect ankle kinematics, therefore due to unsatisfactory results they were abandoned several years ago (Bonasia et al., 2010; DiDomenico et al., 2010; van den Heuvel et al., 2010,). Nowadays TAR implants are non-cemented, two- or three-component, semi-constrained designs with mobile bearing polyethylene (Figure 1.). As short-term and intermediate-term results seem to be acceptable (Besse et al., 2010; Bonnin et al., 2004; Bonnin et al., 2010; Buechel et al., 2004; Doets et al., 2006; Fevang et al., 2007; Haddad et al., 2007; Henricson et al., 2007; Henricson et al., 2010; Hintermann et al., 2004; Hosman et al., 2007; Knecht et al., 2004; Kofoed, 2004; Pyevich et al., 1998; Su et al., 2004; Valderrabano et al., 2004; Wood & Deakin, 2003) it is according to many authors challenging the position of ankle arthrodesis as a gold standard in the treatment of painful ankle arthritis. Koefod and Stirrup (1994) showed in series of 26 patients that results of total ankle replacement were better than ankle arthrodesis.

3.1 Survival of total ankle replacement

Despite acceptable survival reports there are concerns regarding the long-term implant survival as the results of total ankle arthroplasty are generally considered to be inferior compared to total hip or knee arthroplasty. Some centers have reported 5-year survival rates

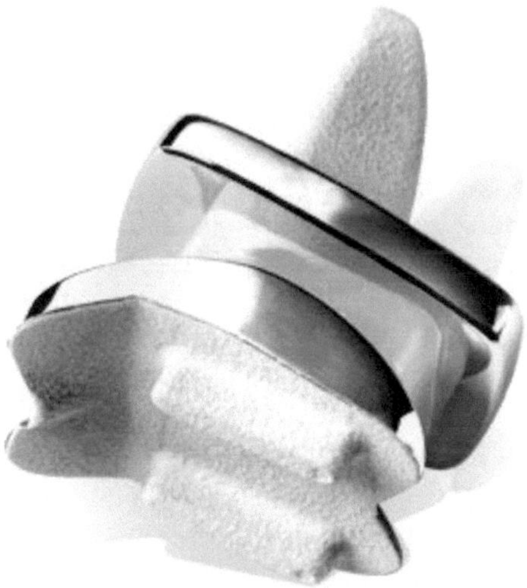

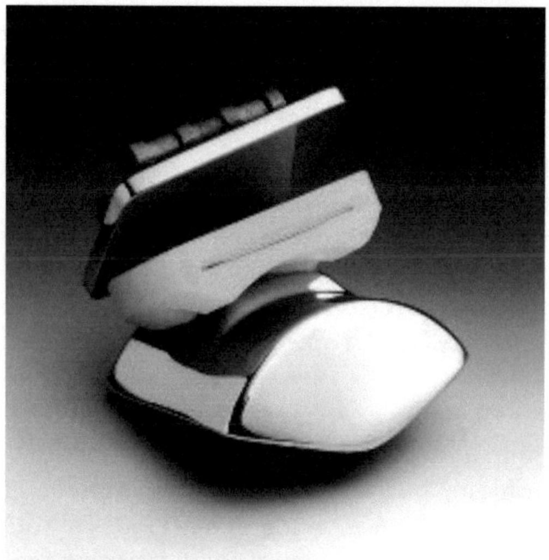

Fig. 1. Ankle Evolutive System (AES) total ankle implant (picture from Biomet Finland Oy) and Scandinavian Total Ankle Replacement (STAR) implant (picture from Anderson, T., Montgomery, F. & Carlsson, Å. (2003). Uncemented STAR total ankle prosthesis: Three to eight-year follow-up of fifty-one consecutive ankles. *J Bone Joint Surg Am*. Vol. 85, No. 7, (July 2003), pp. 1321-1329, 1535-1386).

of 70 % to 93 % (Anderson et al., 2003; Doets et al., 2006; Knecht et al., 2004; San Giovanni et al., 2006; Spirt et al., 2004; Wood et al., 2008; Wood et al., 2009) and 10- to 12-year survival rates even from 85 to 95 % (Bonnin et al., 2010; Buechel et al., 2004; Knecht et al., 2004; Kofoed, 2004). Results from Swedish, Norwegian and Finnish national registries have been slightly inferior with survival rates of 78% to 89% at five years and 62% to 72% at ten years (Fevang et al., 2007; Henricson et al., 2007; Skytta et al., 2010). In studies based on these registers with over 1300 patients altogether, aseptic loosening has been the most frequent reason for revision (31 - 48 %) (Fevang et al., 2007; Henricson et al., 2007; Skytta et al., 2010).

3.2 Total ankle replacement and osteolysis

In Finland the most used TAR implant has been Ankle Evolutive System (AES) (Transystéme, Nimes, France), which has a tibial component with stem and a mobile bearing polyethylene. Before AES the most commonly used TAR implant in Finland was Scandinavian Total Ankle Replacement (STAR) (Waldemar Link, Hamburg, Germany), which has no stem on the tibial component. At 2008 the sale of the AES implant was prohibited in France due to alarming findings regarding osteolytic lesions beside the implant. Therefore our own TAR patients were analyzed and a large amount of osteolysis with AES implants was found. The results were published in Journal of Bone and Joint Surgery British version at 2009 (Koivu et al. 2009). Other reports with similar findings have been published afterwards (Besse et al., 2009; Besse et al., 2010; Kokkonen et al., 2011; Rodriguez et al., 2010).

Alarming percentage of osteolysis has been reported with total ankle arthroplasty before (Doets et al., 2006; Knecht et al., 2004; Pyevich et al., 1998; Schutte & Louwerens, 2008; Su et al., 2004; Valderrabano et al., 2004; Wood & Deakin, 2003). On the other hand, some authors have reported the opposite and bone mineral density has been shown to increase adjacent to hydroxyapatite coated ankle arthroplasty (Zerahn et al., 2000, Zerahn & Kofoed, 2004). Knecht et al. (2004) detected osteolytic lesions in up to 76 % with the Agility Ankle implant (DePuy, Warsaw, IN). However, most of the lesions in their study were small and stable; progression was obtainable in approximately 12 % of all lytic lesions. The authors defined lytic lesions into two different categories by their nature, "expansile" and "mechanical", of which the latter has previously been called "ballooning" lysis (Pyevich et al., 1998). It has been characterised as early-onset and usually non-progressive lesion, when in turn expansile lysis was characterised as late-onset, progressive lesion due to implant wear. In our study the lesions were both early-onset, as first lesions were seen on radiographs one to two years after the operation, and rapidly progressive (Koivu et a., 2009).

3.2.1 Revision surgery for osteolysis

In hip and knee arthroplasty, the implants may be well fixed despite large aggressive granulomatous lesions around the implants (Eskola et al., 1990; Jasty et al., 1986; Nolan and Bucknill, 1992; Santavirta et al., 1990; Tallroth et al., 1989) and some authors consider these lesions and aseptic loosening as different conditions (Santavirta et al., 1990). Few findings in the literature (Knecht et al., 2004; Valderrabano et al., 2004; Wood & Deakin, 2003) and our own results support this theory also in ankle arthroplasty (Koivu et al., 2009). Most of our patients with osteolysis were clinically asymptomatic and the implants have been steadily fixed in revision. To prevent the loosening of the implants, all ankles with marked osteolytic lesions have been revised as has also been suggested by other authors (Besse et al., 2009). At revision surgery, a débridement, allogenous spongious bone grafting and exchange of polyethylene inlay if necessary has been done. Large lytic cavities containing brownish grey granulomatous necrotic material were found around the components, but there was no metallosis in surrounding tissues. In most ankles both tibial and talar components were stable. The histology of the samples of all patients was identical and was interpreted as foreign body reaction. These findings were consistent with previous studies regarding periprosthetic osteolytic lesions (Jasty et al., 1986; Santavirta et. al, 1990, Tallroth et al., 1989).

4. CT of osteolysis related to total ankle replacement

Traditionally patients with total ankle prosthesis are monitored only using radiographs. Anteroposterior (AP) and lateral radiographs are obtained usually at each clinical control visit, in standing position whenever possible (Figure 2.). On radiographs osteolysis has been defined as a new or expanding sharply demarcated lucency adjacent to prosthesis components (Puri et al., 2002). Alarming reports regarding osteolytic lesions around AES total ankle prosthesis (Besse et al., 2009; Besse et al., 2010; Koivu et al., 2009; Kokkonen et al., 2011, Rodriquez et al., 2009) have increased interest in computed tomography in follow-up of total ankle prostheses.

4.1 Methods for decreasing metal artifacts on CT

Every metal implant causes artifacts on CT distorting the normally excellent image quality (Barret & Keat, 2004). The factors that affect artifacts include the composition of the and, orientation of the hardware, acquisition parameters (peak voltage, tube charge, collimation and acquired section thickness), and reconstruction parameters (Lee et al., 2007).

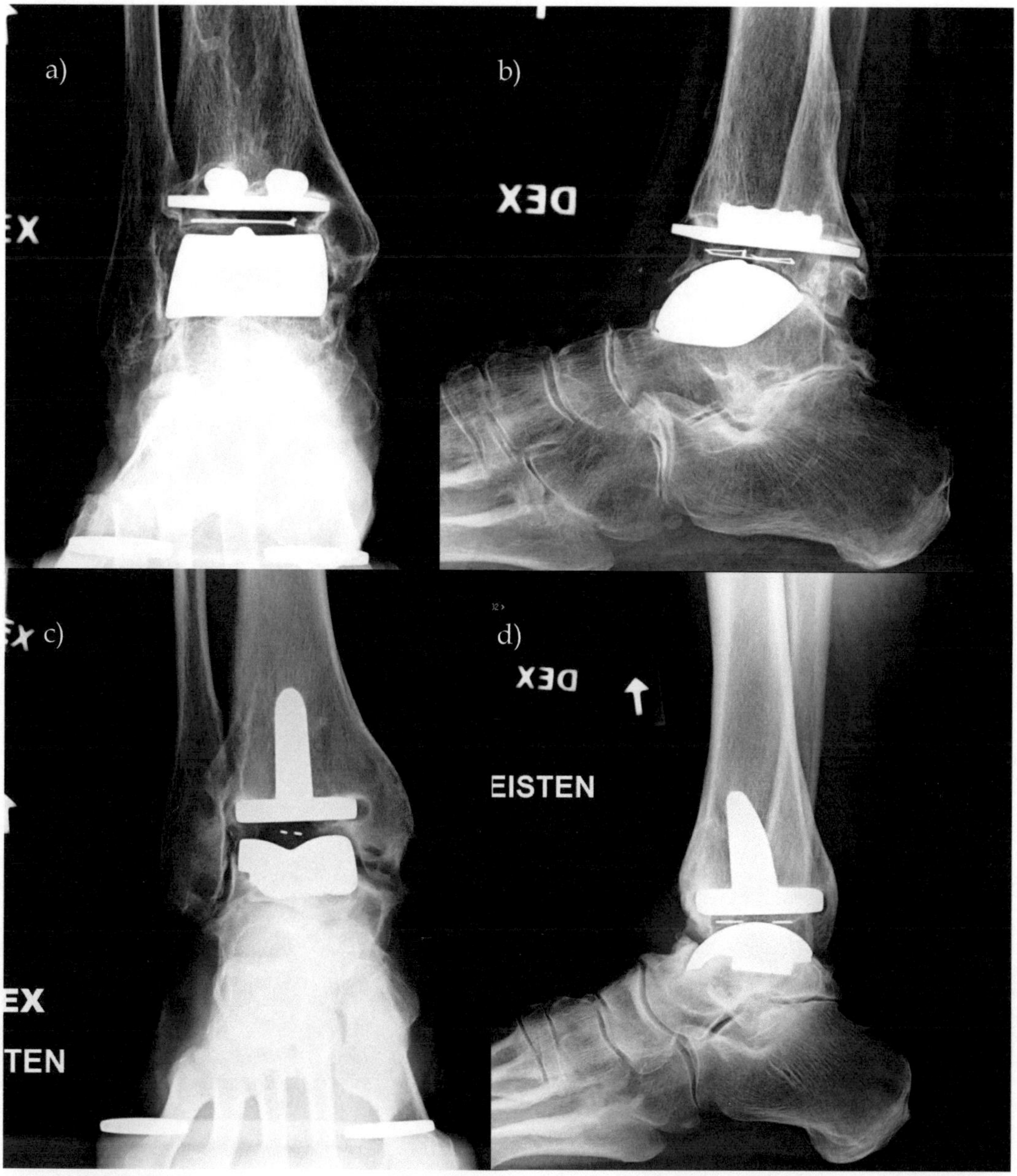

Fig. 2. Radiographs of STAR (a and b) and AES prostheses (c and d) in standing position.

Metal composition, as well as geometry of metal implant and cross-sectional area of the hardware affects the amount of artifacts produced. Titanium causes less artifacts than stainless steel and cobalt-chrome (Lee et al., 2007; Stradiotti et al., 2009). Large metallic components cause bigger artifact than smaller and thinner ones (Lee et al., 2007). To minimize artifacts during scanning the implant should be positioned so that the X-ray beam traverses the smallest possible cross-sectional area of it (Lee et al., 2007; Stradiotti et al., 2009). Artifacts produced can also be reduced by optimizing imaging parameters. A higher

X-ray peak kilovoltage (kVp), a higher tube current (mAs) and lower pitch settings have been shown to diminish artifacts (Lee et al., 2007). Additionally, narrowing collimation reduces metal artifacts. In modern scanners extended CT scale technique (ECTS) can be used when imaging areas with metal implants. This technique allows expansion of the Hounsfield scale from a standard maximum window of 4000 HU to 40 000 HU. This technique is based on the fact that metals have high linear attenuation coefficients that are outside the normal range of reconstructed CT numbers (Lee et al., 2007; Link et al., 2000).

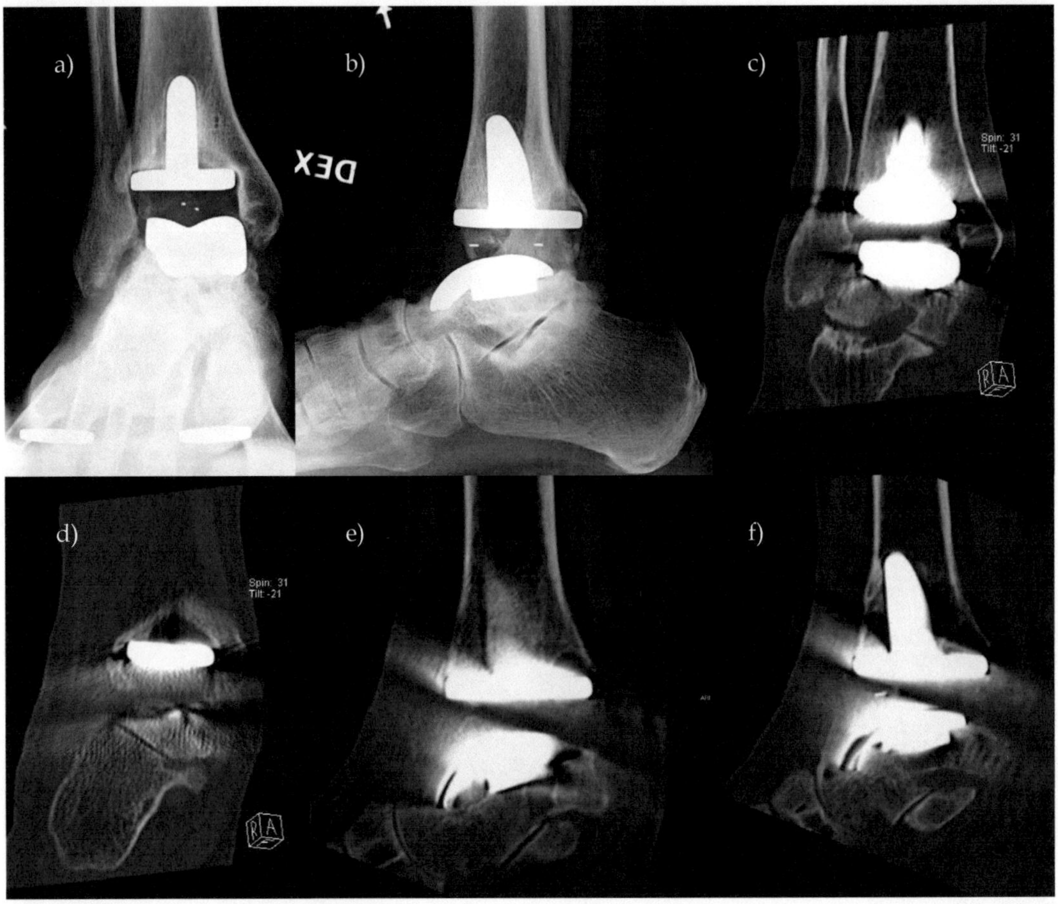

Fig. 3. 47 year-old male with rheumatoid arthritis. Radiographs 14 months after AES TAR (a and b) with osteolytic lesions at least in tibia. Several lesions on CT both in distal tibia and talus 2 years after operation (c-f).

The amount of metal artifacts may be further decreased in the post-prosessing phase when reconstructing images at workstation. Partial volume artifacts are usually best avoided by acquiring thinner sections (Lee et al., 2007), however, the drawback of increased information is increased image noise. During image reconstruction, combining several thin sections to get thicker ones are routinely used to reduce image noise. The increased thickness of the reformatted sections dramatically affects image quality, decreasing the noise and also severity of metal-related artifacts (Lee et al., 2007). Thicker reconstructed images with use of standard or smooth reconstruction filter (kernel) diminish metal artifacts and visible noise on the images (Lee et al., 2007). A novel metal artifact reduction (MAR) image reconstruction algorithm has been tested in some studies with promising results (Liu et al., 2009; Watzke & Kalender, 2004). However, the prosessing time needed for image reconstruction using this method was 2 to 4 hours for each examination, and therefore at least now this program is not suitable for standard clinical use (Liu et al., 2009).

To allow good image quality and possibility to reformat images in any arbitrary plane ankles with metal prostheses need to be imaged using MDCT. During scanning patients are lying supine on a table. The scanned area should cover the whole implant, starting proximal to the tibial component and ending distal to the talar component. In some studies (Hanna et al., 2007; Puri et al., 2002) high kilovoltage (140 kVp) has been used to reduce implant-related artifacts. However, it has also been estimated that there is no additional value attained in using settings more than 120 kVp (Lee et al., 2007). We have used a scan protocol of 120 kVp, metal-artifact reducing extended CT scale algorithm and 0.6 mm slice thickness with 0.4 mm recon increments. Coronal, sagittal and axial images are routinely reformatted from the original data with 2 to 3 mm slice thickness. On CT osteolytic lesions have been defined as well demarcated, periprosthetic lucencies without detectable osseus trabeculae (Hanna et al., 2007). Figures 3 - 6 show examples of TAR implants on CT.

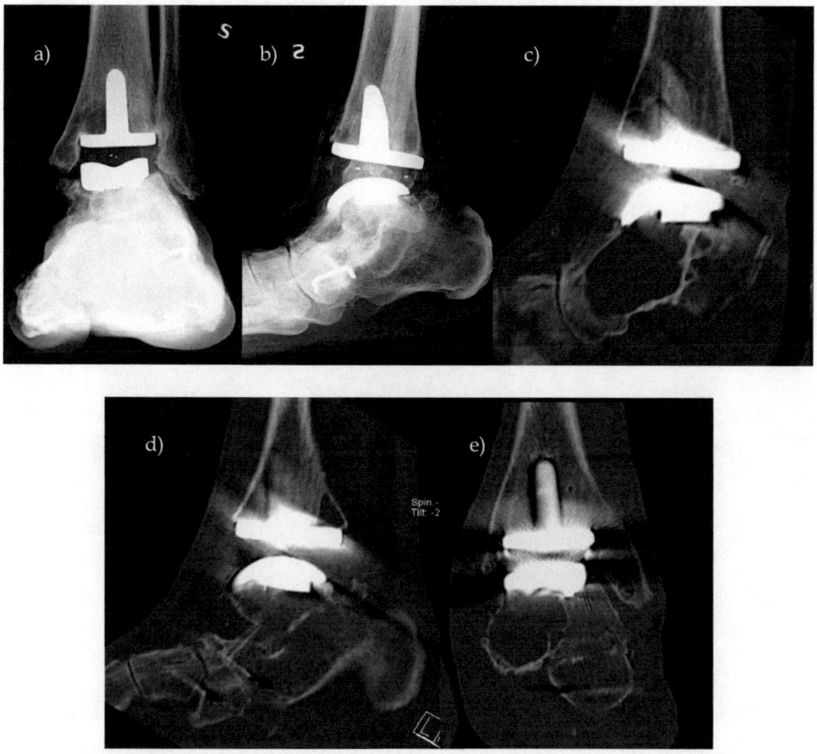

Fig. 4. 67 year-old male with rheumatoid arthritis. 2 years after total ankle replacement osteolytic lesions in distal tibia and suspicion of osteolysis also in talus on radiographs (a and b). On CT images 3 years after AES TAR (c-e) several osteolytic lesions in tibia and one huge lesion with cortical disruption in talus.

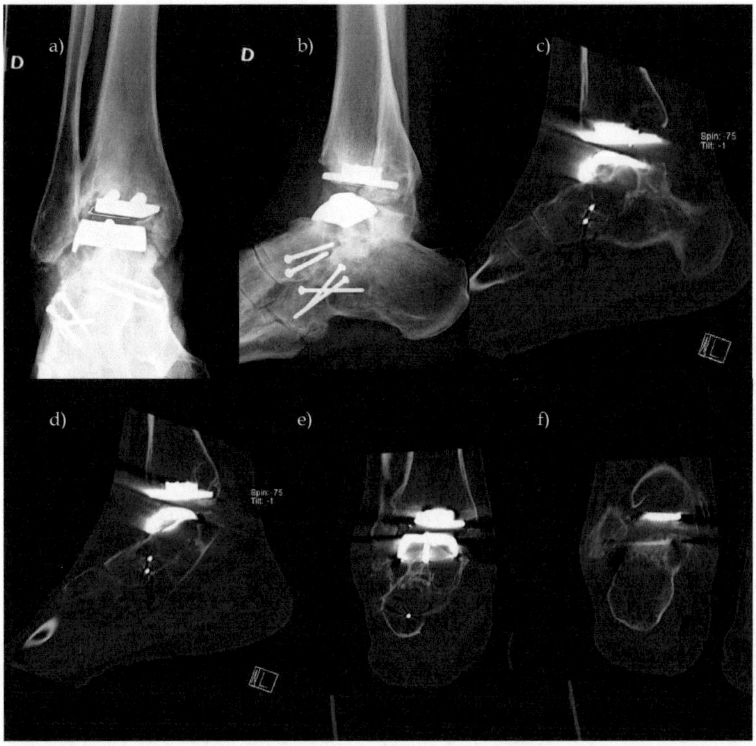

Fig. 5. 32 year-old female with rheumatoid arthritis. Radiographs 8 years after STAR total ankle replacement (a and b). Small osteolytic lesions in distal tibia and suspicion of osteolysis under talar component. On CT (c-f) 7 months after radiographs there were several lesions in tibia and also large lesions in talus.

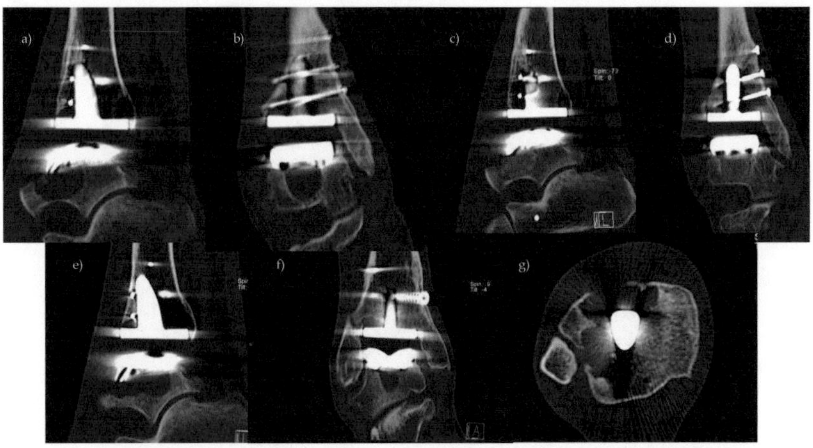

Fig. 6. 53 year-old male with post-traumatic osteoarthritis. On CT (a and b) several osteolytic lesions around AES prosthesis in distal tibia and one large lesion in talus, corrective osteotomy had also been performed. 2 years after TAR large lesion in talus and also one lesion in tibia were filled with allogenous bone grafting (c and d). At one year follow-up there is no visible bone grafting on CT and the osteolytic lesions have enlarged dramatically (e-g).

4.2 Reported appearance of osteolysis on CT

To our knowledge, the first study of total ankle replacement associated osteolysis and CT is where Hanna et al. (2007) studied 17 patients (19 ankles). The implant used in the study was Agility Ankle implant (DePuy, Warsaw, IN) the only second generation prosthesis fully approved by the FDA at that time. Unique to this implant is that fusion of the distal tibiofibular syndesmosis is required to stabilize the tibial component. In this study osteolytic lesions only in distal tibia and fibula were studied. More lesions were detected on CT than on radiographs. The mean size of the lesions on CT was over three times larger than the size on radiographs (Hanna et al., 2007).

Few studies have been published concerning CT of osteolysis related to AES prosthesis (Besse et al., 2009; Rodriquez et al., 2009). In one study with 18 ankles osteolysis was depicted on radiographs in 14 ankles (77 %) while all ankles had osteolytic lesions on CT. In addition, CT was more sensitive to osteolysis than radiographs especially around talar component (Rodriquez et al., 2009). The mean follow-up time in that study was 39.4 months. In another prospective study fifty AES implants in 47 patients were examined. The main cause for ankle replacement was post-traumatic osteoarthritis (50 %). The mean follow-up was 40 months. The clinical results in this study were good in spite of high amount of osteolytic lesions at bone-prosthesis interface. There were tibial osteolytic lesions in 62 % and talar lesions in 43 % of ankles. This study established that radiographs underestimate the size and number of osteolytic lesions when comparing to computed tomography (Besse et al., 2009).

5. Conclusion

Although total ankle replacement has become a noteworthy alternative to arthrodesis in the treatment of destructed upper ankle joint there are still concerns about stability of total ankle prosthesis in long-term follow-up. For example, the medium and long term results are not comparable to total hip and knee replacements. Common complications after total ankle replacement are osteolysis and aseptic loosening (Berquist, 2006; Fevang et al., 2007; Henricson et al., 2007; Pyevich et al., 1998; Skytta et al., 2010; Spirt et al., 2004). More studies of materials and designs of total ankle prosthesis are needed to improve survival of these prostheses.

Previous studies have shown that radiographs give limited information of osteolytic lesions around prosthesis components (Besse et al., 2009; Hanna et al., 2007; Rodriquez et al., 2009). Computed tomography is more accurate method for assessing the presence and extent of osteolytic lesions around TAR (Besse et al., 2009; Hanna et al., 2007; Koivu et al., 2009; Rodriguez et al., 2009). Furthermore, CT should be considered before total ankle replacement to determine the presence of any degenerative cysts or geodes in distal tibia, fibula or talus avoiding to misinterpretantion these lesions later as osteolysis (Figure 7.). In addition, CT is highly useful defining the exact locations of osteolytic lesions in preoperative planning of revision surgery for the failed TAR. We conclude that it is extremely important to remember that patients can have progressing osteolysis without visible osteolytic lesions on radiographs. CT should be included in every TAR patient follow-up scheme to detect these lesions as early as possible.

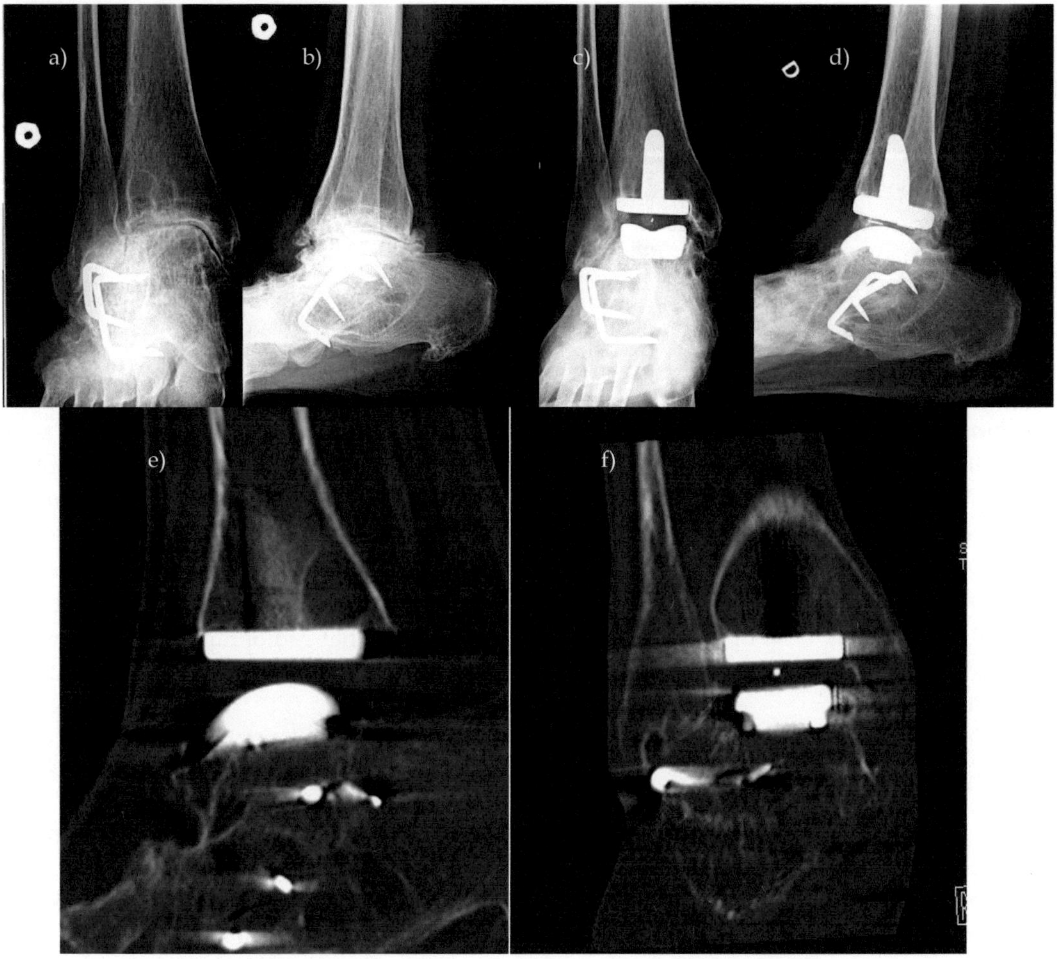

Fig. 7. 58 year-old female with rheumatoid arthritis. Radiographs before (a and b) and after AES TAR (c and d). CT images (e and f) 7 years after TAR. The lesion in postero-lateral tibia was considered as a geode, because it was visible already on preoperative radiographs.

6. References

Anderson, T.; Montgomery, F. & Carlsson, Å. (2003). Uncemented STAR total ankle prosthesis: Three to eight-year follow-up of fifty-one consecutive ankles. *J Bone Joint Surg Am*. Vol. 85, No. 7, (July 2003), pp. 1321-1329, 1535-1386

Barret, J. & Keat, N. (2004). Artifacts in CT: Recognition and Avoidance. *RadioGraphics*, 24, 6, pp. 1679-1691, 0271-5333

Berquist, T. (2006). Imaging of Joint Replacement Procedures. *Radiol Clin N Am*, 44, pp. 419-437, 0033-8389

Besse, J.; Brito, N. & Lienhart, C. (2009). Clinical evaluation and radiographic assessment of bone lysis of the AES total ankle replacement. *Foot Ankle Int.* Vol. 30, No. 10, (October 2009), pp. 964-975, 1071-1007

Besse, J.; Colombier, J; Asencio, J; Bonnin, M: Gaudot, F: Jarde, O; Judet, T; Maestro, M; Lemrijse, T; Leonardi, C; Toullec E & l'AFCP (2010). Total ankle arthroplasty in France. *Orthop Traumatol Surg Res.* Vol. 96, No. 3, (May 2010), 291-303, 1877-0568

Bonasia, D.; Dettoni, F.; Femino, J.; Phisitkul, P.; Germano, M. & Amendola, A. (2010). Total ankle replacement: why, when and how? *Iowa Orthop J.* Vol. 30, pp. 119-130, 1541-5457

Bonnin, M.; Gaudot, F.; Laurent, J.; Ellis, S.;Colombier, J. & Judet T. (2011). The Salto total ankle arthroplasty: survivorship and analysis of failures at 7 to 11 years. *Clin Orthop Relat Res.* Vol. 469, No. 1, (January 2009), pp. 225-236, 0009-921X

Bonnin, M.; Judet, T.; Colombier, J.; Buscayret, F.; Graveleau, N. & Piriou, P. (2004). Midterm results of the Salto Total Ankle Prosthesis. *Clin Orthop Relat Res.* 2004 Vol. 424, (July 2004), pp. 6-18, 0009-921X

Buckwalter, K.; Parr, J.; Choplin, R. & Capello, W. (2006). Multichannel CT Imaging of Orthopedic Hardware and Implants. *Semin Musculoskelet Radiol,* 10, 1, pp. 86-97, 1089-7860

Buechel, F. Sr,; Buechel, F. Jr. & Pappas, M. (2004). Twenty-year evaluation of cementless mobile-bearing total ankle replacements. *Clin Orthop Relat Res.* 2004 Vol. 424, (July 2004), pp. 19-26, 0009-921X

Cahir, J.; Toms, A.; Marshall, T.; Wimhurst, J. & Nolan, J. (2007). CT and MRI of hip arthroplasty. *Clinical Radiology,* 62, pp. 1163-1171, 0009-9260

DiDomenico, L.; Treadwell, J. & Cain, L. (2010). Total ankle arthroplasty in the rheumatoid patient. *Clin Podiatr Med Surg.* 2010 Vol. 27, 2, (April 2010), pp. 295-311, 1558-2302

Doets, H.; Brand, R. & Nelissen R. (2006). Total ankle arthroplasty in inflammatory joint disease with use of two mobile-bearing designs. *J Bone Joint Surg Am.* Vol. 88, No. 6, (June 2006), pp. 1272-1284, 1535-1386

Dumbleton, J.; Manley, M. & Edidin, A. (2002). A literature review of the association between wear rate and osteolysis in total hip arthroplasty. *J Arthroplasty.* Vol 17, No. 5, (August 2002), pp. 649-661, 0883-5403

Eskola, A.; Santavirta, S.; Konttinen, Y.; Hoikka V.; Tallroth, K. & Lindholm, T. (1990). Cementless revision of aggressive granulomatous lesions in hip replacement. *J Bone Joint Surg Br.* Vol. 72, No. 2, (March 1990), pp. 212-216, 1535-1386

Fevang, B., Lie, S.; Havelin, L.; Brun, J.; Skredderstuen, A. & Furnes, O. (2007). 257 ankle arthroplasties performed in Norway between 1994 and 2005. *Acta Orthop.* Vol. 78, No. 5, (January 2007), pp. 575-583, 1745-3674

Haddad, S., Coetzee, J., Estok, R., Fahrbach, K., Banel, D. & Nalysnyk, L. (2007). Intermediate and long-term outcomes of total ankle arthroplasty and ankle arthrodesis. A systematic review of the literature. *J Bone Joint Surg Am.* Vol. 89, No. 9, (September 2007), pp. 1899-1905, 1535-1386

Hanna, R.; Haddad, S. & Lazarus, M. (2007). Evaluation of Periprosthetic Lucency After Total Ankle Arthroplasty: Helical CT Versus Conventional Radiography. *Foot Ankle Int.,* 28, 8, pp. 921-926, 1071-1007

Harris, W. (1995). The problem is osteolysis. Clin Orthop. Vol. 311, (February 1995), pp. 46-53, 0095-8654

Henricson, A., Knutson, K., Lindahl, J. & Rydholm, U. (2010). The AES total ankle replacement: A mid-term analysis of 93 cases. *Foot Ankle Surg.* Vol. 16, No. 2, (June 2010), pp. 61-64, 1268-7731

Henricson, A., Skoog, A. & Carlsson, Å. (2007). The Swedish Ankle Arthroplasty Register. An analysis of 531 arthroplasties between 1993 and 2005. *Acta Orthop*. Vol. 78, No. 5, (January 2007), pp. 569-574, 1745-3674

Hintermann, B., Valderrabano, V., Dereymaker, G. & Dick, W. (2004). The HINTEGRA ankle: rationale and short-term results of 122 consecutive ankles. *Clin Orthop Rel Res*. Vol. 424, (July 2004), pp. 57-68, 0009-921X

Holt, G., Murnaghan, C., Reilly, J. & Meek, R. (2007). The biology of aseptic osteolysis. *Clin Orthop Rel Res*. Vol. 460, (July 2007), pp. 240-252, 0009-921X

Holt, G.; Murnaghan, C.; Reilly, J. & Meek, R. (2007). The Biology of Aseptic Osteolysis. *Clin Orthop*, 460, pp. 240-252, 0095-8654

Hosman, A., Mason, R., Hobbs, T. & Rothwell, A. (2007). A New Zealand national joint registry review of 202 total ankle replacements followed up to 6 years. *Acta Orthop*. Vol. 78, No. 5, (January 2007), pp. 584-591, 1745-3674

Jacobs, J., Roebuck, K., Archibek, M., Hallab, N. & Glant, T. (2001). Osteolysis: Basic science. *Clin Orthop Rel Res*. Vol. 393, (December 2001), pp. 71-77, 0009-921X

Jasty, M., Floyd, W 3rd., Schiller, A., Goldring, S. & Harris W. (1986). Localized osteolysis in stable, non-septic total hip replacement. *J Bone Joint Surg Am*. Vol. 68, No. 6, (July 1986), pp. 912-919, 1535-1386

Jones, L. & Hungerford, D. (1987). Cement disease. *Clin Orthop Rel Res*. Vol. 225, (December 1987), pp.192-206, 0009-921X

Keogh, C.; Munk, P.; Gee, R.; Chan, L. & Marchinkow, L. (2003). Imaging of the Painful Hip Arthroplasty. *AJR*, 180, pp. 115-120, 0361-803X

Knecht, S., Estin, M., Callaghan, J., Zimmerman, M., Alliman, K., Alvine, F. & Saltzman, C. (2004). The Agility total ankle arthroplasty. Seven to sixteen-year follow-up. *J Bone Joint Surg Am*. Vol. 86-A, No. 6, (June 2004), pp. :1161-1171, 1535-1386

Kofoed, H. & Stirrup, J. (1994). Comparison of ankle arthroplasty and arthrodesis. *The Foot*. Vol. 4, No. 1, (March 1994), pp. 6-9, 0958-2592

Kofoed, H. (2004). Scandinavian Total Ankle Replacement (STAR). *Clin Orthop Relat Res*. Vol. 424, (July 2004), pp. 73-79, 0009-921X

Koivu, H., Kohonen, I., Sipola, E., Alanen, K., Vahlberg, T. & Tiusanen, H. (2009). Severe periprosthetic osteolytic lesions after the Ankle Evolutive System total ankle replacement. *J Bone Joint Surg Br*. Vol. 91, No. 7, (July 2009), pp. 907-14, 1535-1386

Kokkonen, A., Ikavalko, M., Tiihonen, R., Kautiainen, H. & Belt, E. (2011). High rate of osteolytic lesions in medium-term followup after the AES total ankle replacement. *Foot Ankle Int*. Vol. 32, No. 2, (February 2011), pp. 168-175, 1071-1007

Konttinen, Y., Zhao, D., Beklen, A., Ma, G., Takagi, M., Kivela-Rajamaki, M., Ashammakhi, N. & Santavirta S. (2005). The microenvironment around total hip replacement prostheses. *Clin Orthop Rel Res*. Vol. 430, (January 2005), pp.28-38, 0009-921X

Lee, M.; Kim, S.; Lee, S.; Song, H.; Huh, Y.; Kim, D.; Han, S. & Suh, J. (2007). Overcoming Artifacts from Metallic Orthopedic Implants at High-Field-Strength MR Imaging and Multidetector CT. *RadioGraphics*, 27, 3, pp. 791-803, 0271-5333

Link, T.; Berning, W; Scherf, S.; Joosten, U.; Joist, A.; Engelke, K. & Daldrup-Link, H. (2000). CT of Metal Implants: Reduction of Artifacts Using an Extended CT Scale Technique. *J Comput Assist Tomogr*, 24, 1, pp. 165-172, 0363-8715

Liu, P.; Pavlicek, W.; Peter, M.; Spangehl, M.; Roberts, C. & Paden, R. (2009). Metal artifact reduction image reconstruction algorithm for CT of implanted metal orthopedic devices: a work in progress. *Sleletal Radiol*, 38, pp. 797-802, 0364-2348

Looney, R.; Boyd, A.; Totterman, S.; Seo, G.; Tamez-Pena, J.; Campbell, D.; Novotny, L.; Olcott, C.; Martell, J.; Hayes, F,; O´Keefe, R. & Schwarz, E. (2002). Volumetric computerized tomography as a measurement of periprosthetic acetabular osteolysis and its correlation with wear. *Arthritis Res*, 4, pp. 59-63, 1465-9905

Nolan, J & Bucknill, T. (1992). Aggressive granulomatosis from polyethylene failure in an uncemented knee replacement. *J Bone Joint Surg Br.* Vol. 74, No. 1, (January 1992), pp. 23-24, 1535-1386

Ohashi, K.; El-Khoury, G.; Bennet, D.; Restrepo, J. & Berbaum, K. (2005). Orthopedic Hardware Complications Diagnosed with Multi-Detector Row CT. *Radiology*, 237, 2, pp. 570-577, 0033-8419

Park, J.; Ryu, K.; Hong, H.; Park, Y.; Chun, Y. & Yoo, M. (2004). Focal osteolysis in total hip replacement: CT findings. *Skeletal Radiol*, 33, pp. 632-640, 0364-2348

Purdue, P., Koulouvaris, P., Nestor, B. & Sculco, T. (2006). The central role of wear debris in periprosthetic osteolysis. *HSSJ*. Vol 2, No. 2, (September 2006), pp. 102-113, 1818-4960

Puri, L.; Wixson, R.; Stern, S.; Kohli, J.; Hendrix, R. & Stulberg, S. (2002). Use of Helical Computed Tomography for the Assessment of Acetabular Osteolysis After Total Hip Arthroplasty. *J Bone Joint Surg Am.*, 84, 4, pp. 609-614, 1535-1386

Pyevich, M., Saltzman, C., Callaghan, J. & Alvine F. (1998). Total ankle arthroplasty: a unique design. Two to twelve-year follow-up. *J Bone Joint Surg Am.* Vol. 80, No. 10, (October 1998), pp. 1410-1420, 1535-1386

Rodriguez, D., Bevernage, B., Maldague, P., Deleu, P., Tribak, K. & Leemrijse, T. (2010). Medium term follow-up of the AES ankle prosthesis: High rate of asymptomatic osteolysis. *Foot Ankle Surg.* Vol. 16, No. 2, (June 2010), pp. 54-60, 1268-7731

Saleh, K., Thongtrangan, I. & Schwarz, E. (2004). Osteolysis: medical and surgical approaches. *Clin Orthop Rel Res.* Vol. 427, (October 2004), pp. 138-147, 0009-921X

San Giovanni, T., Keblish, D., Thomas, W. & Wilson, M. (2006). Eight-year results of a minimally constrained total ankle arthroplasty. *Foot Ankle Int.* Vol. 27, No. 6, (June 2006), pp. 418-26, 1071-1007

Santavirta, S. (2005). Biotribology. *Acta Orthop.* 2005 Oct;Vol. 76, No. 5, (October 2005), pp. 613, 1745-3674

Santavirta, S., Hoikka, V., Eskola, A., Konttinen, Y., Paavilainen, T. & Tallroth, K. (1990). Aggressive granulomatous. *J Bone Joint Surg Br.* Vol. 72, No. 6, (Nowember 1990), pp. 980-984, 1535-1386

Schutte, B. & Louwerens, J. (2008). Short-term results of our first Scandinavian total ankle replacements (STAR). *Foot Ankle Int.* Vol. 29, No. 2, (February 2008), pp. 124-127, 1071-1007

Skytta, E., Koivu, H., Eskelinen, A., Ikävalko, M., Paavolainen, P. & Remes, V. (2010). Total ankle replacement: a population-based study of 515 cases from the Finnish Arthroplasty Register. *Acta Orthop.* Vol. 81, No. 1, (February 2010), pp. 114-118, 1745-3674

Spirt, A., Assal, M, & Hansen, S Jr. (2004). Complications and failure after total ankle arthroplasty. *J Bone Joint Surg Am.* Vol. 86-A, No. 6, (June 2004), pp. 1172-1178, 1535-1386

Stradiotti, P.; Curti, A.; Castellazzi, G. & Zerbi, A. (2009). Metal-related artefacts in instrumented spine. *Eur Spine J*, 18 (Suppl 1), pp. 102-108, 0940-6719

Su, E., Kahn, B. & Figgie, M. (2004). Total ankle replacement in patients with rheumatoid arthritis. *Clin Orthop Relat Res.* Vol. 424, (July 2004), pp. 32-38, 0009-921X

Tallroth, K., Eskola, A., Santavirta, S., Konttinen, Y. & Lindholm, T. (1989). Aggressive granulomatous lesion after hip arthroplasty. *J Bone Joint Surg Br.* Vol. 71, No. 4, (August 1989), pp. 571-575, 1535-1386

Valderrabano, V., Hintermann, B. & Dick, W. (2004). Scandinavian total ankle replacement: a 3.7-year average followup of 65 patients. *Clin Orthop Rel Res.* Vol. 424, (July 2004), pp. 47-56, 0009-921X

van den Heuvel, A., Van Bouwel, S. & Dereymaeker, G. (2010). Total ankle replacement. Design evolution and results. *Acta Orthop Belg.* Vol. 76, No. 2, (April 2010), pp. 150-61, 0001-6462

Walde, T.; Weiland, D.; Leung, S.; Kitamura, N.; Sychterz, C.; Engh, C. Jr.; Claus, A.; Potter, H. & Engh, C. Sr. (2005) Comparison of CT, MRI and Radiographs in Assessing Pelvic Osteolysis. *Clin Orthop*, 437, pp. 138-144, 0095-8654

Watzke, O. & Kalender, W. (2004). A pragmatic approach to metal artifact reduction in CT: merging of metal artifact reduced images. *Eur Radiol*, 14, pp. 849-856, 1756-1175

West, A.; Marshall, T. & Bearcroft, P. (2009). CT of the musculoskeletal system: What is left is the days of MRI? *Eur Radiol*, 19, pp. 152-164, 1756-1175

Wood, P. & Deakin, S. (2003). Total ankle replacement. The results in 200 ankles. *J Bone Joint Surg Br.* Vol.85, No. 3, (April 2003), pp. 334-341, 1535-1386

Wood, P., Prem, H. & Sutton, C. (2008). Total ankle replacement: medium-term results in 200 Scandinavian total ankle replacements. *J Bone Joint Surg Br.* 2008 Vol 90, No. 5, (May 2008), pp. 605-609, 1535-1386

Wood, P., Sutton, C., Mishra, V. & Suneja, R. (2009). A randomised, controlled trial of two mobile-bearing total ankle replacements. *J Bone Joint Surg Br.* Vol. 91-B, No. 1, (January 2009), pp. 69-74, 1535-1386

Zerahn, B. & Kofoed, H.(2004). Bone mineral density, gait analysis, and patient satisfaction, before and after ankle arthroplasty. *Foot Ankle Int.* Vol. 25, No. 4, (April 2004), pp. 208-214, 1071-1007

Zerahn, B., Kofoed, H. & Borgwardt A. (2000). Increased bone mineral density adjacent to hydroxyl-apatite-coated ankle arthroplasty. *Foot Ankle Int.* Vol. 21, No. 4, (April 2000), pp. 285-289, 1071-1007

16

Cardiac Rhythm Management Device Infections: Imaging Examinations to Direct Replacement Timing

Michela Casella et al.*
Cardiac Arrhythmia Research Centre,
Centro Cardiologico Monzino IRCCS, Milan,
Italy

1. Introduction

In this paper we describe the management of ICD (implantable cardioverter defibrillator) carriers who undergo extraction of infected leads and who, in view of the need for same-side reimplantation, are studied with ^{18}F-fluorodeoxyglucose (^{18}F-FDG) positron emission tomography with computed tomography (PET-CT) scan, or with leukocyte technetium-99m hexamethylpropylene amine oxime (^{99m}Tc-HMPAO) scan before reimplantation, in order to rule out a residual infection at the site of original implantation.

2. Case report 1

A 59-year-old man was admitted to our Institution with a three-week history of chills and fever (maximum 39.5°C). He had been implanted previously with a biventricular ICD placed at the left subclavicular region and had undergone repositioning of the right ventricular lead two months before the current hospitalization.
On admission, he had a high erythrocyte sedimentation rate (53 mm/h) and C-reactive protein (45 mg/L); blood cultures were positive for *Staphylococcus hominis* and transesophageal echocardiography visualized a vegetation on the right ventricular lead at the level of the tricuspid valve. Moreover, a chest ^{18}F-FDG PET-CT scan showed enhanced ^{18}F-FDG uptake at the left subclavicular region and along the intracardiac portion of the leads, thus supporting the diagnosis of device infection (figures 1 and 2). For that reason, intravenous antibiotics were started and the patient underwent successful transvenous lead extraction. The post-procedural course was free from complications, with no further evidence of systemic or local infection. After 14 days, an attempt to re-implant a new biventricular ICD from the contralateral side

* Francesco Perna[1], Antonio Dello Russo[2], Gemma Pelargonio[1], Stefano Bartoletti[2], Lucia Leccisotti[1], Ghaliah Al-Mohani[2], Pasquale Santangeli[3], Luigi Di Biase[3], Andrea Natale[3], Fulvio Bellocci[1] and Claudio Tondo[2]
[1]*Catholic University of the Sacred Heart, Rome, Italy*
[2]*Cardiac Arrhythmia Research Centre, Centro Cardiologico Monzino IRCCS, Milan, Italy*
[3]*Texas Cardiac Arrhythmia Institute at St David's Medical Center, Austin, TX, USA*

failed as selective angiography documented total occlusion of the right subclavian vein, whereas the left one was shown to be patent (figures 3 and 4).

At that point, in order to place the new biventricular ICD via the left subclavian vein, we referred the patient for a chest ^{18}F-FDG PET-CT. This showed focal enhanced ^{18}F-FDG uptake in the soft tissues at the left subclavicular region, supporting a diagnosis of residual local infection at the site of the original implantation (figure 5). We thus maintained the patient monitored in the Cardiology Ward, on combined intravenous and oral antibiotic therapy. After 15 more days we repeated a PET-CT scan, which showed normalization of ^{18}F-FDG uptake at the left subclavicular region, where we therefore decided to implant the new biventricular ICD via the left subclavian vein. The patient had no more infection-related symptoms or signs at 1, 3 6 and 12 month follow-up visits.

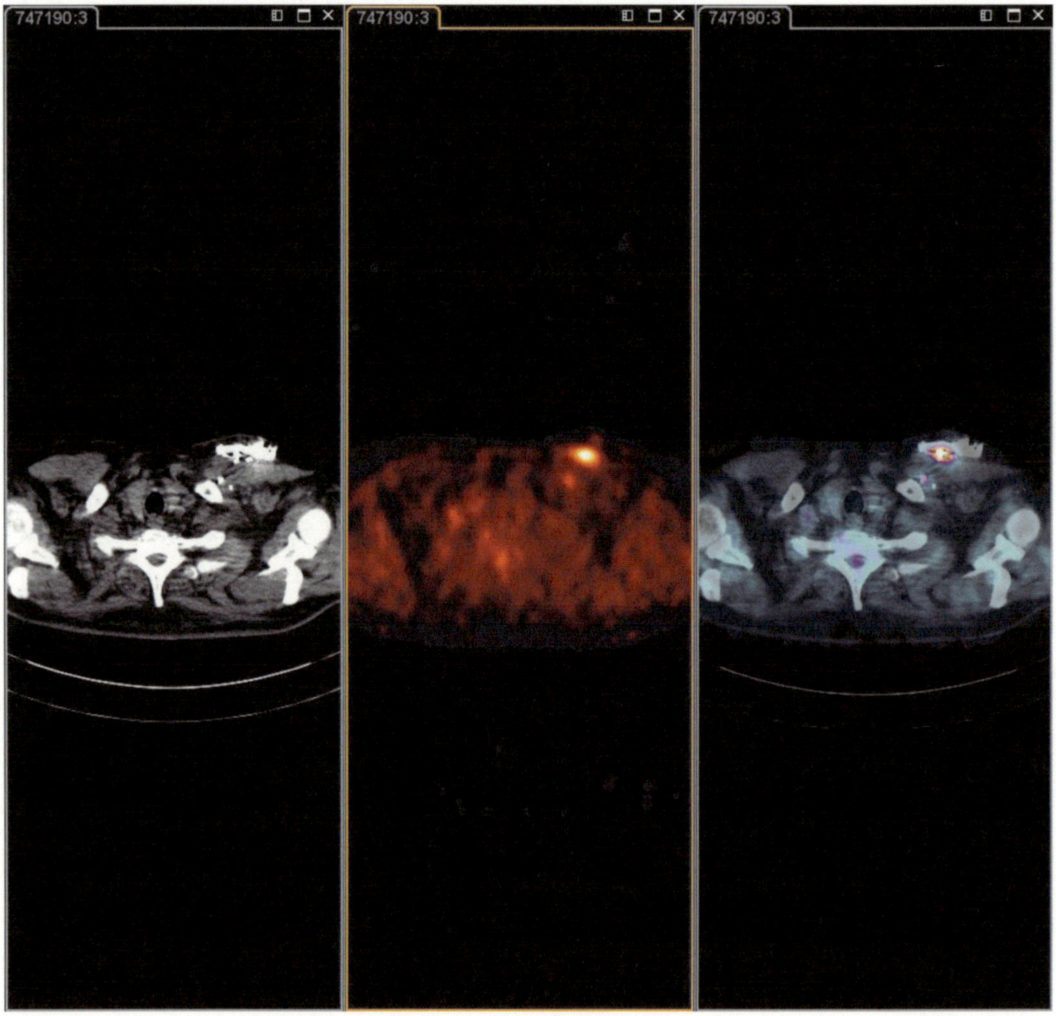

Fig. 1. Chest ^{18}F-FDG PET-CT showing enhanced 18F-FDG uptake within the ICD pocket. Left to right: CT image; PET image; PET-CT merge.

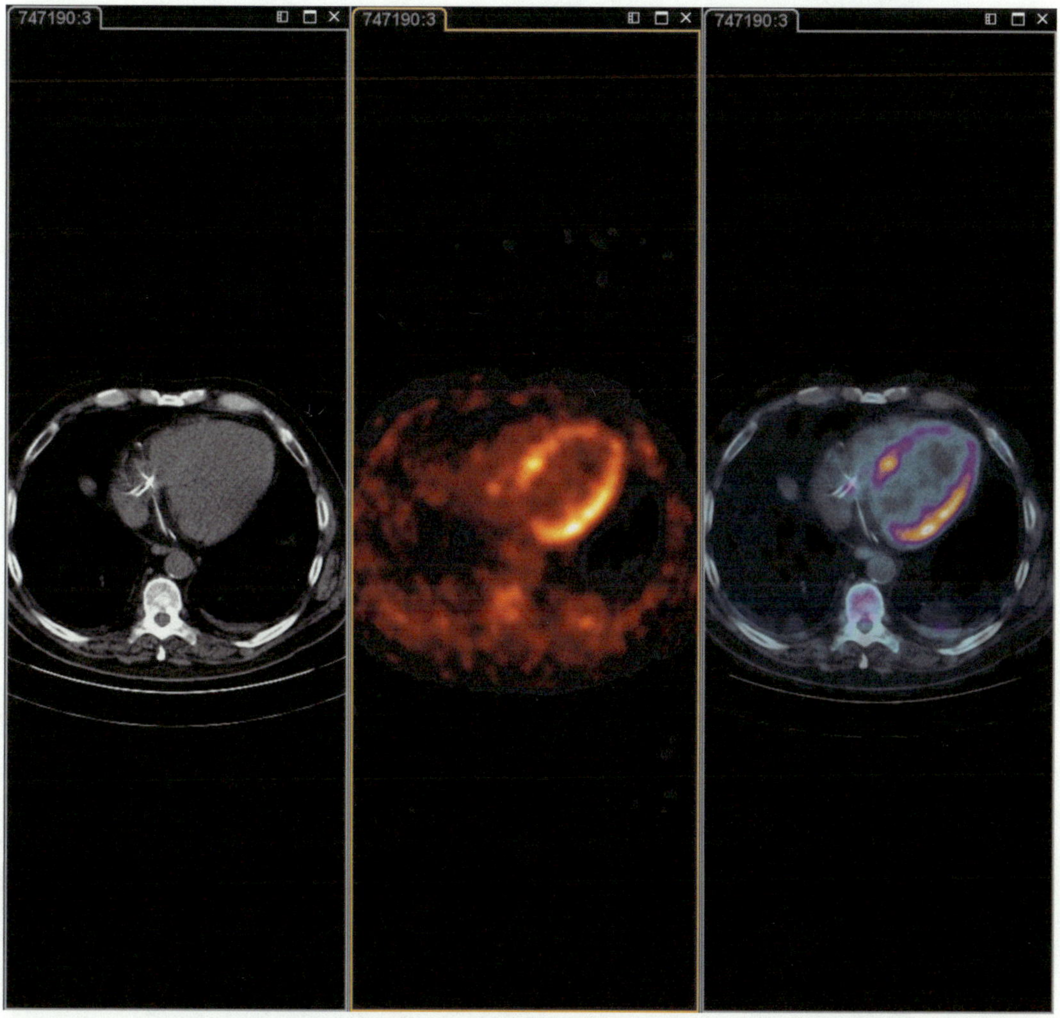

Fig. 2. Chest ^{18}F-FDG PET-CT showing enhanced 18F-FDG uptake along the intracardiac portion of the right ventricular lead running across the tricuspid valve. Left to right: CT image; PET image; PET-CT merge.

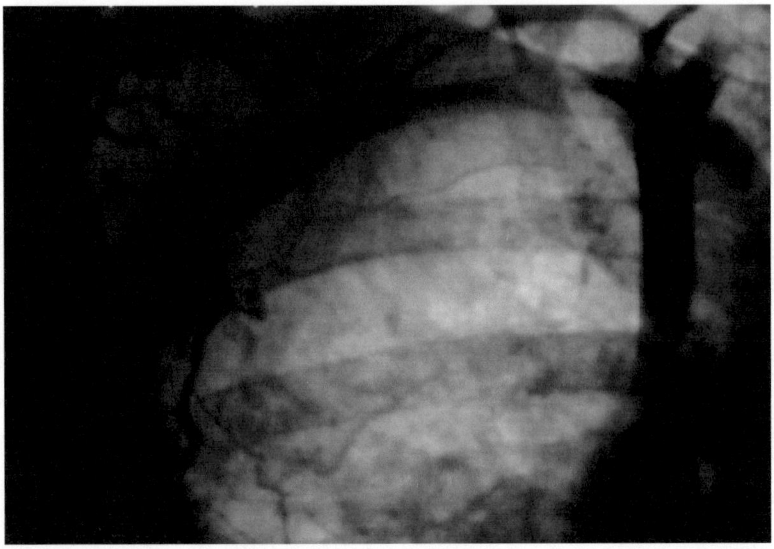

Fig. 3. Selective angiography of the right subclavian vein.

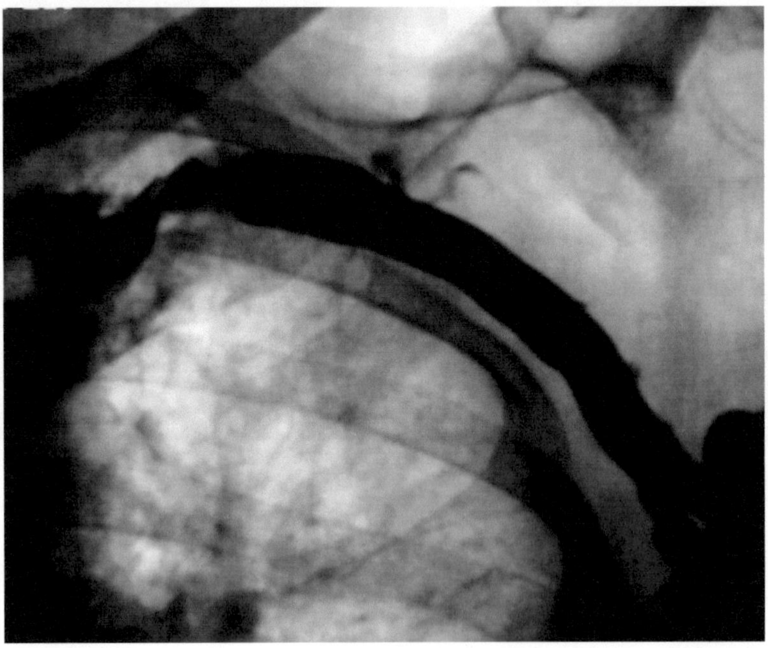

Fig. 4. Selective angiography of the left subclavian vein.

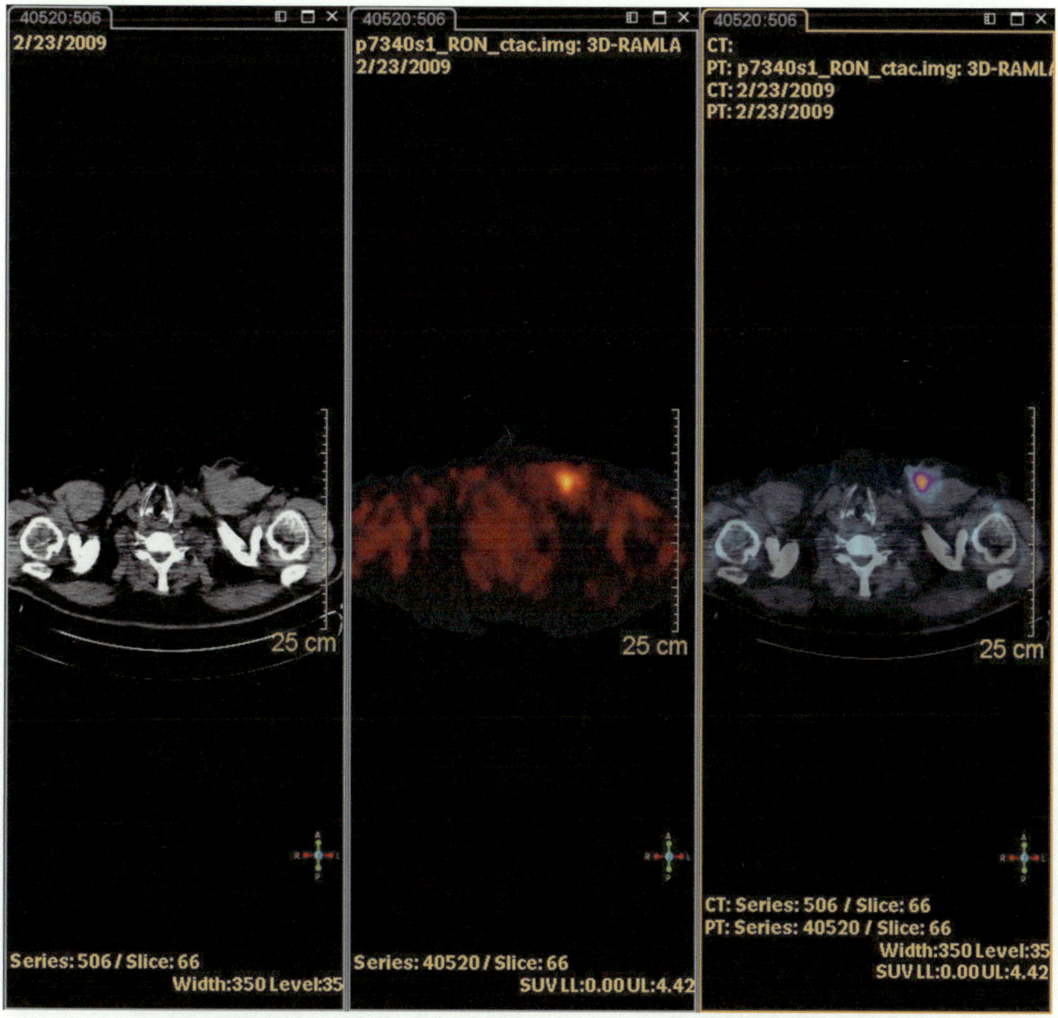

Fig. 5. Chest ^{18}F-FDG PET-CT showing focal 18F-FDG uptake in the subclavicular region after ICD extraction. Left to right: CT image; PET image; PET-CT merge.

3. Case report 2

A 71-year old man with two previous remote myocardial infarctions was admitted to our Institution for ICD lead extraction and reimplantation. He had undergone ablation of sustained ventricular tachycardia in 2000 and was implanted with a bicameral ICD at a left subclavicular site. When the generator was replaced in 2007, the device had become infected and both the generator and leads had to be extracted; the patient was then reimplanted on the right-sided subclavicular site. In April 2010, rising defibrillation impedance prompted a device revision procedure, which however led to a second device infection.

The patient came to our Institution with neither fever nor other symptoms and, after a transoesophageal echocardiogram excluded lead vegetations, he underwent extraction of both generator and leads without complications, followed by antibiotic therapy guided by sensitivity testing from the right-sided ICD pocket.

The issue of ICD reimplantation proved more difficult than initially thought, as the left subclavian vein, though seemingly patent on ultrasound and CT imaging, was shown by angiography to possess only a winding, thread-like residual patency with extensive collateral circulation (figure 6), whereas the right subclavian vein was shown to be fully patent. Therefore the possibility of using the previously infected right-sided subclavicular pocket was then taken into consideration and a ^{99m}Tc-HMPAO labelled leukocyte scan and SPECT was used to evaluate whether residual inflammation was present within the pocket (figure 7). The scan was negative and the new ICD was reimplanted at the right subclavicular site.

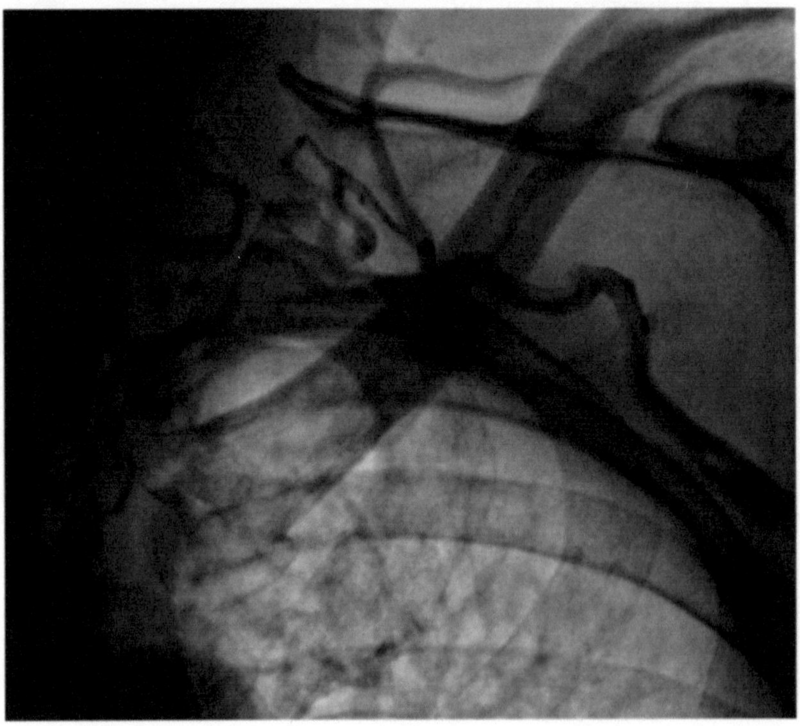

Fig. 6. Selective angiography of the left subclavian vein.

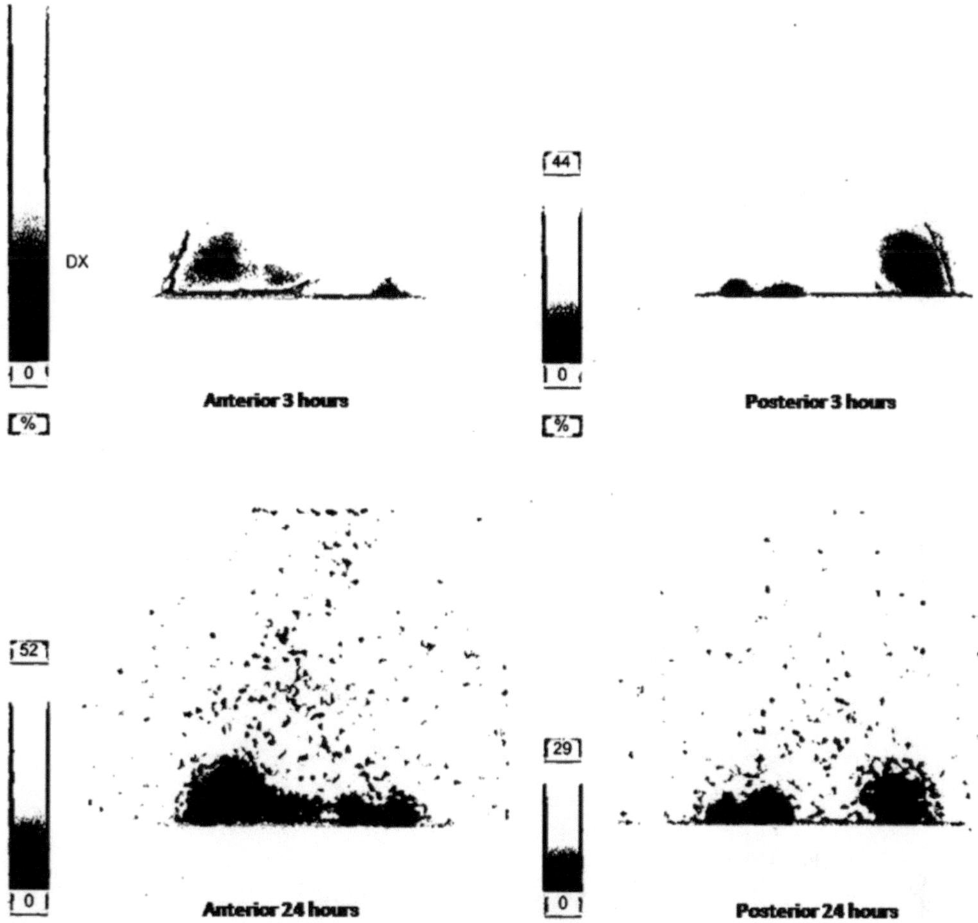

Fig. 7. White blood cell scintigraphy scan, showing no concentration of marked white blood cells at either subclavicular site.

4. Discussion

Generator or lead infection is the most common indication for removal of cardiovascular implantable electronic devices (CIED), and the increasing number of cardiac device implants explains the subsequent rise in the number of such procedures[1,2]. Recent guidelines provide detailed indications for lead extraction due to infection, depending on the involvement of such structures as heart valves, catheter leads, device pocket, or on the presence of sepsis/bacteremia; furthermore, directions about the timing of device reimplantation following infected device removal have been drawn up[3].

However, the authors just recommend not to place a second CIED in the same side as the extracted one and no specific indications have been established when same-side implantation is needed and an epicardial approach is not preferred. This might hold particular importance in patients who need prompt replacement of their device, for example because of stimulation-dependence or severe conduction disturbance.

To the purpose of safely implanting a CIED at the same site of the explanted one, an imaging investigation able to diagnose subclinical infection involving the subcutaneous soft tissues would be desirable. Few diagnostic tools have been specifically studied with the aim to detect residual infection at the sites of removed generator and leads, and the decision to reimplant is mainly based upon the absence of clinical signs or symptoms and on laboratory tests (mostly blood cultures) showing no sign of a local or systemic inflammatory/infectious process after a predetermined period of time[3].

FDG-PET and PET-CT scan have been used in the past decade in the diagnosis of patients with infection and inflammatory disorders, such as fever of unknown origin[4,5]. Combined FDG-PET and CT imaging has the potential to determine the sites of infection or inflammation with high precision, and it proved unaffected by significant metal-related artifacts due to CIED in phantom and patient studies (with an exception for ICD coils in one study)[6-8]. Possible limitations of this diagnostic technique are the spatial resolution (although our system achieves a 4 mm resolution after merging the two imaging modalities) and the possible occurrence of high-density material-related artifacts, which we avoided by comparing the combined images to the pre-acquired FDG-PET scan alone[9].

FDG-PET has been used in a previous report to detect a suspected pocket and lead infection and to opt for pacemaker removal in a patient with no other signs of infection detectable on clinical and instrumental examinations; in that case, PET scan showed a faint non-specific uptake in the empty pocket after pacemaker removal[10]. However, the ^{18}F-FDG uptake pattern can help to reliably distinguish between a healing scar-related signal and an infection-related one. In another published image, PET-CT was used to investigate a suspected foreign-body infectious endocarditis in a patient with an implanted ICD and a recent purulent discharge from the device pocket, that had been treated with antibiotics, and it detected an infection concerning both the wire line from the device up to the right atrium and the catheter within the coronary sinus[11].

Leukocyte ^{99m}Tc-HMPAO scan is also used for the visual diagnosis of infectious and inflammatory processes,[12-14] based on the principles that white blood cells concentrate in site of ongoing inflammation. The use of this technique is well-documented for the diagnosis of infection of endovascular prostheses such as grafts and stents[15-16] and of left ventricular assist devices[17], while there is scarcer evidence in CIED infections. Ramackers and colleagues reported in 1995 the use of ^{99m}Tc-HMPAO labelled granulocyte scan with SPECT imaging for the detection and follow-up of recurrent infective endocarditis in a patient equipped with a pacemaker.[18] In that case, the patient's conditions excluded the possibility of lead extraction, so the SPECT scan was used not only to diagnose the infection, but also to document disappearance of inflammation after adequate antibiotic therapy, despite no significant change on echocardiography. Howarth and colleagues reported in 1998 the use of ^{99m}Tc-HMPAO labeled leukocyte scan to demonstrate infection of pacing leads in a patient with a cardiac pacemaker.[19] In that case, initial gallium- and technetium-labeled leukocyte scans were negative, but repeat ^{99m}Tc-HMPAO scan after five weeks allowed to localize the septic focus, an infected thrombus along the pacing leads in the subclavian and brachiocephalic veins. Lead extraction was necessary before the patient's conditions could improve. A more recent publication used indium-111 leukocyte scan with SPECT for much the same purpose.[20]

We used the PET-CT scan and marked leukocytes scan after lead extraction to rule out a residual infection in the region of previous implantation, in order to feel safer in performing such a procedure and to set the date for ICD reimplantation. While there is no evidence on the relative advantages of one over the other in CIED infections, the two techniques described in our case reports have been compared for the diagnosis of infection of an aortic graft in a single case report, in which it was observed that ^{18}F-FDG PET-CT was able to diagnose the infection, whereas ^{99m}Tc-HMPAO labelled leukocyte scan was not.[21]

Given the continuous advances in technology and the absence of other reliable diagnostic tests, this approach may prove to be the study of choice in the foreseeable future for precise localization of involved sites and as a tool to direct CIED replacement timing.

5. References

[1] Voigt, A. Shalaby, A. Saba. Rising Rates of Cardiac Rhythm Management Device Infections in the United States: 1996 through 2003. JACC 2006; 48(3): 586–97.

[2] Smith MC, Love CJ: Extraction of Transvenous Pacing and ICD Leads. PACE 2008; 31: 736-752.

[3] Wilkoff BL, Love CJ, Byrd CL, Bongiorni MG, Carrillo RG, Crossley GH 3rd, Epstein LM, Friedman RA, Kennergren CE, Mitkowski P, Schaerf RH, Wazni OM. Transvenous lead extraction: Heart Rhythm Society Expert consensus on facilities, training, indications, and patient management: this document was endorsed by the American Heart Association (AHA). Heart Rhythm 2009; 6(7): 1085-104.

[4] Basu S, Chryssikos T, Moghadam-Kia S, Zhuang H, Torigian DA, Alavi A. Positron Emission Tomography as a Diagnostic Tool in Infection: Present Role and Future Possibilities. Semin Nucl Med 2009; 39: 36-51.

[5] Keidar Z, Gurman-Balbir A, Gaitini D, Israel O. Fever of Unknown Origin: The Role of 18F-FDG PET/CT. J Nucl Med 2008; 49: 1980–1985.

[6] Townsend DW. Positron Emission Tomography/Computed Tomography. Semin Nucl Med 2008; 38: 152-166.

[7] DiFilippo FP, Brunken RC. Do Implanted Pacemaker Leads and ICD Leads Cause Metal-Related Artifact in Cardiac PET/CT? J Nucl Med 2005; 46: 436–443.

[8] Kaneta T, Takanami K, Wakayama Y, Sato A, Higano S, Fukuda H, Yamada S, Takahashi S. High-density materials do not always induce artifacts on PET/CT: what is responsible for the difference? Nucl Med Commun 2007; 28(6): 495-9.

[9] Li TR, Tian JH, Wang H, Chen ZQ, Zhao CL. Pitfalls in positron emission tomography/computed tomography imaging: causes and their classifications. Chin Med Sci J 2009; 24(1): 12-9.

[10] Vos FJ, Bleeker-Rovers CP, van Dijk APJ, Oyen WJG. Detection of pacemaker and lead infection with FDG-PET. Eur J Nucl Med Mol Imaging 2006; 33:1245.

[11] Khamaisi M, Medina A, Mazouz B, Bocher M. Imaging coronary sinus infection in pacemaker electrode with [18F]-Fluorodesoxyglucose positron emission tomography. J Cardiovasc Electrophysiol, 2008; 19: 1327-1328.

[12] de Vries EF, Roca M, Jamar F, Israel O, Signore A. Guidelines for the labelling of leucocytes with (99m)Tc-HMPAO. Inflammation/Infection Taskgroup of the European Association of Nuclear Medicine. Eur J Nucl Med Mol Imaging. 2010; 37(4): 842-8.

[13] Peters AM, Osman S, Henderson BL, Kelly JD, Danpure HJ, Hawker RJ, et al. Clinical experience with 99mTc-hexamethylpropyleneamineoxime for labelling leukocytes and imaging inflammation. Lancet. 1986; 8513: 946–949.

[14] Roddie ME, Peters AM, Danpure HJ, Osman S, Henderson BL, Lavender JP, et al. Inflammation: imaging with Tc-99m HMPAO-labeled leukocytes. *Radiology.* 1988; 166: 767–772

[15] Liberatore M, Misuraca M, Calandri E, Rizzo L, Speziale F, Iurilli AP, Anagnostou C. White blood cell scintigraphy in the diagnosis of infection of endovascular prostheses within the first month after implantation. Med Sci Monit. 2006; 12(3): MT5-9.

[16] d'Ettorre G, Ceccarelli G, Zaffiri L, Falcone M, Mastroianni CM, Venditti M, Vullo V. Infectious aortitis and spondylodiscitis in patients with endovascular stents. Minerva Med. 2009; 100(2): 167-70.

[17] Litzler PY, Manrique A, Etienne M, Salles A, Edet-Sanson A, Vera P, Bessou JP, Hitzel A. Leukocyte SPECT/CT for detecting infection of left-ventricular-assist devices: preliminary results. J Nucl Med. 2010; 51(7): 1044-8.

[18] Ramackers JM, Kotzki PO, Couret I, Messner-Pellenc P, Davy JM, Rossi M. The use of technetium-99m hexamethylpropylene amine oxime labelled granulocytes with single-photon emission tomography imaging in the detection and follow-up of recurrence of infective endocarditis complicating transvenous endocardial pacemaker. Eur J Nucl Med. 1995; 22(11): 1351-4.

[19] Howarth DM, Curteis PG, Gibson S. Infected cardiac pacemaker wires demonstrated by Tc-99m labeled white blood cell scintigraphy. Clin Nucl Med. 1998; 23(2): 74-6.

[20] Squires S, Juweid M. Visualization of infected cardiac pacemaker leads by SPECT In-111 leukocyte imaging. Clin Nucl Med. 2005; 30(8): 584-5.

[21] Gardet E, Addas R, Monteil J, Le Guyader A. Comparison of detection of F-18 fluorodeoxyglucose positron emission tomography and 99mTc-hexamethylpropylene amine oxime labelled leukocyte scintigraphy for an aortic graft infection. Interact Cardiovasc Thorac Surg. 2010; 10(1): 142-3.

17

Comparison of Patient Localization Accuracy Between Stereotactic X-Ray Based Setup and Cone Beam CT Based Setup on Intensity Modulated Radiation Therapy

Naoki Hayashi et al.*
School of Health Sciences, Fujita Health University
Japan

1. Introduction

1.1 Background and objectives

Radiotherapy aims to deliver a radiation dose to the tumor which is high enough to kill all tumor cells. Daily patient localization variation, internal organ motion and deformation have long been a concern for radiotherapy. To account for these variations and to make sure adequate target coverage, margins for each direction are added around clinical target volume (CTV) to define a planning target volume (PTV). However, the larger margins may increase the irradiated volume. Nowadays, image-guided radiation therapy (IGRT) is used to accurate the patient localization and to deliver the radiation correctly under monitoring the respiratory motion. Recently, there are available several IGRT technologies such as kilo-voltage (kV) and megavoltage (MV) X-ray imaging, on-board kV and MV computed-tomography (CT), in-room conventional CT, and ultrasound systems. These images are most frequently used for image-guidance: positioning of the patient or target position is evaluated by a comparison of the acquired images with the planning CT or digitally reconstructed radiography (DRR) related to the planning CT. With IGRT, the dose for tumor cells is able to be escalated because that for normal tissue becomes reduced. The principle and merits of these technologies are reported by many investigators and defined in American Association of Physicists in Medicine Report.

The NovalisTx (NTX), this is manufactured by BrainLAB (Heimstetten, Germany), is a dedicated to high precision radiotherapy system that offers a versatile combination of advanced technologies for treatment of tumors and other anatomical targets (Fig. 1). NTX is equipped with a 2.5 mm high-definition multi-leaf collimator and special patient localization system for precise tissue targeting (Fig. 1). The patient localization system distinguishes into 3 systems: BrainLAB 6D system, an on-board imager (OBI) based cone

---

* Hitoshi Takagi[2], Shinichi Hashinokuchi[2], Hiroshi Fujiwara[2],
Hidetoshi Kobayashi[3], Fumitaka Itoh[3], Yumi Oie[3] and Hideki Kato[1]
[1]*School of Health Sciences, Fujita Health University*
[2]*Department of Radiology, Ogaki Municipal Hospital*
[3]*School of Medicine, Fujita Health University, Japan*

beam computed tomography (CBCT), and an electrical portal imaging device (EPID) based megavoltage portal vision systems (MVPV).

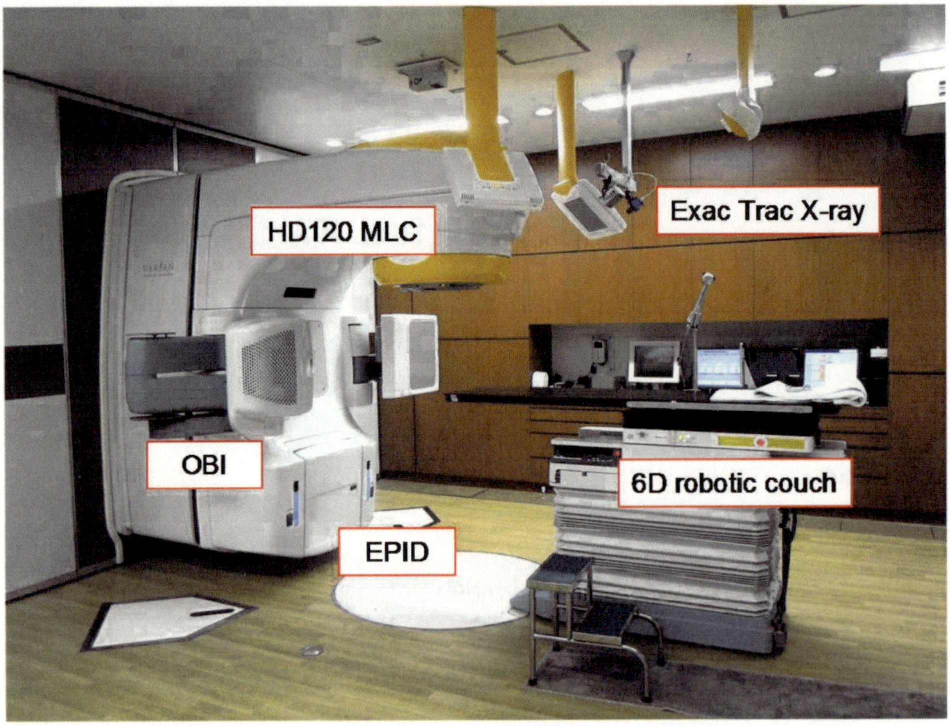

Fig. 1. Overview of Novalis Tx.
NTX is dedicated to high precision radiotherapy in combination with image-guided technology.

BrainLAB 6D system consists of ExacTrac X-ray 6D (ETX) and precise robotic couch system. ETX system is one of the commercially available patient positioning devices. ETX system combines an infrared (IR)-based tracking system with a X-ray-imaging-based system. Two IR cameras are fixed to the ceiling. Two kV X-ray beams are projected from the two X-ray tubes in oblique directions for the purpose of verifying patient localization. The procedure for patient setup with the ETX system consists of three steps: in step one, the initial patient setup according to the IR body markers is performed. Normally, the IR body markers are placed asymmetrically on the patient's body surface. The placement of each IR marker is detected by two IR cameras, and then the IR based patient localization is completed by the automatic robotic couch movement. In step two, two X-ray images are taken and compared with a DRR by specific registration software. The DRR is reconstructed by the planning CT. The specific registration software is able to be compared with DRR to calculate the patient localization accuracy in three translational directions and three rotational angles. In step three, X-ray image-based patient localization is completely corrected by the automatic robotic couch movement.
The OBI is mounted on the gantry of the linear accelerator via controlled arms in a direction orthogonal to the therapeutic beam direction. The OBI consists of a kV-X-ray source and a flat-panel detector using amorphous silicon detector. The OBI provides three acquisition

modes: 2D radiographic acquisition, 2D fluoroscopic image acquisition, and 3D CBCT. When the gantry rotates around the patient with the kV-X-ray source, volumetric data are acquired as CBCT images. The transverse images are reconstructed by the specific application software when the X-ray projected data are acquired. The CBCT images are ganarated from 360 to 655 kV-photon beam projections. There are six CBCT settings available in the system: Low-dose Head, Standard-dose Head, High-quality Head, Pelvis Spotlight, Pelvis, and Low-dose Thorax. The operator should select optimal setting when CBCT acquisition. The CBCT images are able to be compared with the planning CT to evaluate the patient localization accuracy in three translational directions and one rotational angle. The patient localization errors are then corrected by shifts of the treatment couch.

The MVPV provides a 2D image using megavoltage photon therapeutic beam and also is capable of EPID based portal dosimetry QA to accurately. Clinical users are able to use them for patient localization and can select the procedure optimally case by case. After acquisition of clinical image with the device, the image fused with the digital reconstructed radiography and/or CT images for treatment planning. It is very important for high precision radiotherapy to verify the accuracy of image fusion in this procedure. After the verification, the patient will be moved to optimal position with robotic couch system. This procedure is routine step of high precision radiotherapy with NTX system.

The purpose of this study is to evaluate setup discrepancies measured with ETX system and CBCT for patients under treatments of intensity modulated radiation therapy (IMRT) for prostate cancer.

2. Materials and methods

In this study, the phantom-based study as for fundamental evaluation and the patient study as for clinical evaluation were performed. For fundamental study, an anthropomorphic phantom was put on intentional positions. Next, the images obtained with ETX and CBCT systems to evaluate the accuracy of each imaging systems. For clinical study, five patients with prostate cancer were analyzed retrospectively. The patients were immobilized by vacuum pillow system and localized with ETX and CBCT each other. The patient localization discrepancies were evaluated statistically with the calculated values in each modality.

2.1 Fundamental study

Before patient study, we performed the phantom study using anthropomorphic phantom (Fig. 2). The phantom was modified for bone, soft-tissue, and other heterogeneity with various shapes and effective atomic numbers simulating human body.

A micro spherical ball with a diameter of 5 mm was inserted to center of the phantom. Several IR markers were placed on the surface of the phantom asymmetry. The phantom without specific localizer was scanned by multi-detector CT (Asterion: Toshiba Medical Corporation, Tokyo, Japan) with slice-thickness of 1 mm. The i-plan treatment planning workstation (BrainLAB, Heimstetten, Germany) was used to design a treatment plan from these CT scans. A round-shaped target was defined at center of the micro spherical ball. The target was defined as the planning target volume (PTV). The intentional treatment plan had a single perpendicular beam from gantry angle of 0 degree with an isocenter located at center of PTV. The coordinate of the target was transferred to ETX and CBCT application for the purpose of performing IGRT technology.

The phantom localization procedure is shown in Fig. 3. Firstly the phantom was subliminal localized using the IR markers on the surface of the phantom. Secondly the ETX-based phantom localization was performed. After the ETX-based phantom localization, another two oblique X-ray images with ETX were acquired as the localization error of ETX. Thirdly CBCT images were acquired with a slice thickness of 1 mm. The CBCT images were compared with the planning CT to verify the localization errors using online 3D registration in review software (AM workstation, Varian Medical Systems, Palo Alto, USA). The calculated errors were used as the localization error between ETX and CBCT systems. These procedures were repeated 20 times.

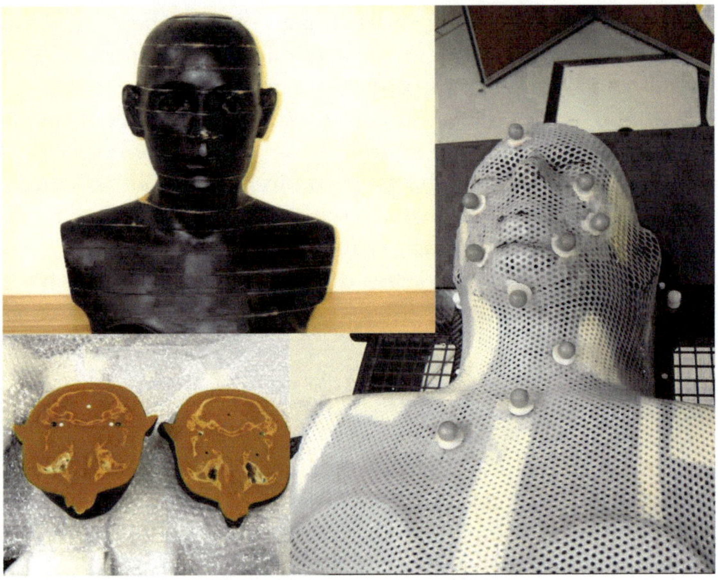

Fig. 2. A phantom for fundamental experiment.
A sphere ball of 5mm diameter was inserted to phantom. IR markers were put on the phantom.

2.2 Patient study

From September 2010 to March 2011, five patients with prostate cancer were selected for this study. All patients received IMRT treatment using NTX unit. The patients were immobilized by the vacuum cushion on the couch in a natural supine position. A planning CT image set of each patient was acquired using a CT simulator (Asteion 4, Toshiba Medical Systems, Tokyo) with a slice thickness of 2 mm. The treatment plans were designed by i-plan workstation. CTV includes prostate and seminal vesicles. The organ-at risk includes bladder and rectum.

As well as the fundamental study, IGRT techniques were used for the patient localization. The workflow of the patient localization is shown in Fig. 3. Firstly the patients subliminal localized firstly by IR markers on the surface of the patients as the skin-based setup procedure. Secondly two oblique X-ray images were acquired to carry out ETX-based patient localization. After ETX-based patient localization, another pair of two oblique X-ray images with ETX was acquired to calculate the patient localization discrepancy of ETX. Thirdly CBCT images were acquired with a slice thickness of 1 mm. In this study, no shifts were applied in between CBCT and the last pair of two X-ray images to be easier for comparison of patient position. The CBCT images were compared with the planning CT to verify the patient localization errors using online 3D registration in Varian's review software. All registrations were compared bone matching with target matching settings. The calculated errors were used as the patient localization error between ETX and CBCT systems. These procedures were performed for all patients in every fraction.

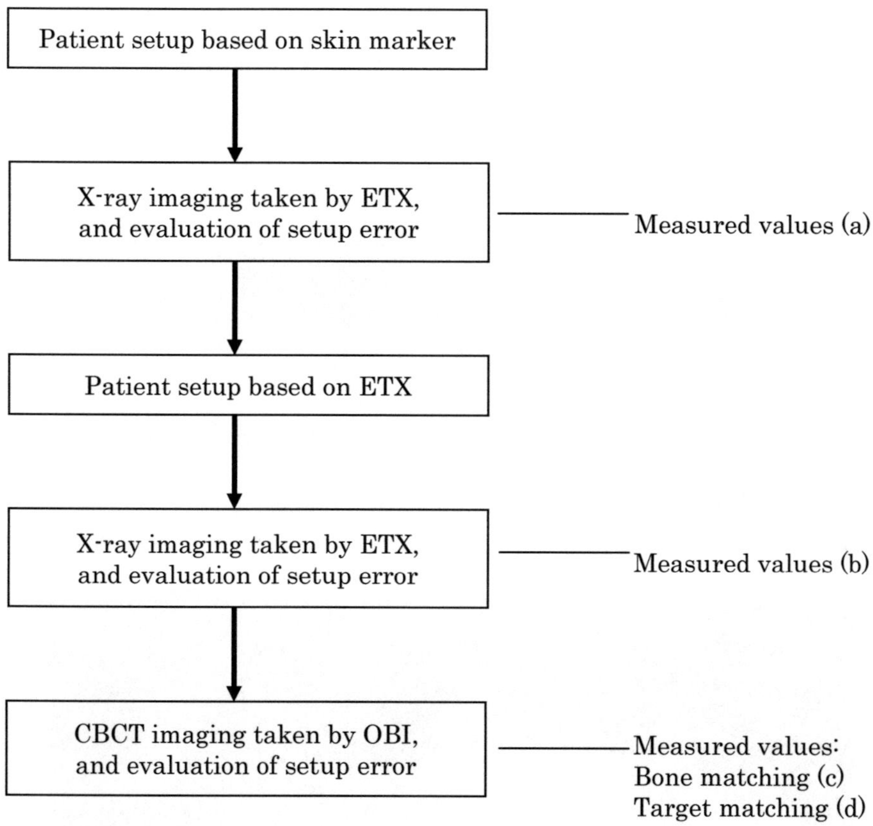

Fig. 3. Procedure of patient localization and evaluation for setup errors.

In Fig. 3, the measured values of (a), (b), (c), and (d) were transacted as the discrepancies of IR (skin)-based, 2D X-ray -based, CBCT-based referring to bony structure, and CBCT-based referring to the target, respectively. The values on the verification software were statistically analyzed.

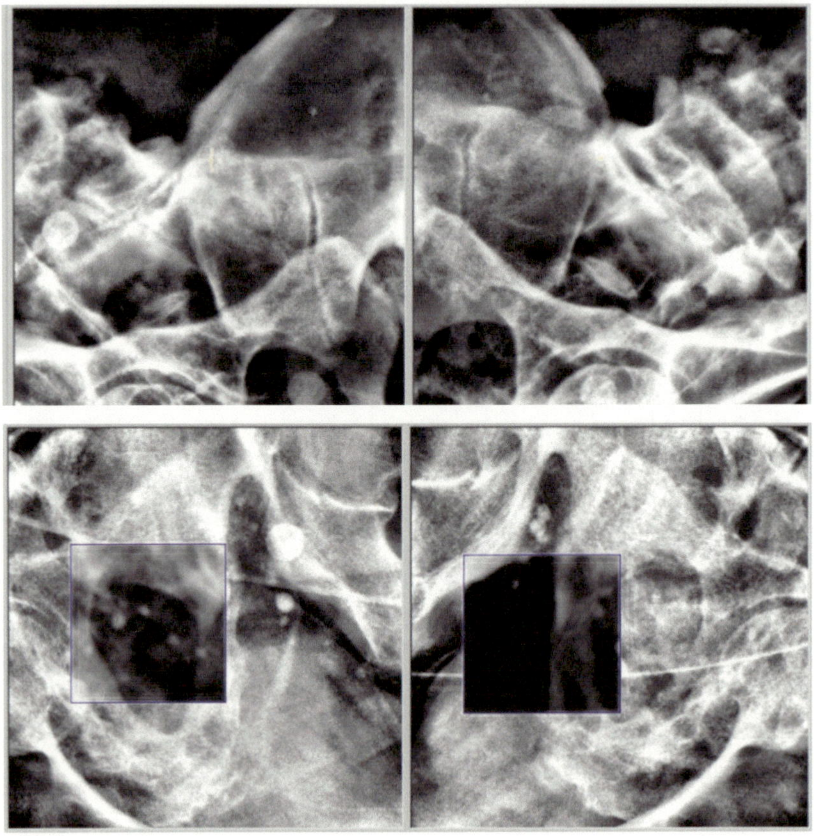

Fig. 4. The patient localization by ETX system.
Superior figure shows the snapshot of 2D oblique X-ray images.
Inferior figure shows the comparison of X-ray image (outer-ROI) and DRR (inter-ROI).

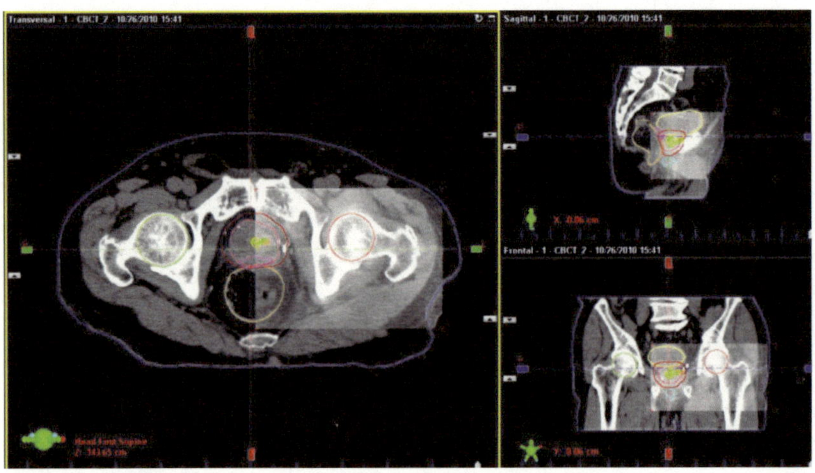

Fig. 5. CBCT guided patient registration using AM software.
The CBCT image (inter-ROI) was acquired to compare with the planning CT (Outer-ROI).

3. Results

This study indicates that the discrepancies between ETX and CBCT imaging systems for IMRT of prostate cancer. The results of fundamental examination indicate that translational and rotational discrepancies between ETX and CBCT were less than 0.8 mm and 0.5 degree, respectively. This means NTX system provides high precision radiotherapy and these values satisfied the tolerance of mechanical accuracy which described in American association of physicists in medicine (AAPM) task group 142.

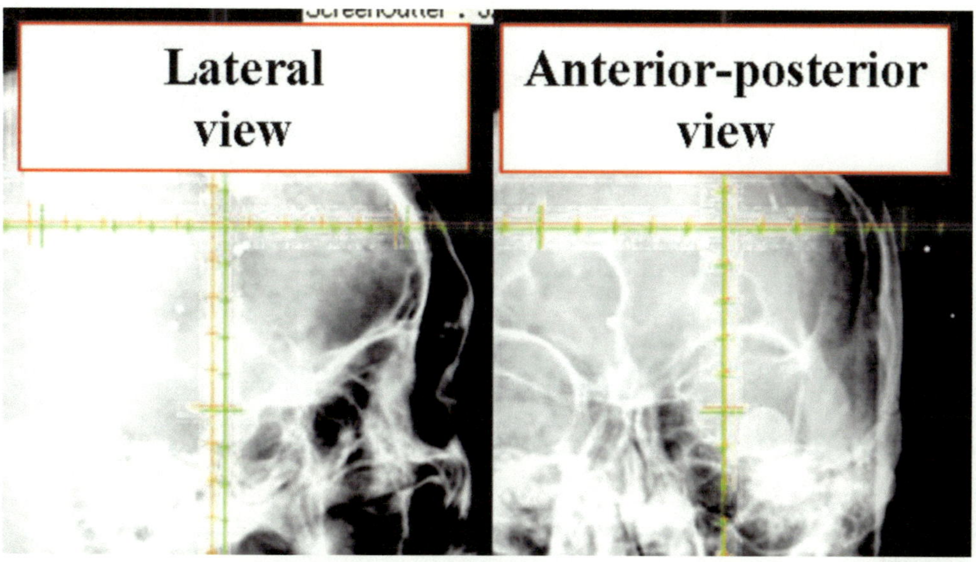

Fig. 6. OBI guided patient registration using AM software.

The results of clinical study are shown in Table 1 and 2. The setup discrepancies in translational error between skin-based setup and bony structure-based setup were measured respectively as -0.28±3.85 (mm) vertically, 147±4.48 (mm) longitudinally, -1.24±2.17 (mm) laterally shifts. The angle errors between those were less than 1 degree in all directions.

The setup discrepancies in translational error between ETX and CBCT setup referring to bony structure were measured respectively as -0.14±0.18 (mm) vertically, 0.00±0.18 (mm) longitudinally, -0.04±0.12 (mm) laterally shifts. There is no significant angle error between those setup methods. The setup discrepancies in translational error between ETX and CBCT setup referring to target structure were measured respectively as -2.04±3.26 (mm) vertically, 0.80±1.13 (mm) longitudinally, -1.01±2.12 (mm) laterally shifts. There is no significant angle error between those setup methods. With these values, the setup discrepancies in translational error between CBCT setup referring to bony structure and that referring to target structure were calculated as 2.11±3.30 (mm) vertical, 0.80±1.15 (mm) longitudinally, 1.03±2.09 (mm) laterally shifts and -0.50±0.27 (degree) rotational angle.

			Direction	Sample	Average ± SD	Maximum	Minimum
ETX	Skin	Shift (mm)	Vertical	150	-1.21±3.74	6.53	-11.05
			Longitudinal	150	1.55±4.63	14.53	-10.33
			Lateral	150	-0.83±2.27	5.55	-8.59
		Angle (degree)	Vertical	150	0.46±1.00	2.99	-1.93
			Longitudinal	150	0.32±0.83	3.53	-2.87
			Lateral	150	0.59±1.50	5.52	-2.32
	Bone	Shift (mm)	Vertical	142	-0.93±0.76	0.99	-4.28
			Longitudinal	142	0.01±1.09	2.15	-2.19
			Lateral	142	0.40±0.89	3.13	-2.30
		Angle (degree)	Vertical	142	0.50±0.98	3.04	-1.94
			Longitudinal	142	-0.06±0.22	0.77	-0.86
			Lateral	142	0.07±0.41	3.19	-0.94
	Skin vs Bone	Shift (mm)	Vertical	142	-0.28±3.85	7.44	-10.87
			Longitudinal	142	1.47±4.48	15.48	-9.91
			Lateral	142	-1.24±2.17	4.76	-10.61
		Angle (degree)	Vertical	142	-0.03±0.20	1.39	-1.04
			Longitudinal	142	0.35±0.92	4.01	-2.43
			Lateral	142	0.52±1.45	4.45	-2.48

Table 1. Overall analysis of setup errors evaluated by ETX

			Direction	Sample	Average ± SD	Maximum	Minimum
CBCT	Bone match	Shift (mm)	Vertical	137	-0.14±0.18	0.5	-0.6
			Longitudinal	137	0.00±0.18	0.4	-0.4
			Lateral	137	-0.04±0.12	0.3	-0.4
		Rotation (degree)		137	0.10±0.21	1.0	-1.0
	Target match	Shift (mm)	Vertical	114	-2.04±3.26	7.6	-3.8
			Longitudinal	114	0.80±1.13	2.4	-1.4
			Lateral	114	-1.01±2.12	3.3	-2.5
		Rotation (degree)		114	-0.80±0.50	1.0	-1.00
	Bone vs Target	Shift (mm)	Vertical	114	2.11±3.30	7.1	-3.2
			Longitudinal	114	0.80±1.15	2.5	-1.6
			Lateral	114	1.03±2.09	2.3	-2.2
		Rotation (degree)		114	-0.50±0.27	1.0	-1.0

Table 2. Overall analysis of setup errors evaluated by CBCT

4. Discussions

The geometric and localization accuracy between ETX and CBCT systems was compared by determining the subliminal localization errors. For the evaluation of geometrical accuracy and patient localization accuracy, the phantom examination and clinical patient's examination were performed, respectively.

In clinical situation, ETX and CBCT images are majorly applied to the patient localization before treatment. These are useful to be close to origin of the coordinate of PTV. In addition, it is possible to monitor the intra-fraction organ motion if we use them during treatment. The advantages of ETX are easier registration with bone matching, short-time patient localization, and low imaging dose compared to CBCT. The advantages of CBCT are the availability of 3D image information, and visualization of soft-tissue and/or target such as pelvis lesion. In addition, there is an opportunity for online re-planning and adaptive radiation therapy. With careful consideration and strategy of image guidance in radiation therapy, each modality has been widely adopted to provide real-time geometric and anatomic information with the patient in treatment position.

However, the disadvantage of ETX and CBCT systems is an excessive radiation dose when used routinely in radiation therapy. The concomitant dose should be carefully considered and recorded when designing treatment imaging process in order to remain faithful to the radiology principle of "As Low As Reasonably Achievable (ALARA)". Because the evaluation of cumulative imaging dose is non-trivial problem, a separate AAPM Task group 75 has produced a report analyzing the radiation dose delivered during IGRT. According to the report, the imaging dose of ETX and for body lesion was 0.551 mGy. On the other hand, the imaging dose of CBCT for pelvis lesion was 60 mGy as $CTDI_{air}$. Song et al. (2008) investigated the CBCT imaging dose in comparison of Elekta XVI system and Varian OBI CBCT systems. They summarized that the average dose for XVI system ranged from 0.1 to 3.5 cGy with the highest dose measured in prostate region. The average dose for the OBI system ranged from 1.1 to 8.3 cGy with the highest dose measured. The reason of this difference was the availability of half-scan in XVI system. Therefore there is no significant change of imaging dose between different vendor's CBCT systems. Operator of CBCT should select optimal setting of

The general acceptable imaging dose management is represented by the acronym ALALA. We should use IGRT devices with acceptable effective dose without reducing the image information. For diagnostic image, the relationship between exposure condition and image quality is trade it off. To gain high contrast for the image, the expose dose should be increased. In IGRT, the beam alignment information derived from images used for the targeting of tumors is less dependent on image quality because it is dependent on imaging frequency to observe the constancy of patient localization before/during treatment. In radiotherapy process, a large number of the images will yield smaller errors in dose alignment. On the other hand, a large number of the images will add more imaging radiation dose to normal tissue. The frequency and settings of IGRT process should be optimized with considering the relationship between imaging dose and the benefit such as obtaining the alignment error.

There are three modalities for IGRT including ETX, CBCT and EPID in NTX system. Hence, the localization accuracy using NTX is able to increase. This characteristic advantage of NTX can reduce the safety margin adding to CTV.

When initial corrections of the patient localization were done only with the ETX system, it is sometimes not sufficient to answer the question whether the localization of PTV is correct or not because ETX system is only possible to detect bone and/or high contrast marker in 2D-to-3D matching. The patient localization using CBCT system can be performed based on both bony and soft-tissue matching.

However, this study was a preliminary evaluation of patient localization accuracy of multi-modality IGRT in prostate cases. Therefore the number of samples was not enough to construct the evidence. Additional evaluation with more patients and further images should be analyzed to ensure the usefulness and organ motion. In addition, this evaluation included only prostate cases. It would be exciting to extend this evaluation to other regions.

5. Conclusions

Image guidance with various technologies is recently applied to radiotherapy. The characteristic advantage of each technology provides the accurate patient localization with guidance of body surface, bony and target structures. Accuracy of CT scanning for treatment planning might be consequently sure to construct the accurate coordinate scale of image guidance for patient localization. Furthermore,

The ETX system provides speedy patient localization with high precision and accuracy. However, it will not detect the soft tissue movement. For accurate patient localization in IMRT for prostate cancer, it requires to obtain clear images with each device and to fuse each image correctly. The optimal selection of imaging device is important and leads to reduce setup margins.

6. References

Tanyi JA, Summers PA, McCracken CL, Chen Y, Ku LC, et al. (2009). Implications of a high-definition multileaf collimator (HD-MLC) on treatment planning technique for stereotactic body radiation therapy (SBRT): a planning study. *Radiat Oncol* 2009, 4, 22.

Murphy MJ, Balter J, Balter S, BenComo JA, Das IJ, et al. (2007). The management of imaging dose during image-guided radiotherapy: Report of the AAPM Task Group 75. *Med Phys*, 34, 4041-4063.

Thongphiew D, Wu QJ, Lee WR, Chankong V, Yoo S, et al. (2009). Comparison of online IGRT techniques for prostate IMRT treatment: Adaptive vs repositioning correction. *Med Phys*, 36, 1651-1662.

Richter A, Hu Q, Steglich D, Baier K, Wilbert J, et al. (2008). Investigation of the usability of conebeam CT data sets for dose calculation. *Radiat Oncol*, 2008, 3 42.

Tyagi N, Lewis JH, Yashir CM, Jiang SB, Mundt AJ, at al. (2011). Daily online cone beam computed tomography to assess interfractional motion in patients with intact cervical cancer. *Int J Radiat Oncol Biol Phys*, 80, 273-280.

Tryggestad E, Christian M, Ford E, Kut C, Le Y, et al. (2011). Inter- and Intrafraction patient positioning uncertainties for intracranial radiotherapy: A study of for frameless thermoplastic mask-based immobilization strategies using daily cone-beam CT. *Int J Radiat Oncol Biol Phys*, 80, 281-289.

Song W, Kamath S, Ozawa S, Ani SA, Chvetsov A, et al. (2008). A dose comparison study between XVI® and OBI® CBCT systems. *Med Phys*, 35, 480-486.

Martin MJ, Bayley A, Bristow R, Chung P, Gospodarowicz M, et al. (2009): Image guided dose escalated prostate radiotherapy still room to improve. *Radiat Oncol* 2009, 4, 50.

Hong LX, Chen CC, Garg M, Yaparpalvi R, Mah D. (2009). Clinical experiences with onboard imager kV images for linear accelerator-based stereotactic radiosurgery and radiotherapy setup. *Int J Radiat Oncol Biol Phys*, 73, 556.

Sorberg TD, Selch MT, Smathers JB, Desalles AA. (1998). Fractionated stereotactic radiotherapy: rationale and methods. Med Dosim, 23, 209-19.

Part 5

Applications

18

CT-Scanning in Forensic Medicine

Peter Mygind Leth
University of Southern Denmark
Denmark

1. Introduction

The forensic community has in general been slow to implement the modern diagnostic imagining modalities, partly due to unawareness of its potentials and probably also for financial reasons. Now CT and other imagining techniques such as magnetic resonance imaging are however gaining access to forensic medicine, as an increasing number of forensic institutes install CT-and even MR-scanners (1-6). A research group from the University of Bern and their international partners in the socalled *virtopsy-project* has been leading in this development (7, 8).

Investigation of deseased is of importance for several different reasons, including jurisprudence, science, education and quality control. The traditional methods of investigation have been an external examination of the body at the inquest, often followed by an autopsy. The autopsy techniques have been developed to a high standard during many hundred years, but have some obvious limitations: certain parts of the body are not always investigated, especially in the limbs, the back and the neck, and the autopsy procedure disturbs the normal anatomy. Some may have ethical or religious objections (9). The number of autopsies seems to be declining in many countries (10) and have long since ceased to be the main focus for pathological departments.

Modern diagnostic imaging techniques will therefore be of increasing importance in the investigation of the dead in the future. There are important differences between clinical and forensic postmortem radiology (11). Movement artefacts or radiation overdose is not a problem in the latter. Contrast administration requires specialized techniques (12, 13) and are not yet routinely used. Internal lividity, intravascular clots and gasformation from decomposition may cause interpretational problems (figure 1 - 2) (14). Furthermore, knowdledge of forensic pathology, especially forensic traumatology, is needed for the interpretation. The focus of the forensic investigation is different from clinical practise and includes consideration of the injury mechanism. A forensic radiologist must thus be educated in both radiology and forensic pathology and preferrably work in co-operation with the pathologist who performs the autopsy (15).

CT may be used before the medicolegal inquest to broaden the basis for decision about autopsy, or it may be used as an adjunct to autopsy in all cases or in selected cases. If available, CT should be performed in trauma cases, including gunshots, in battered child cases and in identifications. Postmortem CT has some obvious limitations compared to autopsy. The visual sensations are of inferior quality with less resolutions and no colour, and other senses such as touch and smell are not used. It is difficult to obtain material for microscopy or microbiology. CT-guided biopsies of organs or mass lesions may however be obtained when autopsy is not consented (16).

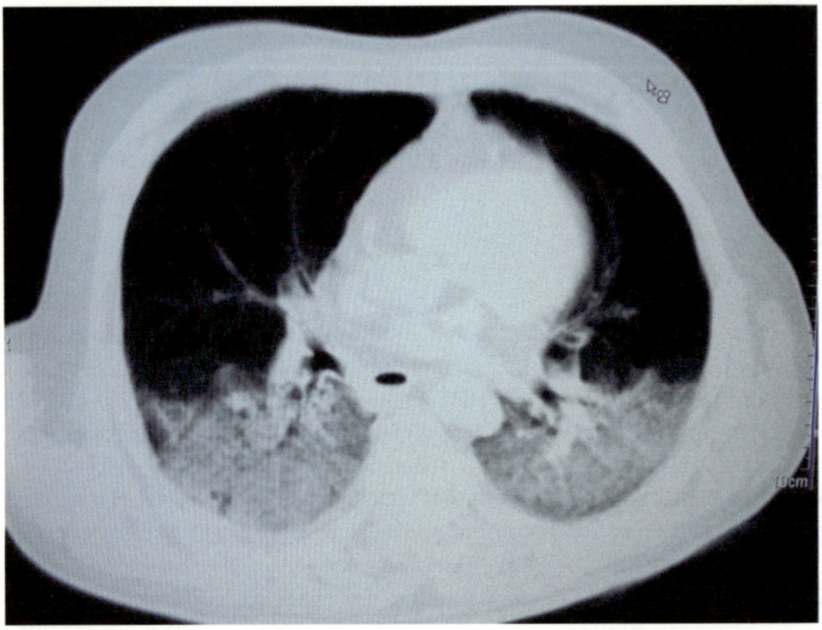

Fig. 1. Transversal CT-image of thorax with internal lividity in the lungs.

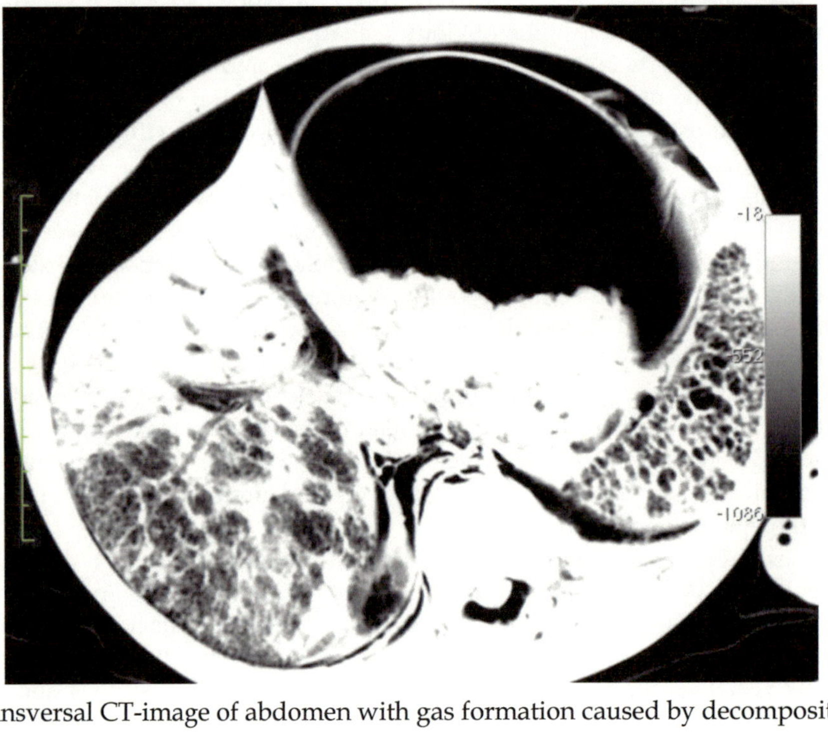

Fig. 2. Transversal CT-image of abdomen with gas formation caused by decomposition.

2. Equipment

Forensic facilities with a large wordload will need an efficient multislice helical scanner. In smaller institutions a less expensive CT-scanner may suffice if the equipment is used primarily as an adjunct to autopsy.

The scanoperator should preferably be a fulltime radiographer, but in our experience it is possible for a forensic technician to operate the equipment in routine cases after appropriate training and supervision.

The equipment should be installed next to the morgue and the workstation in or next to the autopsy room, for easy access to the CT images. CT images can also be sent to a smartphone or an iPad. Some forensic centers coorperate with clinical radiological centers and utilize their staff and equipment.

The CT-images may be stored on a variety of storage media, such as an external harddisk or on CDs. The CT diagnoses may be registered according to standardised systems. We use ICD-diagnoses for non-trauma diagnoses and AIS for trauma diagnoses (17-19).

3. Determination of identity

Bodies may be unrecognizeable due to external factors such as fire, severe trauma or putrefaction. In these cases, CT may be of great help in establishing the identity. The identification process is based on a comparison of postmortem and antemortem descriptions and may be registered on Interpol identification forms. These contain general characteristics of the deseased such as sex, age estimate, height and hair colour, and some specific characteristics such as tatoos, scars and implants. Of particular importance are odonthology, fingerprints and DNA-profile. Most of the relevant sections in the Interpol forms can be filled out from the CT investigation (20) which has the additional benefit of providing a permanent objective record of the findings. Some characteristics such as the shape of the nose or ears may be even better appreciated from CT-images because of their "neutral" apperance (figure 3). Superimposition on portrait photos in photoshop is also possible. CT makes an anthropological assessment of the bones possible without defleshing, providing information of height from the length of the long bones, of age and of sex. Implants, such as prosthetic implants or artificial heart valves are easily found (figure 4). Sometimes antemortem X-rays may yield important clues to the identity, but are often not available until after the autopsy. If a volume of digitalized X-ray information from a post mortem CT-scanning is available, then it is easy to reconstruct an X-ray in the correct projection for comparison (21). The individual unique shape of the frontal sinus is among the features that may be used for identification based on X-ray-photos (22).

CT has been used for disaster victim identification. In Great Britain mobile CT-units have been deployed to the autopsy area for a major road traffic accident (23, 24), and in Australia CT has been used with great success in the Victoria bushfire disaster (25). CT substitutes the three traditionally used types of X-ray imaging: plain X-rays, fluoroscopy, and dental radiographs. Special software is needed for the latter.

4. Traffic fatalities

Postmortem examination of traffic fatalities serves as a quality check of treatment and diagnosis and provides information for accident profylaksis. A combination of CT and

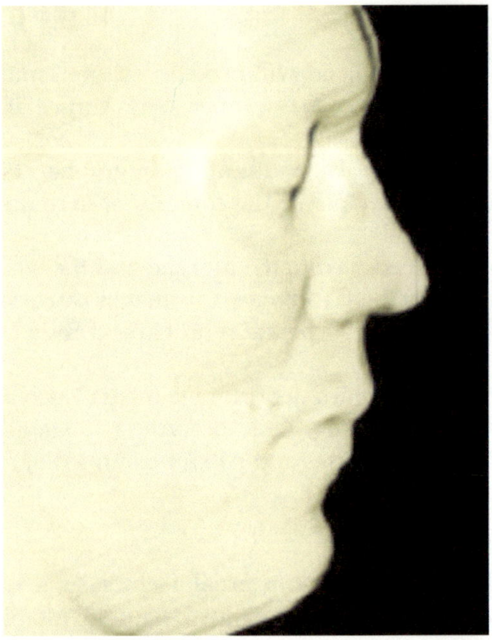

Fig. 3. Face eyes, nose and mouth of unidentified man seen in profile. 3D CT reconstruction.

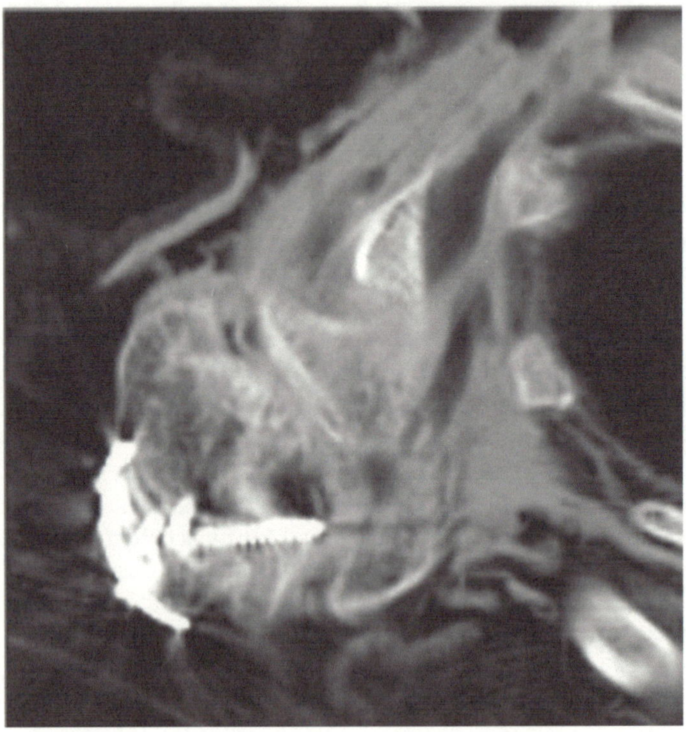

Fig. 4. Implant in humerus. Such CT finding may be of importance in the identification process. Unidentified man found in ditch.

autopsy gives the most accurate information, but if an autopsy is not possible for legal or ethical reasons a CT scanning should be performed. The trauma diagnoses could be registered according to the abbreviated injury scale for easy comparison among trauma centers (19).

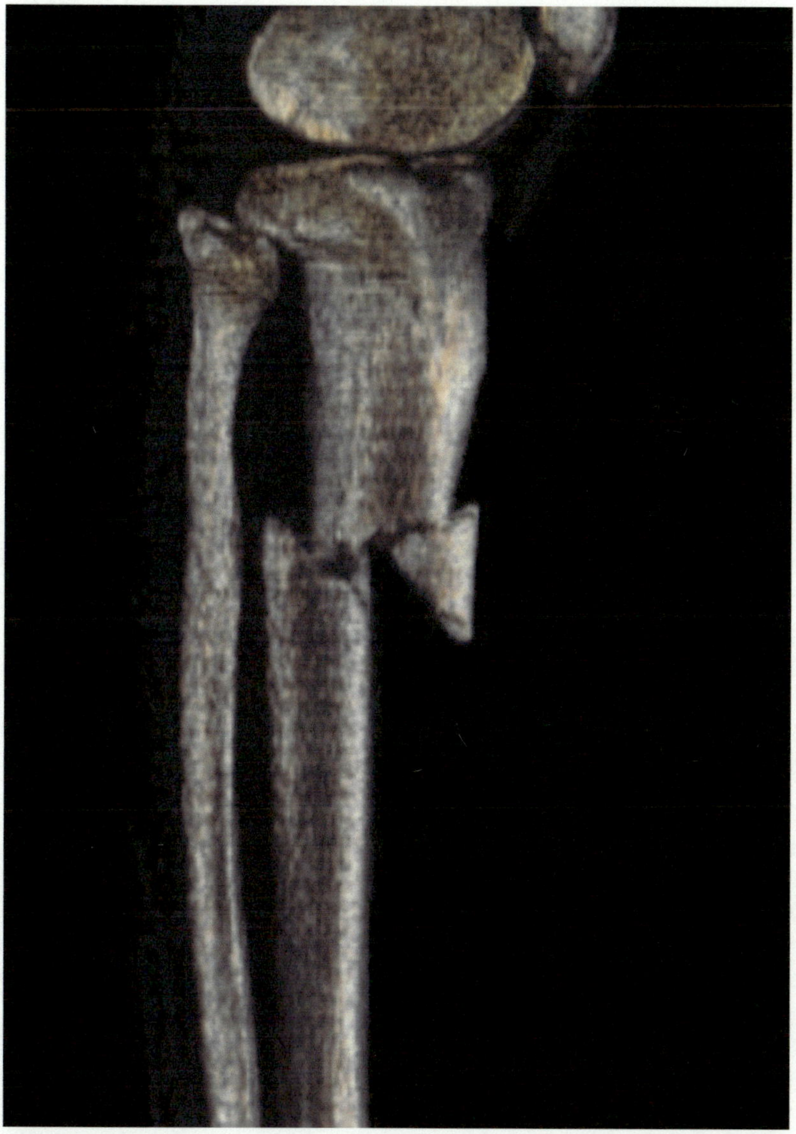

Fig. 5. Tibia with intermediary fragment caused by anterior impact. 3D CT reconstruction. Pedestrian hit by car.

It is possible to identify injury patterns characteristic of specific accident scenarios (figure 5). Frontal car chrashes, which are the most common type of motor vehicle accidents, will for example cause the unrestrained driver or front seat passenger to be propeled forward causing first an extension of the lumbar spine and a slide forward with knee impact against the fascia, and then a move upwards and forwards of the body with impact of the crown against the roof frame and of the chest against the steering wheel/dashboard, and finally a foreward flexion of the cervical or thoracic spine with a final strike of the head against the windshield or the pillars. The resulting lesions appear from table 1. A more exhaustive text should be sought for a detailed description of the various accident types and their characteristic injury patterns (26). Many factors will contribute to modify the classical injury patterns. Airbags may cause severe head, neck and chest injuries in the unrestrained driver or front seat passenger (27). If the victim is ejected from the car, all kinds of injuries can be seen. In selected cases it may therefore be advisable to confer the case with the car inspector, and if possible to inspect the wreckage and the accident scene in order to make the proper clinico-pathological correlations.

Hit-and-run cases present a special challenge. In such cases it is of particular importance to obtain a volume of digitalized CT-data as this permits later comparisons with characteristics of the vehicle. The virtopsy group has applied photogrammetry for such comparisons (28).

Region	Injuries
Head and neck	Skull fractures, pneumoencephalon intracranial hematoma, cerebral contusion and laceration, brainstem damage, fractures of cervical vertebrae, atlanto-occipital dislocation, transection of cervical cord
Chest	Fracture of sternum and ribs, haemopneumothorax, lung laceration, heart laceration, aorta rupture
Abdomen	Laceration of liver, spleen, mesentery/omentum,
Extremities	Fractures of pelvis, femur with dislocation of hip joints, patella, tibia, fibula and metatarsal bones

Table 1. Injuries found in driver and front seat passenger in frontal crashes

5. Gunshot cases

The use of radiology in the investigation of firearm fatalities has been a standard practice since the discovery of X-rays. However CT offers significant advantages over plain film X-rays (29, 30). CT cannot replace all the information that an autopsy can provide, and at present CT should be considered an adjunct to the forensic autopsy.

This chapter contains information about CT used in cases of firearm fatalities, but a more detailed description of weapon types and ammunition should be sought in a more comprehensive text (31).

The primary aim of the radiological examination is to localize the projectiles and fragments, to determine the bullet tracks and to evaluate extent of damage caused, with the ultimate aim to reconstruct the event. The absence of foreign material suggests that the projectile may have traversed the body and exited. The evaluation is much easier done in 3D CT-images than in 2D plain radiographs. It is easy to create an overview of the distribution of pellets in shotgun lesions and to localize projectiles or fragments from single projectile gunshot lesions. It is also possible to localize the entrance and exit wounds, to determine the bullet tracts, fracture patterns and other major lesions, and in contrast to dissection this may be obtained without disturbing the normal anatomy. Gunshot residues in and around the entrance wound can be detected by routine clinical CT which is of use in the forensic investigation of surviving victims where an inspection of the bandaged entrance wound is not possible (32). When a projectile passes a flat bone, typically the cranium, a conical shaped injury with socalled "bevelling" is seen to the inside of the entrance wound and outside to the exit wound, easily identifiable on CT. Sometimes a projectile strikes the skull and deflects away without entering the cranial cavity. This may result in a socalled "keyhole" injury with both internal and external bevelling.

When a projectile penetrates the body, it delivers energy to the tissues. The amount of destruction is proportional to the amount of energy delivered. A projectile produces a permanent channel in its path (figure 6) and produces a temporary radial displacement of tissues. High velocity projectiles produce a very large temporary cavity that may cause tissue damage at a distance from the the permanent wound track. The resultant radiological picture depends on the elasticity of the tissue in question. In liver and brain there will be considerable organ disruption whereas lung tissue better tolerates the lateral displacement.

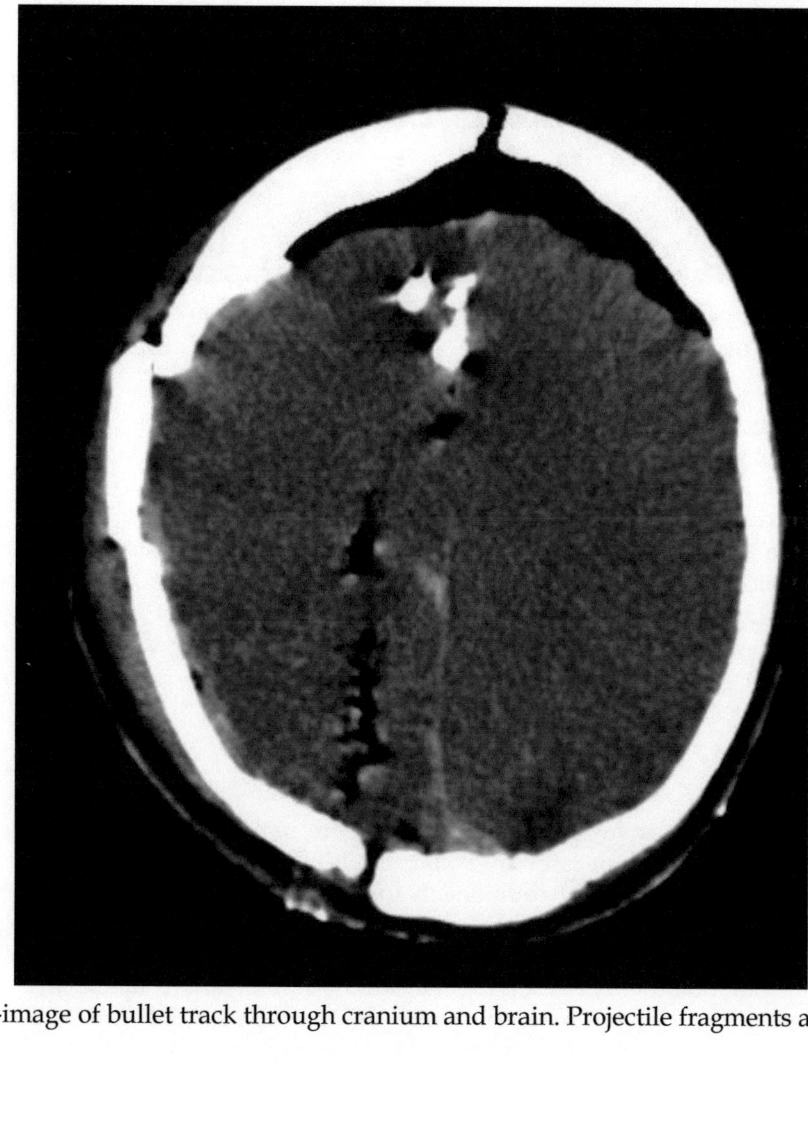

Fig. 6. CT-image of bullet track through cranium and brain. Projectile fragments are seen. Suicide.

Projectiles may cause injury to vessels resulting in haemothorax, haemopericardium (figure 7) or intraperitoneal bleeding. Pellets may enter the bloodstream and travel to a distant site - a socalled projectile embolus. The vascular injuries are not easily visualized by post-mortem CT since contrast medium is not used routinely.

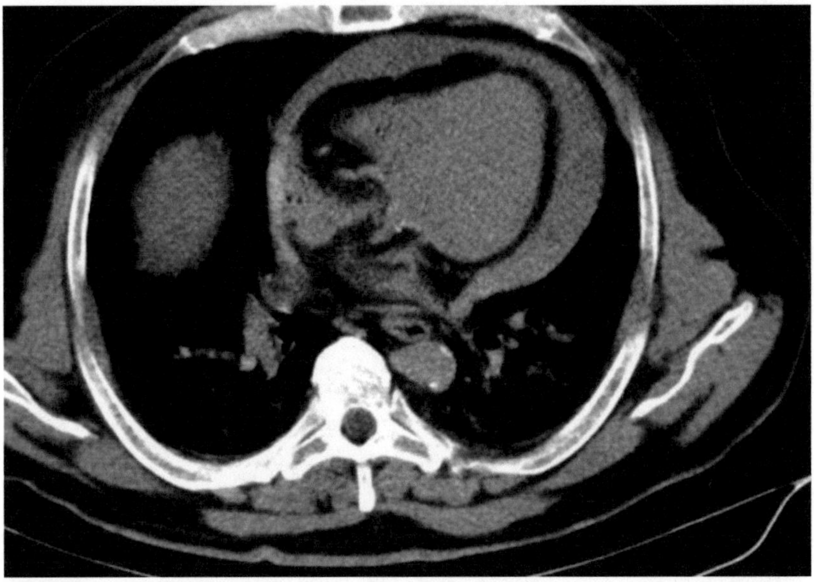

Fig. 7. CT-image displaying haemopericardium caused by a lesion of a coronary artery by a projectile track through the thorax

A shotgun produces a conical stream of pellets that disperse over an ever widening area at increasing distance. Close range shotgun lesions may contain pieces of wadding in addition to the pellets, but the wadding is not identifiable on CT. In shotgun lesions the shot angle can be illustrated by marking the entrance wounds and the pellets in different colours.

CT allows discrimination between foreign objects that differ in radio absorption, such as glass fragments from a shot fired through a window or metal fragments from passage through the door of a vehicle. Retrieval and analysis of such fragments may be of importance in reconstructing the event and in determining the location of the crime scene (29).

CT may provide important additional information in cases where the visual evaluation is difficult due to severe decomposition or charring.

The high-quality, neutral CT-images reduce the need for autopsy photographs in court.

6. Terror bombs

The types of explosives involved in terror attacks are remotely controlled explosives and suicide bombers. The explosives often contain multiple shrapnel fragments such as nails, bolts, small metal balls and other components to increase the damage. These fragments can easily be found by CT, and subsequently secured for technical investigation. The injuries are classified into three catagories. Primary blast injuries are caused by the shock wave (blast wind) and include pulmonary hemorrhage, gastrointestinal hemorrhage and perforation of the eardrums. Secondary injuries are caused by objects propelled outward by the explosion. They include penetrating injuries and orthopedic impact injuries. Tertiary injuries occur when the victims are thrown against solid objects by the blast wind. CT allows a quick overview of the fracture systems and injuries to internal organs. Information about the scene is essential for the evaluation of the CT and autopsy findings. In terror-bombing caused by a suicide terrorist, it is often possible to identify the suicide bomber based on the pattern of lesions which of course is of great importance to the police investigation (33, 34).

7. Stab wounds

Stab wounds are often encountered in forensic practice. The main forensic issues are number and location of wounds, stab channel depth and direction, wound morphology and indicators of thrust force. The ultimate issues are reconstruction of the event, type of weapon used and estimation of permanent injury and life danger. CT can detect a high percentage of stab wounds, and it is often possible to determine the depth and direction of the wound channel (35). The information gained from CT is often more reliable than can be obtained from dissection or probing. These invasive techniques change the anatomy whereas CT shows the undisturbed anatomy. However, caution should be exerted when measuring the channel depth in soft tissues since the channel may collapse, resulting in too short a measurement. It must also be emphasized that not all stab wound can be visualized on CT, especially if there are many closely grouped wounds and if the wounds are superficial. It is therefore important to correlate CT findings with the findings at the external examination. These problems may be overcome with scanners with better resolution or by optimizing the scanning technique (35). CT can easily detect skeletal injuries. These are important since they are indicators of thrust force. Instillation of contrast medium in the stab wound tract has been investigated experimentally (figure 8) (36).

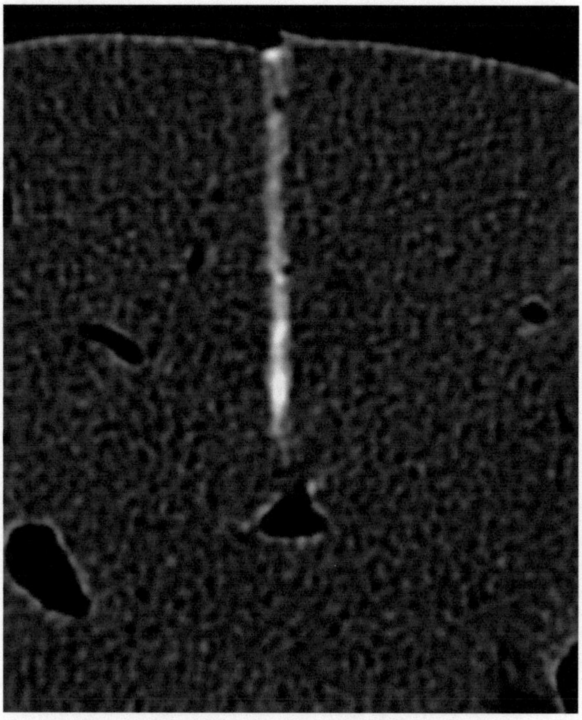

Fig. 8. Stab channel in liver tissue filled with contrast medium.

8. Blunt trauma to the head and neck

Facial fractures are very common in forensic pathology, but are often overlooked at autopsy if the soft tissues of the face are not dissected. Fractures of the cranial vault and base can usually be visualized on CT, although not with the same degree of precision as can be obtained by autopsy (37). CT allows massive cranial fractures to be viewed in situ (figure 9) which can be of importance in homicide cases where a comparison with a blunt weapon may be needed. With dissection the cranial fragments tend to fall apart. Intracranial haemorrhages are easily detected by CT and the volume measured. Figure 10 illustrates a cerebral haemorrhage in a severly decomposed body. At the autopsy the brain was completely liquified and it was impossible to localize and measure the haemorrhage.

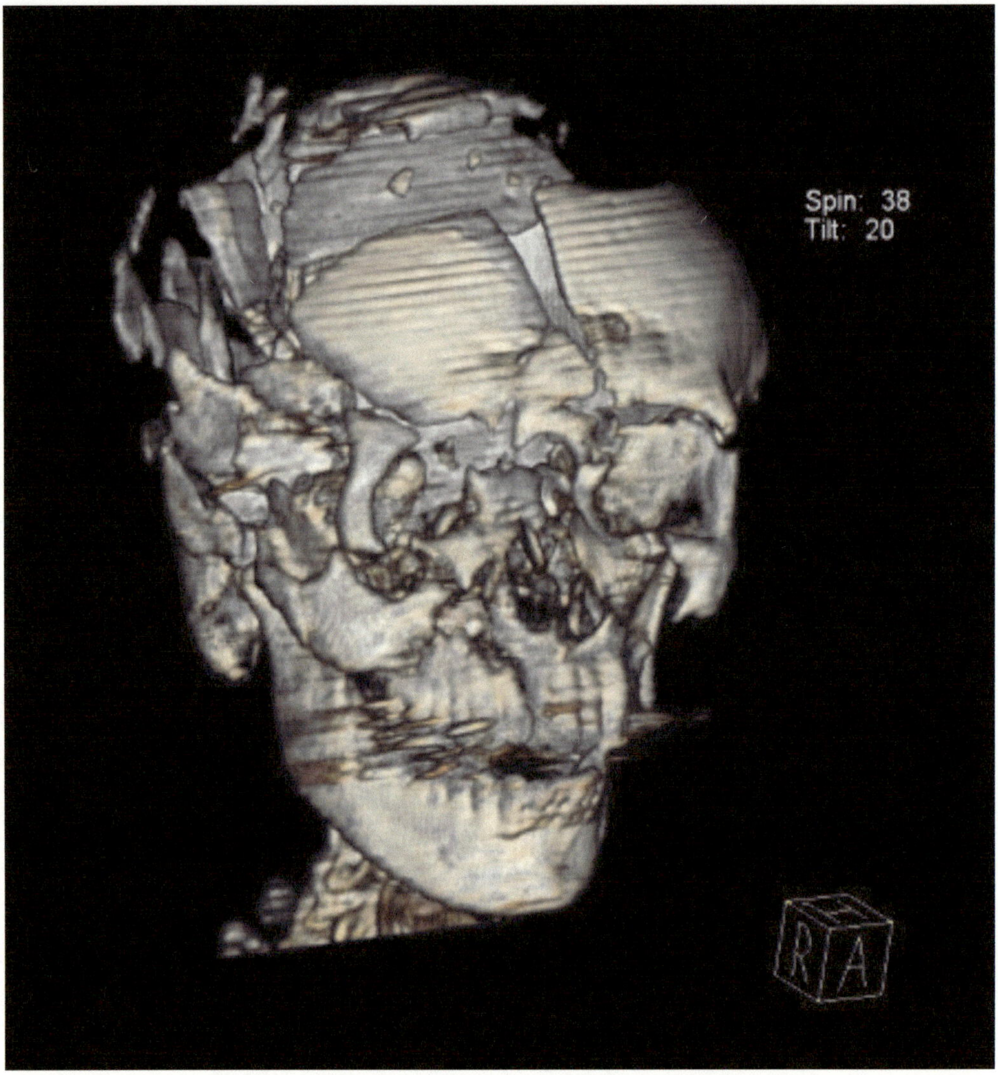

Fig. 9. CT-image displaying extensive fractures of cranium and facial bones. Car driver, traffic accident.

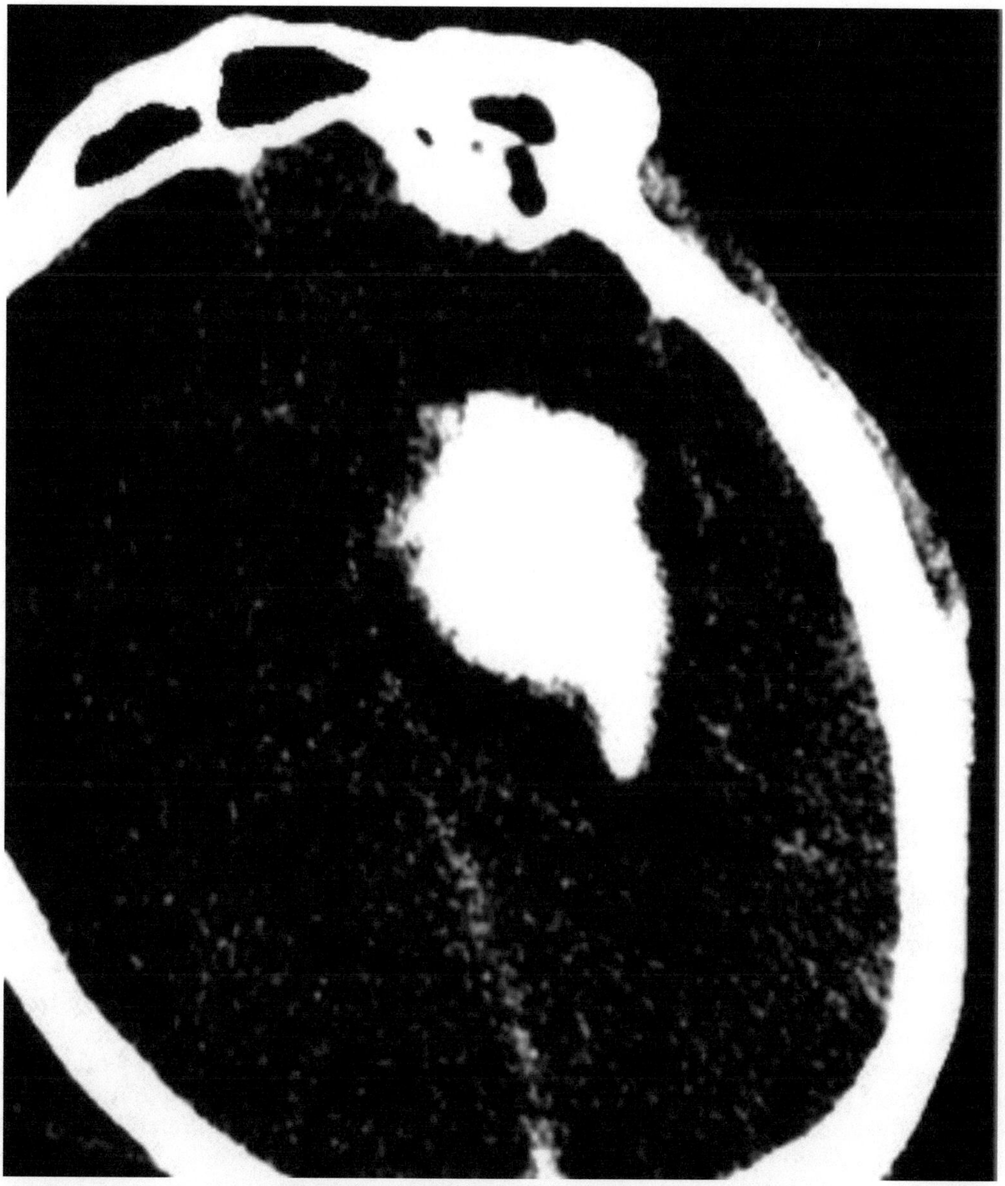

Fig. 10. Transversal CT-image of the head. An intracerebral haemorrhage is clearly visible. Severely decomposed body scanned inside the body bag.

Fractures in the cranio-cervical region are relatively common, but are sometimes overlooked at autopsy, and it may be difficult to evaluate the degree of spinal stenosis. CT makes this evaluation much easier, but does not depict small hemorrhages, contusions or necroses of the spinal cord or brain (38, 39).

Hanging, ligature strangulation and manual strangulation are of great forensic importance. Strangulation marks on the neck are detectable by CT and provide a permanent record of the shape that can not be obtained by any other means. Some soft tissue lesions such as subcutaneus, lymph node and intramuscular haemorrhage can be detected by CT, but minor bleedings are not found (40, 41). Hyoid, thyroid and cricoid fractures are usually found. Pneumomediastinum and cervical emphysema have been described in hanging cases and are probably a vital reaction caused by attempted breathing (42).

9. Drowning

In wet drownings aspiration of water to the lungs is seen in 60 % of cases, and more fluid is found in the main bronchi and trachea than normally seen postmortem. Pleural effusion and fluid in ventricle, duodenum and paranasal sinuses are also common findings. A reduced bronchial-arterial coefficient is a sign of bronchospasm (43). Reduction of the blood density (Houndsfield Units) in the right heart chamber is indicative of haemodilution (44). The body fat of cadavers that have been in the water for a long time becomes transformed to an insoluble soap called adipocire. The extent of adipocire formation can be determined by CT and can be used to give a crude estimate of the postmortem interval (45).

10. Burnt bodies

Bodies damaged by fire must be investigated in order to secure the identity and to establish the cause and mode of death. It is important to determine if the deceased was alive when the fire started, to find injuries and secure samples for toxicology (including CO and cyanide from fire smoke). CT is of help in determining the identity and to detect projectiles in victims shot and then torched. CT can not detect soot in the airways (an important vital sign). A socalled pseudohaematoma, which is a postmortem heath-caused epidural hematoma, is easily identified by CT. It transverses the cranial suture lines in contrast to a true epidural hematoma.

CT are very useful in determining the number of individuals and getting an overview in cases of multiple fire deaths (25).

11. Child abuse

Radiology has played a significant role in the forensic investigation of physical abuse of children since John Caffey's landmark paper of 1946 (46). Abusive head trauma is the leading cause of death from child abuse. Skeletal injuries are important markers of trauma mechanism and frequency.

The injuries should as a general rule be evaluated in connection with the presenting story, which in cases of child abuse is inconsistent with the injuries found. Multiple fractures and fractures of varying age are highly suspicious of child abuse. Relevant differential diagnoses should be considered (47). In cases of fatal child abuse, a thorough radiological examination should be performed (48). CT raw data should be kept permanently.

Cranial fractures are not in themselves highly suggestive of child abuse, but the level of suspicion should increase with complex skull fractures. Child abuse with intracranial injury includes subarachnoid and subdural hemorrhage, intracerebral and intracerebellar haemorrhage, and brain edema. It has been discussed whether intracranial injuries can be caused by shaking alone or if an impact of the head is also needed (49).

Smaller children subjected to abuse are sometimes grabbed around the chest and shaken resulting in posterior fractures of the ribs whereas older children are held by the extremities. Rib fractures are rarely seen as a result of resuscitation. Socalled bucket handle metafysal fractures are virtually pathognomonic of child abuse. These injuries are usually seen in nonambulatory small children and are located at the distal humerus, knee or ankle. Twisting and pulling may cause subperiostal haemorrhage which subsequently calcifies and shows up on radigraphs as either a subtle thin line or of more massive proportion depending on the degree of bleeding. Diaphyseal spiral fractures caused by a twisting force are highly suggestive of abuse, especially in children who do not yet walk, but transverse long bone fracture may also be seen. Hand fractures are highly suspicious, except for fractures of the distal phalanx of the fingers from closing doors. Scapular fractures are also suspicious. They involve the acromion or less commenly the blade. Clavicle fractures may be seen as a perinatal fracture, but rarely as a result of child abuse.

12. Various other CT findings

Postmortem CT can document the position of catheters, tubes or drains prior to the autopsy which can be of great importance in medical malpractise cases.

CT is well suited to detect abnormal gas collections such as pnemothorax, pneumomediastinum, pneumoencephalon and air embolism (figure 11). Air embolism may occur in various forensic settings such as head trauma (50), diving accidents, stab wounds, gunshot wounds and traumatic pneumothorax. In cases of massive airembolism right heart failure may occur. Hypoxic brain death is also possible due to vascular obstruction in the cerebral vessels. Diagnosing air embolism at autopsy is difficult. One method involves aspiration of air from the right heart chamber, a method that allows a chemical analysis of the aspired air. Postmortem CT readely displays the amount and distribution of gas in the vascular system and in the cardiac chambers, but does not allow a chemical characterization of the gas. The distribution of the gas may indicate if the presence of gas is caused by air embolism or putrefaction.

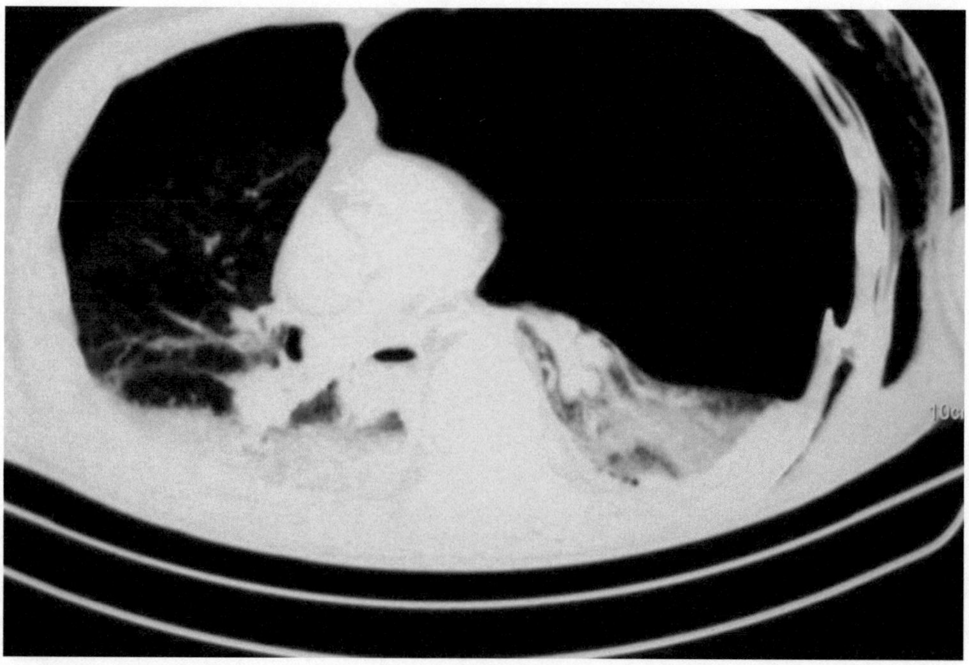

Fig. 11. Transversal CT-image of a pressure pneumothorax with displacement of the heart, rib fractures and subcutaneous emphysema. Man trampled by Icelandic horse.

Autopsy determination of fatal hemorrhage as the cause of death depends on sparsity of lividity and on the amount of blood in the vessels. This is a highly subjective method. It has been suggested that a quantitative estimation of blood loss may be possible by CT measurement of the diameter of major vessels (51).

13. Natural deaths

A large proportion of medico-legal deaths are of natural origin. At our department natural deaths comprise a third of the autopsy workload. These cases include sudden unexpected deaths, suspected malpractice cases, individuals found dead under suspicious circumstances and others. The findings are not in principle different from similar cases known from clinical radiology, but there are as already mentioned, some important differences in technique (no contrast medium), post-mortem changes of the body and not least the purpose of the investigation. In most cases it is not possible to replace the autopsy with a CT-scanning. Too many diagnoses will be missed without autopsy, and it is much easier to obtain sufficient and suitable material for histology and microbiology at an autopsy. However CT provides important additional information. Internal fluid collections such as hydrothorax and ascites (5) are easily found and quantified. It is possible to evaluate degree of displacement of internal structures which is not so easily done at autopsy (figure 12).

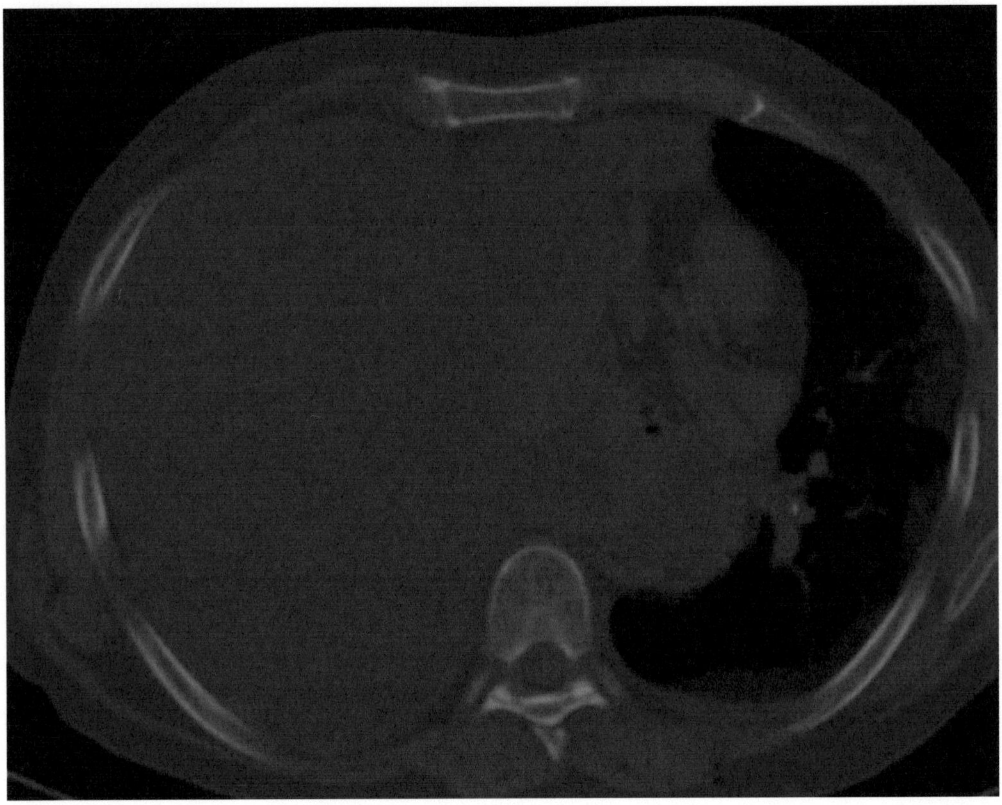

Fig. 12. Transversal CT-image of thorax with severe hydrothorax in the right pleural cavity causing displacement of the heart to the left.

14. Future developments

A Swiss group has developed a method for post-mortem angiography based on an oily contrast agent (52) introduced through the femoral artery and vein. Samples for toxicology must be taken before the angiography is performed, but since the oily contrast agent remains in the vessels biopsies for histology can be taken later. It is also possible to perform an autopsy, although the organs become somewhat slippery. The method seems to be particular useful for detection of postsurgical bleeding, and it is likely that it will become an important tool in the future.

Jacobsen et al (53) have suggested using finite element analysis on the volume of digitalized data from a fractured skull for biomechanical approximation of the injury mechanism and involved forces. The idea is to remove the fracture digitally and then perform digital simulations of various blunt impacts. Such experiment has hitherto used standard cranial models, but the CT data allow an individualized model to be used. The calculations are very demanding, and not yet practically possible without a supercomputer, but it is certainly an original idea to use CT-data for other purposes than imaging.

Another future application could be cinematographic analysis of a whole body and its surroundings for reconstruction of a crime or an accident. Various scenarios could be tested to see if certain bullet paths or fracture systems could be recreated under different conditions. This would be very useful, not least in analysis of trauma mechanisms in traffic accidents.

Computerized tomography and other methods for acquisition of a digitalized data volume from bodies will undoubtedly play an increasing role in forensic medicine in the future.

15. References

[1] Leth PM. Computerized tomography used as a routine procedure at postmortem investigations. Am J Forensic Med Pathol. 2009 Sep;30(3):219-22.

[2] Poulsen K, Simonsen J. Computed tomography as routine in connection with medico-legal autopsies. Forensic Sci Int. 2007 Sep 13;171(2-3):190-7.

[3] Rutty GN, Morgan B, O'Donnell C, Leth PM, Thali M. Forensic institutes across the world place CT or MRI scanners or both into their mortuaries. J Trauma. 2008 Aug;65(2):493-4.

[4] O'Donnell C, Rotman A, Collett S, Woodford N. Current status of routine post.mortem CT in Melbourne, Australia. Forensic Sci Med Pathol. 2007;3:226-32.

[5] Yamazaki K, Shiotani S, Ohashi N, Doi M, Kikuchi K, Nagata C, et al. Comparison between computed tomography (CT) and autopsy findings in cases of abdominal injury and disease. Forensic Sci Int. 2006 Oct 16;162(1-3):163-6.

[6] Thomsen AH, Jurik AG, Uhrenholt L, Vesterby A. An alternative approach to Computerized Tomography (CT) in forensic pathology. Forensic Sci Int. 2009;183:87 - 90.

[7] Thali MJ, Yen K, Schweitzer W, Vock P, Boesch C, Ozdoba C, et al. Virtopsy, a new imaging horizon in forensic pathology: virtual autopsy by postmortem multislice computed tomography (MSCT) and magnetic resonance imaging (MRI)--a feasibility study. J Forensic Sci. 2003 Mar;48(2):386-403.

[8] The Virtopsy Approach. Thali MJ, Dirnhofer R, Vock P, editors: CRC Press; 2009.

[9] Davis GJ, Peterson BR. Dilemmas and solutions for the pathologist and clinician encountering religious views of the autopsy. South Med J. 1996 Nov;89(11):1041-4.
[10] Ayoub T, Chow J. The conventional autopsy in modern medicine. J R Soc Med. 2008 Apr;101(4):177-81.
[11] Christe A, Flach P, Ross S, Spendlove D, Bolliger S, Vock P, et al. Clinical radiology and postmortem imaging (Virtopsy) are not the same: Specific and unspecific postmortem signs. Leg Med (Tokyo). 2010 Sep;12(5):215-22.
[12] Pøhlsgaard C, Leth PM. Post-mortem CT-coronary angiography. Scandinavian Journal of Forensic Science. 2007;13:8-9.
[13] Ross S, Spendlove D, Bolliger S, Christe A, Oesterhelweg L, Grabherr S, et al. Postmortem whole-body CT angiography: evaluation of two contrast media solutions. AJR Am J Roentgenol. 2008 May;190(5):1380-9.
[14] Jackowski C, Thali M, Aghayev E, Yen K, Sonnenschein M, Zwygart K, et al. Postmortem imaging of blood and its characteristics using MSCT and MRI. Int J Legal Med. 2006 Jul;120(4):233-40.
[15] O'Donnell C, Woodford N. Post-mortem radiology--a new sub-speciality? Clin Radiol. 2008 Nov;63(11):1189-94.
[16] Aghayev E, Thali MJ, Sonnenschein M, Jackowski C, Dirnhofer R, Vock P. Post-mortem tissue sampling using computed tomography guidance. Forensic Sci Int. 2007 Mar 2;166(2-3):199-203.
[17] International Statistical Classification of Diseases and Related Health Problems 10th Revision : WHO.
[18] Abbreviated Injury Scale 2005: Association for the Advancement of Automotive Medicine.
[19] Leth PM, Ibsen M. Abbreviated Injury Scale Scoring in Traffic Fatalities: Comparison of Computerized Tomography and Autopsy. J Trauma. 2010;68(6):1413-6.
[20] Sidler M, Jackowski C, Dirnhofer R, Vock P, Thali M. Use of multislice computed tomography in disaster victim identification--advantages and limitations. Forensic Sci Int. 2007 Jul 4;169(2-3):118-28.
[21] Pfaeffli M, Vock P, Dirnhofer R, Braun M, Bolliger SA, Thali MJ. Post-mortem radiological CT identification based on classical ante-mortem X-ray examinations. Forensic Sci Int. 2007 Sep 13;171(2-3):111-7.
[22] Reichs KJ. Quantified comparison of frontal sinus patterns by means of computed tomography. Forensic Sci Int. 1993 Oct;61(2-3):141-68.
[23] Rutty GN, Robinson CE, BouHaidar R, Jeffery AJ, Morgan B. The role of mobile computed tomography in mass fatality incidents. J Forensic Sci. 2007 Nov;52(6):1343-9.
[24] Rutty GN, Robinson C, Morgan B, Black S, Adams C, Webster P. Fimag: the United Kingdom disaster victim/forensic identification imaging system. J Forensic Sci. 2009 Nov;54(6):1438-42.
[25] O'Donnell C, Iino M, Mansharan K, Leditscke J, Woodford N. Contribution of postmortem multidetector CT scanning to identification of the deceased in a mass disaster: Experience gained from the 2009 Victorian bushfires. Forensic Sci Int. 2010 Aug 4.
[26] Saukko P, Knight B. Tranportation Injuries. Knight's Forensic Pathology. London: Arnold; 2004.

[27] Sato Y, Ohshima T, Kondo T. Air bag injuries--a literature review in consideration of demands in forensic autopsies. Forensic Sci Int. 2002 Aug 28;128(3):162-7.

[28] Thali MJ, Braun M, Buck U, Aghayev E, Jackowski C, Vock P, et al. VIRTOPSY--scientific documentation, reconstruction and animation in forensic: individual and real 3D data based geo-metric approach including optical body/object surface and radiological CT/MRI scanning. J Forensic Sci. 2005 Mar;50(2):428-42.

[29] Andenmatten MA, Thali MJ, Kneubuehl BP, Oesterhelweg L, Ross S, Spendlove D, et al. Gunshot injuries detected by post-mortem multislice computed tomography (MSCT): a feasibility study. Leg Med (Tokyo). 2008 Nov;10(6):287-92.

[30] Jeffery AJ, Rutty GN, Robinson C, Morgan B. Computed tomography of projectile injuries. Clin Radiol. 2008 Oct;63(10):1160-6.

[31] Di Maio VJM. Gunshot Wounds: Practical Aspects of Firearms, Ballistics, and Forensic Techniques1999.

[32] Stein KM, Bahner ML, Merkel J, Ain S, Mattern R. Detection of gunshot residues in routine CTs. Int J Legal Med. 2000;114(1-2):15-8.

[33] Shaham D, Sella T, Makori A, Appelbum L, Rivkind AI, Bar-Ziv J. The role of radiology in terror injuries. Isr Med Assoc J. 2002 Jul;4(7):564-7.

[34] Benjaminov O, Sklair-Levy M, Rivkind A, Cohen M, Bar-Tal G, Stein M. Role of radiology in evaluation of terror attack victims. AJR Am J Roentgenol. 2006 Sep;187(3):609-16.

[35] Schnider J, Thali MJ, Ross S, Oesterhelweg L, Spendlove D, Bolliger SA. Injuries due to sharp trauma detected by post-mortem multislice computed tomography (MSCT): a feasibility study. Leg Med (Tokyo). 2009 Jan;11(1):4-9.

[36] Bolliger SA, Preiss U, Glaeser N, Thali MJ, Ross S. Radiological stab wound channel depiction with instillation of contrast medium. Legal Medicine. 2010;12(1):39-41.

[37] Jacobsen C, Lynnerup N. Craniocerebral trauma - Congruence between post-mortem computed tomography diagnoses and autopsy results A 2-year retrospective study. Forensic Sci Int. 2010 Jan 30;194(1-3):9-14.

[38] Yen K, Sonnenschein M, Thali MJ, Ozdoba C, Weis J, Zwygart K, et al. Postmortem multislice computed tomography and magnetic resonance imaging of odontoid fractures, atlantoaxial distractions and ascending medullary edema. Int J Legal Med. 2005 May;119(3):129-36.

[39] Fenger-Gron J, Kock K, Nielsen RG, Leth PM, Illum N. Spinal cord injury at birth: a hidden causative factor. Acta Paediatr. 2008 Jun;97(6):824-6.

[40] Yen K, Thali MJ, Aghayev E, Jackowski C, Schweitzer W, Boesch C, et al. Strangulation signs: initial correlation of MRI, MSCT, and forensic neck findings. J Magn Reson Imaging. 2005 Oct;22(4):501-10.

[41] Leth PM, Christensen MR. Computerized tomography used for investigation of homicide victims. Scandinavian Journal of Forensic Science. 2010;in print.

[42] Aghayev E, Yen K, Sonnenschein M, Jackowski C, Thali M, Vock P, et al. Pneumomediastinum and soft tissue emphysema of the neck in postmortem CT and MRI; a new vital sign in hanging? Forensic Sci Int. 2005 Oct 29;153(2-3):181-8.

[43] Christe A, Aghayev E, Jackowski C, Thali MJ, Vock P. Drowning--post-mortem imaging findings by computed tomography. Eur Radiol. 2008 Feb;18(2):283-90.

[44] Levy AD, Harcke HT, Getz JM, Mallak CT, Caruso JL, Pearse L, et al. Virtual autopsy: two- and three-dimensional multidetector CT findings in drowning with autopsy comparison. Radiology. 2007 Jun;243(3):862-8.

[45] Jackowski C, Thali M, Sonnenschein M, Aghayev E, Yen K, Dirnhofer R. Adipocere in postmortem imaging using multislice computed tomography (MSCT) and magnetic resonance imaging (MRI). Am J Forensic Med Pathol. 2005 Dec;26(4):360-4.

[46] Caffey J. Multiple fractures in the long bones of infants suffering from chronic subdural hematoma. Am J Roentgenol Radium Ther. 1946 Aug;56(2):163-73.

[47] Pandya NK, Baldwin K, Kamath AF, Wenger DR, Hosalkar HS. Unexplained fractures: child abuse or bone disease? A systematic review. Clin Orthop Relat Res. 2011;469(3):805-12.

[48] Adamsbaum C, Mejean N, Merzoug V, Rey-Salmon C. How to explore and report children with suspected non-accidental trauma. Pediatr Radiol. 2010 Jun;40(6):932-8.

[49] Christian CW, Block R, Neglect CCA. Abusive Head Trauma in Infants and Children. Pediatrics. 2009 May;123(5):1409-11.

[50] Adams V, Guidi C. Venous air embolism in homicidal blunt impact head trauma. Case reports. Am J Forensic Med Pathol. 2001 Sep;22(3):322-6.

[51] Aghayev E, Sonnenschein M, Jackowski C, Thali M, Buck U, Yen K, et al. Postmortem radiology of fatal hemorrhage: measurements of cross-sectional areas of major blood vessels and volumes of aorta and spleen on MDCT and volumes of heart chambers on MRI. AJR Am J Roentgenol. 2006 Jul;187(1):209-15.

[52] Grabherr S Fau - Djonov V, Djonov V Fau - Yen K, Yen K Fau - Thali MJ, Thali Mj Fau - Dirnhofer R, R D. - Postmortem angiography: review of former and current methods. AJR Am J Roentgenol. 2007;188(3):832-8.

[53] Jacobsen C, Bech BH, Lynnerup N. A comparative study of cranial, blunt trauma fractures as seen at medicolegal autopsy and by computed tomography. BMC Med Imaging. [Comparative Study Evaluation Studies]. 2009;9:18.

19

Use of X-Ray Computed Tomography (CT) in UK Sheep Production and Breeding

L. Bünger et al.*
Sustainable Livestock Systems Group,
Scottish Agricultural College, Edinburgh
UK

1. Introduction

The aim of this chapter was to review the use of computed tomography (CT) in UK sheep breeding to improve carcass composition and elements of meat quality, as well as the use of CT scanning as a benchmarking system for faster and cheaper carcass evaluation for use both in practise for the livestock industry and for furthering research aims.

This paper will review some of the work carried out at the Scottish Agricultural College (SAC) in collaboration with Biomathematics & Statistics Scotland (BioSS) in the last 14 years. The work investigated the use of CT scanning alongside ultrasound scanning (US) in a synergistic approach to benefit the UK sheep industry by improving the breeding value of terminal sire (meat) rams. *In vivo* measurements via CT of body composition of the top ranking male selection candidates (pre-selected by their US - measured backfat and muscle depth) are used to enhance the accuracy of selection decisions regarding carcass quality and more recently, also some components of meat quality. CT-derived information provides both directly measured traits for use in the breeding process as well as serving as a bench-marking system for the validation of other techniques such as Video image analysis (VIA) or ultrasound scanning. It also has real potential to replace the "Gold Standard" of carcass evaluation which has always been used in past, which is the dissection of carcass tissues into component parts.

Initially, we will characterise UK sheep breeding and the need to accurately and precisely measure body and carcass composition of breeding animals or their close relatives with the aim of improving the quality of slaughter lambs.

UK sheep industry. There are around 15 million breeding ewes in the UK (www.defra.gov.uk/evidence/statistics/foodfarm/general/auk/latest/excel/index.htm), half of which are purebred and half are crossbred, with hill and lowland areas each containing around 40% of the ewes and upland areas the remaining 20% (Pollott & Stone, 2006). The UK sheep industry is characterised by a stratified structure, which has evolved over many years to best utilise the available land and to match breeds or crosses to different systems. The stratified system has different selection goals within each strata and makes use of specialised sire and dam breeds and crosses and exploits both the complementarities of breeds for crossing e.g. longwool (litter size, milk) x hill (hardiness, intermediate mature

* J.M. Macfarlane, N. R. Lambe, J. Conington, K. A. McLean, K. Moore, C.A. Glasbey[1] and G. Simm
[1]*Biomathematics & Statistics Scotland, King's Buildings, Edinburgh, Scotland*

size) and heterosis for maternal traits, survival, growth and carcass traits. On the hill land, characterised by harsh climatic and nutritional environment, most sheep are purebred hardy breeds which have evolved and been selected to have good maternal and survival characteristics. After about 4 or 5 lamb crops in the hill areas, these hill breed ewes are often drafted down to less harsh upland areas. Here they are crossed with longwool sires (e.g. Bluefaced Leicester) and while the F1 crossbred males are sent to slaughter, the resulting F1 crossbred females (Mules) are used in commercial flocks in upland and lowland environments. These crossbred females are then mated with sires from terminal sire breeds (e.g. Texel, Suffolk, Charollais). Terminal sire breeds are mainly bred for high lean growth. Their matings with Mule sheep produce slaughter progeny. Of the lambs slaughtered in the UK for meat production, 71% are sired by terminal sire breeds (Pollott & Stone, 2006). In the UK there are approximately 13.9 million sheep slaughtered per year (Figure 1) indicating the importance of the genetic quality of the terminal sire breeds as on average, they contribute half of the genes of all lambs slaughtered in the UK. Terminal sire breeds are numerically small but as they sire the majority of slaughter lambs in the UK, they have a large impact on the genetics of the national lamb crop. Genetic selection in these breeds focuses on growth and carcass traits, which is an effective way to improve carcass quality.

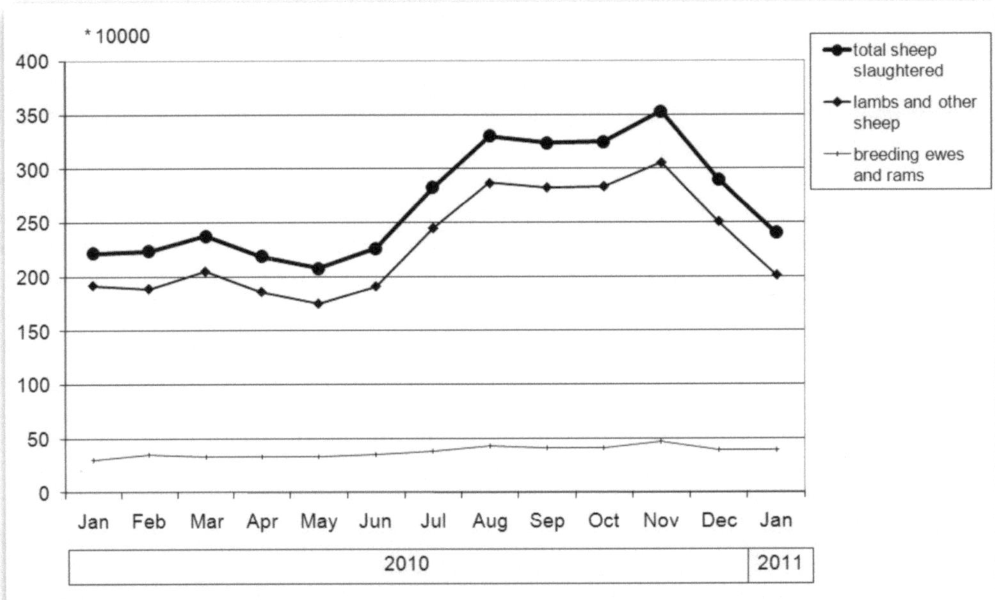

Data: http://www.defra.gov.uk/evidence/statistics/foodfarm/food/slaughter/documents/slaughpn.pdf

Fig. 1. UK average weekly sheep/lambs slaughterings (Thousand Head)

Current genetic improvement programs in the main UK terminal sire breeds are based on index selection for improved lean tissue growth including as selection criteria live weight and US-measured fat and muscle depths and, more recently (since 2000), traits measured using CT. The Lean Index was developed and experimentally tested by SAC (Simm & Dingwall, 1989, Simm *et al.*, 2002) and employed by Signet (National genetic evaluation service for cattle and sheep) in response to consumer demand for lean meat. The breeding objective was to increase carcass lean weight whilst minimising any associated rise in fatness. Impressive rates of genetic gain have been achieved in UK terminal sire breeding programs through selection on this Lean Index as shown for example by Macfarlane and Simm (2007).

In the present commercial circumstances, the need for selective breeding decisions is as important as ever. Sheep producers can only maintain their businesses by producing lambs that meet market specifications, in terms of carcass weight and carcass quality (currently assessed mainly via fat class and conformation). Allied to this is the need to monitor production costs to ensure lambs are produced efficiently, and ensure the flock will generate a positive financial return.

A lamb's potential to produce a quality carcass is ultimately limited by its genetic potential. Breeders therefore need to make long-term plans to invest in the right breeding stock for their enterprise, both initially and for its further development, with a focus on production traits such as growth and carcass composition, but also considering traits such as meat quality, disease resistance, easy care (e.g. lambing ease), and lamb survival.

2. *In vivo* measurement of body composition and meat quality

2.1 Body composition assessed by CT

Researchers in animal science have for a long time sought an accurate and reliable method of measuring *in vivo* body composition, mainly with the aim to improve and manage carcass composition. Improving carcass composition can be done by manipulating the environment, primarily through quantity and quality of nutrition (Emmans *et al.*, 2000). However, there are strong reasons why significant emphasis should be put on altering the genetic potential of animals for growth and development of their carcass tissues. Traditional selection, whereby the best animals are kept as parents for the next generation, offers permanent, cumulative gains that fit well within a sustainable livestock production system (Simm, 1998, Hill *et al.*, 2000). Coupled with modern statistical approaches to breeding scheme design and genetic analysis, substantial genetic gains are possible (Simm, 1998). Modern breeding methods also provide the most economic way to select for improvements in a suite of traits (Amer *et al.*, 2007), and methods that are not invasive (unlike physical dissection or slaughter) are highly valuable tools for breeding programs.

There are many technologies available (e.g. reviewed by Speakman, 2001) to measure body composition and they differ in accuracy, reliability and cost. For example, ultrasound scanners, originally used in diagnostic medicine for humans, have been adapted in the last 20-30 years for use on farm animal species with considerable success. Although this technology is still developing and in widespread use, researchers require more accurate methods of evaluating carcass composition. CT is a more sophisticated diagnostic tool, which offers comprehensive and reliable information. It is a non-invasive imaging technology that was also initially developed for use in human diagnostic medicine. CT uses X-rays to generate cross-sectional, two-dimensional images of the body and each image is acquired by rapid rotation of the X-ray tube 360° around the body of the animal. The object being scanned is divided up into spatially consecutive, parallel sections, the data from which are then summed up to produce total estimates of the different tissues in the carcase (Krause, 1999). The amount of radiation transmitted through the body depends on the attenuation rate of the X-rays, which differ between the various tissue types according to their relative densities. With CT, a computer stores a large amount of these attenuation values, which are registered by one or multiple arrays of detectors (single slice and multi slice scanners), from a selected region of the body. This allows the spatial relationship of the radiation-absorbing structures within it to be determined. The image obtained consists of a matrix of attenuation values which are depicted in various shades of grey, thereby creating a spatial image of the scanned object (Wegener, 1993).

Considering that as recently as 1979, Hounsfield and Cormack received the Nobel Prize for their pioneering work in developing this technology for its use in human medicine, the progress in diagnostic developments since then have been impressive. In the early 1980's the potential of CT for use in animal production research was recognized in Norway, pioneered by a team of researchers led by H. Skjervold, and the Agricultural University of Norway who acquired a Siemens Somatom 2 computer tomograph and began development work. Their results indicated that CT had considerable potential for predicting carcass composition in live animals (e.g. Allen & Leymaster, 1985). This increase in accuracy was expected to lead to potentially large increases in rates of genetic improvement (Simm & Dingwall, 1989). However, because of its limited accessibility and relatively high cost, initially it was not widely used in animal breeding and veterinary medicine. Accessibility has since improved and this has increased the need for expertise in the use of this technique in animals (Rivero et al., 2005). CT now has a wide range of applications and is well documented in the literature. CT scanning of live farm animals (mainly sheep and pigs) for breeding purposes has been used commercially in New Zealand, Hungary, Norway and the UK. Some other countries focussed on the use of CT (or MRI) for post mortem scanning of pig carcasses (e.g. Denmark, France, Germany, Norway).

Experimental studies carried out at SAC in the UK from 1997 to 2000 established the best way to incorporate CT scanning for carcass traits into terminal sire breeding programs in the UK (Young *et al.*, 2001; Macfarlane *et al.*, 2009c). CT provides accurate predictions of tissue weights because of a direct relationship between X-ray attenuation and tissue density. Suitable software procedures to extract and quantify the areas of the different tissues in the cross-sectional images were developed using mathematical algorithms for image analysis (Glasbey & Young, 2002). This involves two main steps: 1) segmentation to remove non-carcass portions of the images; and 2) measurement of tissue areas in the segmented images. The complexity of removing the internal organs and to identify tissue boundaries makes the segmentation challenging and time-consuming if done manually. Automatic procedures have recently been developed (Glasbey & Young, 2002; Navajas *et al.*, 2006a). Using software (STAR: **S**heep **T**omogram **A**nalysis **R**outines, Figure 2) developed at SAC and BioSS (Mann *et al.*, 2008), both steps can be performed automatically and therefore more quickly (Figure 3).

Cross-sectional CT scans taken at 3 specific anatomical locations identified from a longitudinal topogram scan (Figure 4, left) provide images from which measurements of lean, fat and bone areas are derived and then used to very accurately predict the weight of lean, fat and bone in the whole carcass. For example, the accuracy of CT based predictions (R^2) for muscle, fat and bone weights in the carcass from a small number of CT scans (3 reference scans, Figure 4) varies between breeds, with the highest R^2 values in meat breeds of 0.99, 0.98 and 0.89 for fat, muscle and bone, respectively, with accuracies in Scottish Blackface sheep just slightly lower (Young *et al.*, 2001). This reference scanning approach was developed with the aim of maximising accuracy of prediction of tissue weights while holding scanning time as short as possible to minimise cost and animal welfare implications. Development of this approach required considerable initial calibration trials in which CT predictions were bench-marked against dissected tissue weights, and where the number of required cross-sectional images and their location were optimised. This provided breed-specific prediction equations, which are still used in CT scanning of commercial ram selection candidates.

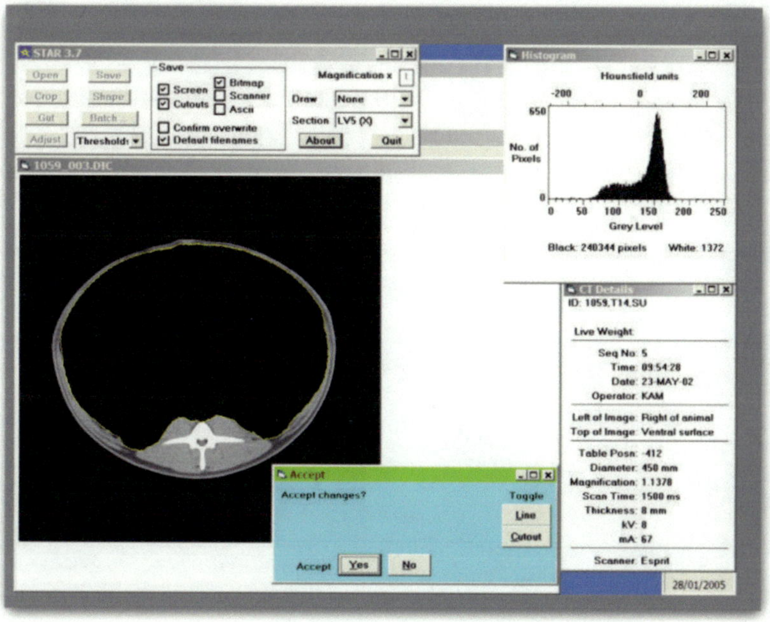

Fig. 2. Screenshot- Software STAR (Sheep tomogram analysis routines) to analyse CT images

Fat is shown as dark grey (less dense), muscle light grey (intermediate density) and bone as white (more dense)

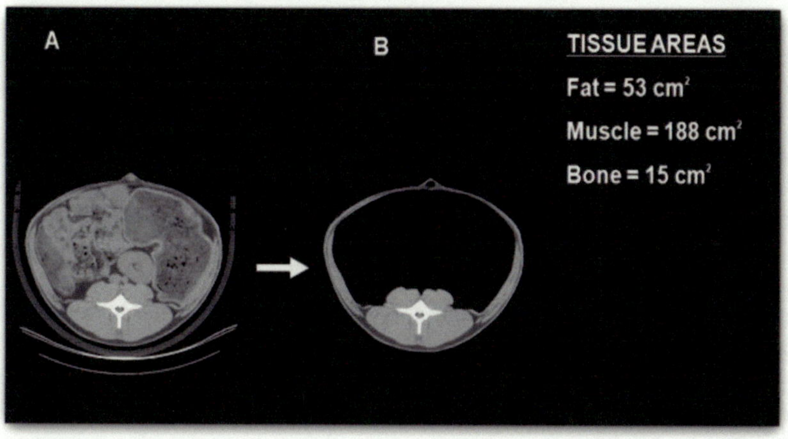

Fig. 3. Cross sectional images at Lumbar vertebra 5 before (A) and after (B) segmentation using STAR software

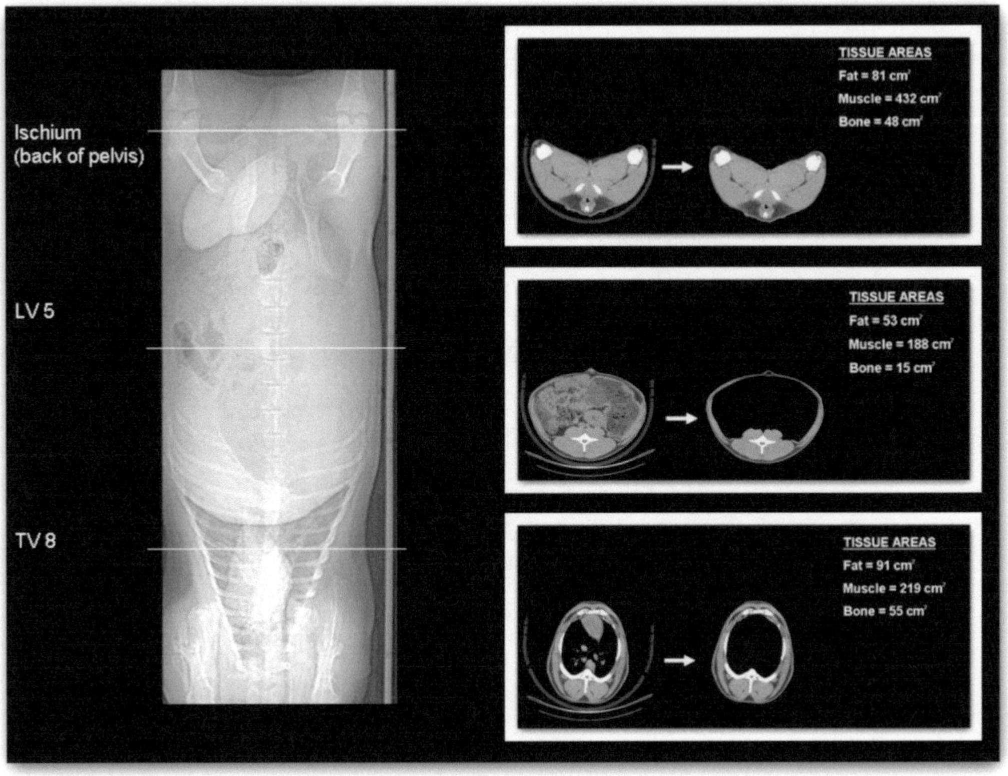

Fig. 4. Reference scanning method showing a longitudinal 2D scan (topogram, left) and cross sectional images at 3 anatomical landmarks and the corresponding tissue areas (right)

2.2 CT based 3D assessment of tissue volumes and weights

An alternative approach to reference scanning (Figure 4) is the *Cavalieri method* in which 15 to 20 cross-sectional, contiguous images are obtained, evenly spaced along the carcass. The volume of each tissue is then calculated from the total area of each tissue from cross-sectional scans multiplied by the inter-scan distance (e.g. Roberts *et al.*, 1993). This provides a direct measure of tissue volumes and weights, which can easily be calculated by multiplying the volume with the specific tissue densities. Both methods (reference scan and *Cavalieri*) show similar accuracies in sheep but require very different time (and therefore economic) inputs for generating the images and interpreting the results. However, if automatic procedures are in place, the *Cavalieri method* is the preferred method as it does not require breed-specific prediction equations or adaptation to allow for changes in a breed over time. Currently, mainly for economic reasons, the reference scan approach is the main method used to provide *in vivo* predictions of carcass composition in sheep breeding programs using CT in the UK.

In addition to carcass composition, CT can also be used to measure *in vivo* muscularity (muscle shape) (Jones *et al.*, 2002). Muscularity is of interest as an objective description of the shape of a carcass, a muscle or a muscle group, which is largely independent of the level of fatness in the carcass. Estimates of muscularity have been undertaken for different muscle regions (loin area and hind leg) and for the whole carcass using the corresponding 2D cross-sectional images and related measurements of the bone length (Jones *et al.*, 2002). These "semi-3D"-muscularity measures have moderate to high heritabilities (0.30-0.60; Jones *et al.*, 2004) indicating that muscularity traits measured by CT can be effectively used in two-stage selection programs for sheep.

Muscularity of the hind leg (Gigot shape) and the loin region (eye muscle) (Figure 5) are currently incorporated into breeding programs for terminal sire sheep in the UK.

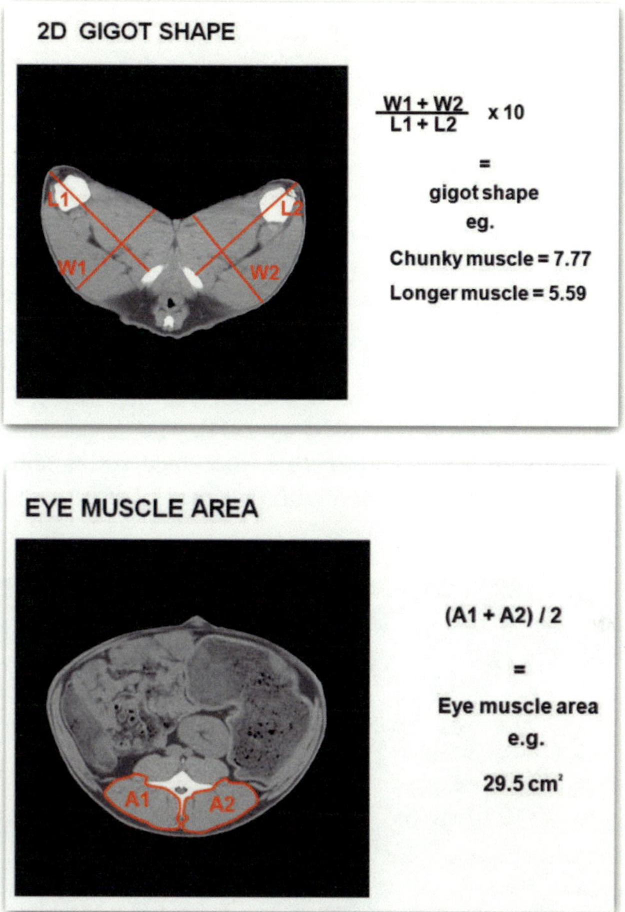

Fig. 5. Description of the shape of the Gigot at the Ischium (above) and measurements of the area of the eye muscle (below, loin or M. longissimus thoracis et lumborum)

Spiral CT scanning (SCTS). In 2002 SAC obtained a new CT scanner (Siemens, SOMATOM Esprit) capable of spiral (or helical) CT scanning. It is a single slice scanner and takes one slice or image as the X-ray beam makes a complete rotation around the animal. Very recent scanners are 64 slice CT scanners, which can take up to 64 slices or images in one rotation. The more detectors a CT Scanner has, the more slices per rotation it is able to acquire and the addition of more detector rows enables the scanner to visualise more anatomy in a shorter amount of time and in greater detail.

SCTS is a rather recent imaging technology which takes a series of images of an object in a similar arrangement to that of a spring or coil. It provides cross-sectional images at intervals of as little as about 1mm (depending on the type of scanner) along the body, which contain a wealth of information. Earlier CT scanners had the X-ray source, which moved in a circular fashion to acquire a single 'slice'. Once the slice had been completed, the scanner table would move to position the animal for the next slice. In the spiral scanner however, the X-ray tube is attached to a freely rotating gantry which rotates continuously in one direction whilst the table on which the animal is lying, is smoothly moved through the gantry.

One major advantage of spiral scanning compared to the traditional 'shoot-and-step approach' is speed, which permits the use of higher resolution acquisitions in the same study time. In addition, the data obtained from SCTS is also well-suited for 3D imaging (Figure 6) allowing volumes and dimensions of the body and of the skeleton to be measured. Recent work has further increased the opportunity to describe muscularity traits. New 3D- muscularity indices for the hind leg and lumbar region in sheep were derived based on the assessment of skeletal dimensions and muscle volumes and mass. Assessments of muscle mass and skeletal dimensions by CT enabled the development of new muscularity measures. Compared to previous CT muscularity indices, the accuracy was much higher with the new index in the hind leg (correlations between CT and dissection indices of 0.89 vs. 0.51). The accurate measurement of femur length by CT used in the new hind leg index made an important contribution to the higher accuracy of this index. The improvement in accuracy was smaller for the loin region (0.55 vs. 0.44). The association of CT muscularity indices and carcass quality in Texel and Scottish Blackface lambs showed that improved muscularity is not phenotypically correlated with detrimental effects on carcass composition (Navajas *et al.*, 2007).

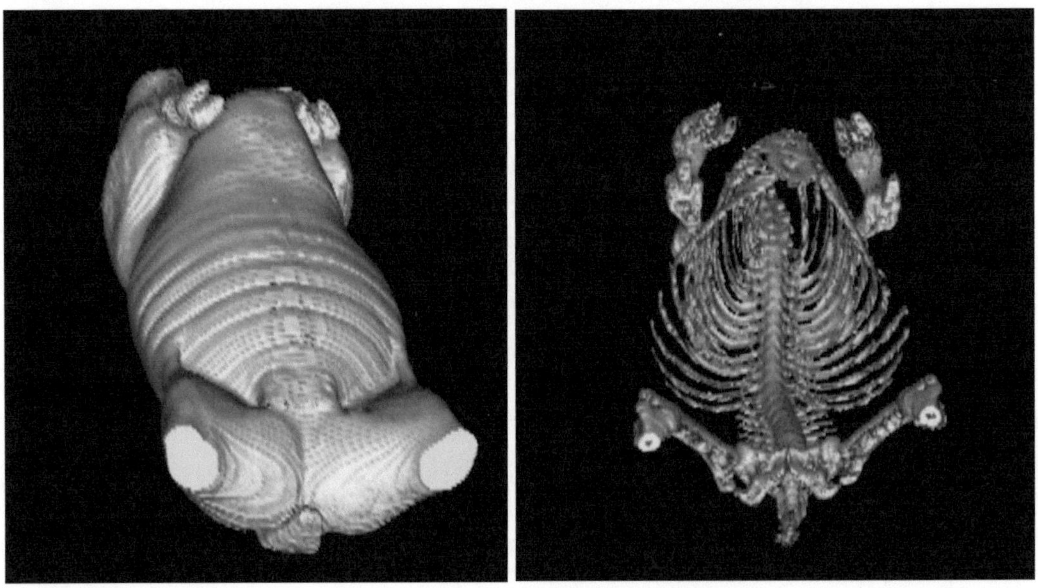

Fig. 6. 3D- reconstruction of the body (left) and skeleton (right) of a live sheep using cross sectional images taken with 8mm distance. A smaller slice distance would make the images smoother and increases the accuracy of dimensional measurements

CT measured muscularity indices provide an alternative method to improve carcass conformation and leanness, using measurements that at a constant weight are independent of fatness (Navajas *et al.*, 2006a; 2007). The heritabilities of the 3D muscularity indices assessed using CT were moderate to high in Texel (h^2= 0.38 to 0.92) and Scottish Blackface (h^2 = 0.42 to 0.78) breeds (Navajas *et al.*, 2006c). This study provided the first estimates of heritabilities for 3D-muscularity indices in Scottish Blackface and Texel sheep. Although the values should be used with caution due to the large standard errors, these estimates show the potential for genetic improvement of muscularity of the whole carcass and of regions with high priced cuts (hind leg and lumbar region). The improvement of muscularity in different regions of the carcass may require the utilisation of different CT indices as selection criteria in an index in these breeds.

SCTS allows rapid, direct estimation of volumes and densities, and therefore weights, of the tissues in the body/carcass and could therefore be used as a "gold standard" for benchmarking other methods of body/carcass quality evaluation. Recently at SAC and BioSS, developments of the STAR software have enabled weights and composition of joints of a carcass to be accurately measured from data captured on a live animal (Macfarlane et al., unpublished). This is done by dividing up the total body spiral scans from a live animal into regions corresponding to carcass joints using anatomical landmarks corresponding to the cuts made by butchers in commercial lamb carcass butchery. This could in future provide sheep breeders with information on direct value of the carcass of the animals being CT scanned.

2.3 Other CT based traits of interest to sheep breeding and production

Muscle density and intramuscular fat (IMF). In pigs, efforts have recently been made to increase IMF level because there is some concern that pork from intensely selected, modern lean lines of pigs may have poorer eating quality compared to the fatter genotypes, and this is resulting in reduced consumer satisfaction. At the same time, published data indicate that visible fat content is a major determinant of purchase intent, with consumers preferring leaner pork. These modern very lean pigs have very low levels of intramuscular fat, and thus exhibit very low levels of marbling in their muscles, which is considered a major contributor to the palatability of pork for both domestic and export markets. IMF levels correlate highly with marbling, with greater juiciness, more desirable flavour, greater tenderness and better overall palatability (Murray *et al.*, 2004). A similar study (Fernandez *et al.*, 1999) on the relationship between IMF and pork eating quality showed that this relationship is not linear, as the willingness to eat and purchase the meat were influenced by IMF level and the perception of texture and taste was enhanced with increased IMF levels. This indicates that the acceptability of pork may be improved by increasing IMF level up to a certain threshold. IMF levels higher than 3.5%, were associated with a high risk of meat rejection due to visible fat and the authors pointed out that the positive effect of increased IMF probably holds only true as long as it is not associated with an increase in the level of intermuscular fat, the fat between the muscles. This indicates that IMF should be targeted by selection on optimum values and should be always measured alongside other fat depots.

In sheep there is also increasing concern about low IMF levels especially for terminal sire breeds, and in this context it is of interest that CT scanning can not only provide useful information for carcass composition in terms of tissue volumes and weights and traits describing muscle shape, but the measured muscle densities are valuable in predicting the

IMF content. This is important, as breeding attempts to reduce carcass fatness may also lead to a correlated reduction in IMF content which is of particular concern as IMF makes an important contribution to meat eating quality, including tenderness, juiciness and flavour. The difficulties of measuring meat quality traits in live breeding animals has meant that they are rarely included in breeding programs. However, recent research has shown a link exists between CT-measured muscle density and IMF content (Young *et al.*, 2001, Macfarlane *et al.*, 2005, 2009b, Karamichou *et al.*, 2006, Navajas *et al.*, 2006b). It is anticipated that this will allow *in-vivo* selection for IMF; however, work is still required on the best way in which to incorporate this trait into breeding programs that also aim to reduce overall carcass fatness.

CT-measured tissue depletion and repletion. Repeated CT scanning of Scottish Blackface ewes of differing reproductive status (pre-mating, pre-lambing, mid-lactation, at weaning [around 18 weeks of age] and at pre-mating the following year) has been used to investigate tissue depletion and repletion. Ewes with higher levels of muscle are more productive than their fatter counterparts (Lambe *et al.*, 2003). The ability to mobilise both muscle and fat depots to fuel lactation for growing lambs leads to heavier lambs and fewer lambs lost before weaning. However, ewes that mobilise larger amounts of their own body tissues are more likely to die, or be culled from the flock, compared to ewes that do not mobilise their body fat and muscle reserves. In other words, ewes that 'look after number one' (themselves) rear poorer and fewer lambs relative to those who 'give it their all', yet they are most likely to be in good condition themselves and survive throughout the year (Figure 7). These results indicate a biological trade-off when it comes to animal performance and produces a bit of a dilemma for the breeders - which type of ewe do they want? Higher-producing, but shorter-living, or lower-producing and longer-living? The answer to that question depends very much on the relative economic returns for ewes that are culled from the flock, compared to the prices obtained for lambs. The results suggest that keeping females in the breeding flock because they maintain their own condition throughout the year, may be have a negative impact on the number and weights of lambs reared to weaning. As long as ewes that have lost condition over summer can regain it before mating in the autumn, they are likely to be the more productive individuals, although they may need to be culled sooner than other ewes in the flock. For the pedigree breeder, the simple answer to this dilemma is to know which animals in their flock have better overall productive performance compared to others, *via* the use of selection indices. The indices used by hill breeds in the UK produce higher scores for animals that carry genes for rearing heavier litters to weaning *and* genes for better ewe longevity. For the commercial producer, buying high index rams to produce female replacements will result in a ewe flock with these preferred combinations of genes and so will minimise the risks associated with the known biological trade-offs. In conclusion, CT can help to identify suitable types of ewes for use in different systems.

CT-measured pelvic dimensions and dystocia. The estimated mean neonatal lamb mortality rate in the UK is approximately 10% (Binns *et al.*, 2002) and the large number of lambs lost early in life has a negative impact on both animal welfare and on the profitably of sheep farming. Lambing difficulty is one of the main causes of lamb losses. It can affect both lamb survival and maternal ability, which are being actively selected for in modern sheep breeding. Many lambing difficulties are due to the disproportionate size of the lamb and ewe. This can be the result of a large lamb, a small pelvic opening, or both. Attempts to measure pelvic dimensions by external measurements have been shown to be impracticable,

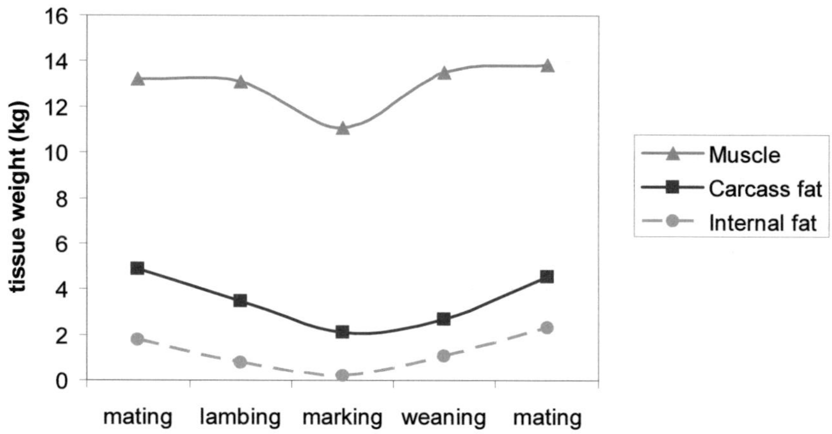

The 'giver': Ewes losing and gaining more fat and muscle are likely to wean more and better lambs, but may survive less years in the flock

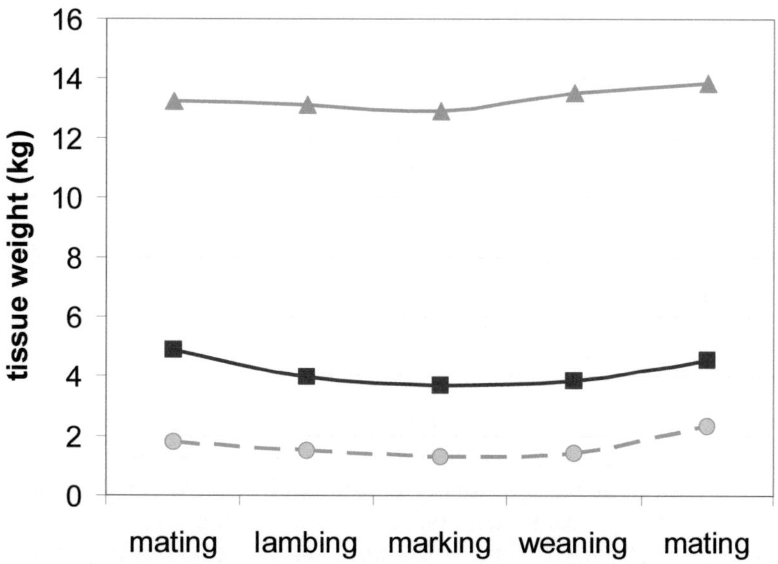

The 'taker': Ewes losing and gaining less fat and muscle may survive longer, but at the cost of weaning fewer or poorer lambs

Fig. 7. CT-measured tissue weights in a longitudinal study on Scottish Blackface ewes.

although the use of X-ray measured pelvic dimensions showed that an incompatibility in size between the maternal pelvis and the lamb at birth is largely responsible for the need for repeated assistance at birth (Mcsporran & Fielden, 1979). The availability of SCTS has substantially increased the opportunities to measure pelvic dimensions and to derive new selection traits based on CT measured 3D-pelvic dimensions to breed for low dystocia (Bilbe *et al.*, 2005).

CT-measured spine characteristics. The loin muscle is one of the higher priced cuts of meat and commercially one of the most important muscles. The muscle runs the length of the spinal column; hence spine characteristics (lengths of spine, number of vertebrae) should relate to the length of the loin and possibly the number of lamb chop cuts that can be obtained from a lamb carcass. Recently, a project to measure spine characteristics using longitudinal CT scans topograms (Figure 4, left) has been instigated to determine the extent to which number of vertebrae and other spinal characteristics are under genetic control. (Donaldson *et al.*, 2011).

Use of CT to evaluate the phenotypic effects of muscling genes. The advent of genomics provides new opportunities for improving carcass and meat quality through the selection of animals carrying favourable genes and/or quantitative trait loci (QTL; region of DNA that is associated with a particular phenotypic trait). For example, such a QTL had been identified previously in the UK increasing muscle growth in Texel sheep (Texel Muscling QTL, *TM-QTL,* Walling *et al.*, 2004). CT has been used to help comprehensively evaluate the effects of TM-QTL, MyoMAX and LoinMAX on carcass traits in UK sheep breeds and as such has been a valuable tool to provide information on the suitability of these QTL/genes for use in commercial sheep breeding programs (Macfarlane *et al.*, 2009a, Masri *et al.*, 2010)

Use of CT to calibrate video image analysis (VIA) of carcasses online in abattoirs. Internationally there is a move from subjective carcass classification to objective instrumental grading. Any instrumental grading systems must be able to predict carcass conformation and composition with a high level of accuracy and at commercial speed for a value based marketing system (*VBMS*) to be effective (Cross & Whittaker, 1992; Belk *et al.*, 1998). CT could certainly provide the required information from carcasses but would be too expensive and too slow to cope with high slaughter-line speeds, but it can serve as a bench-marking system for other suitable systems. The most promising and suitable technology developed in recent years is *VIA* (e.g. Stanford *et al.*, 1998; Hopkins *et al.*, 2004). This provides a non-invasive system operating at normal chain speeds and enables automatic acquisition of data on carcasses from the side and/or back view. It can be integrated into a slaughter line and can deal with high line speeds. Such *VIA* systems (Figure 8) can provide continuously objective electronic information on conformation and fat class, weight and yield of the most valuable cuts, and can also be used to derive immediate sort criteria. Such systems seem 'future proof' as they can easily be combined or augmented with individual carcass identification systems for traceability and possibly with other suitable systems, for the measurement of crude fat content, colour and textural properties indicative for carcass and meat eating quality. Different *VIA* systems have been studied outside the UK, mostly in beef cattle, to predict on-line carcass value and by the use of additional systems also aspects of meat eating quality (e.g. Cannell *et al.*, 2002; Shackelford *et al.*, 2003; Steiner *et al.*, 2003; Vote *et al.*, 2003, Allen & Finnerty, 2001; Allen, 2005). While there are also a few studies on instrumental grading of lamb carcasses (Hopkins, 1996, Stanford *et al.*, 1998, Brady *et al.*, 2003; Hopkins *et al.*, 2004, Cunha *et al.*, 2004), none of them had been applied to UK conditions for lamb carcasses until very recently. This work in the UK has shown that VIA under abattoir conditions and at a line speed of 800 lambs/h was capable of improving the prediction of primal meat yields compared to the current MLC EUROP carcass classification system. VIA could therefore be used as the basis of a VBMS as it accurately and precisely reflects the value of a sheep carcasses (Rius-Vilarrasa *et al.*, 2009b). Other work from our group allowed also the estimation of heritabilities for VIA-measured traits in sheep.

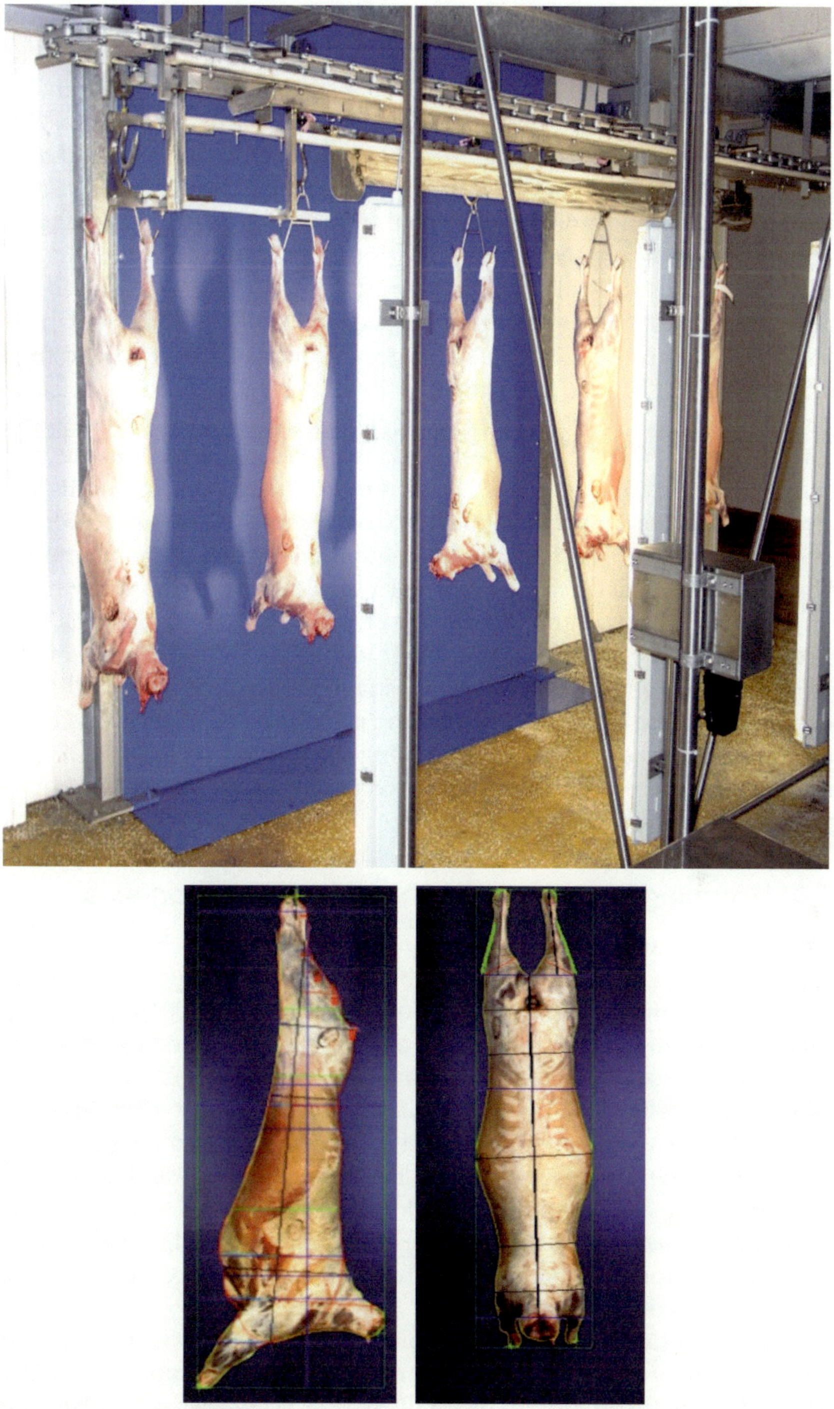

The VIA System is based on two cameras taking images from the side and back of each carcass and special image processing software.

Fig. 8. Video image analysis of lamb carcasses with an E+V Technology VSS2000 system.

Heritabilities for VIA-predicted primal weights were low to moderate (0.08 to 0.26) and had a high repeatability (>0.9), suggesting that including VIA information in breeding programs would be useful to improve carcass quality. Estimated genetic correlations indicated that it is possible to increase primal meat yield without increasing overall carcass fatness (Rius-Vilarrasa *et al.*, 2009a). This work demonstrated the potential that in the near future estimated primal weights and other measures of saleable meat yield could also be used as a measure of carcass quality in the UK abattoirs. In follow-up studies this dataset was also used to estimate genetic parameters for a number of additional carcass measures (carcass weight, MLC-fat class, MLC-conformation, primal joint weights predicted using MLC-fatclass, and several carcass linear and area measures obtained by VIA). Heritability estimates for subjective carcass traits (MLC-fat class and primal joint weights predicted using MLC-fat class) were low (0.05–0.17), and using them in breeding programs would lead to a lower response to selection for improved carcass quality. However, heritability estimates for objective carcass traits (VIA based linear and area measurements on the carcass) were moderate to high (0.20–0.53), suggesting that the use of these traits in genetic improvement programs could lead to a faster response to selection for improved carcass conformation and to a change of the primal joint tissue distribution within the carcass (Rius-Vilarrasa *et al.*, 2010). VIA, with its automated data capture, if combined with electronic identification of individual animals, could offer a significant opportunity to record very accurate information on carcass characteristics from lambs with the possibility of feeding this information into genetic evaluations, thereby increasing the accuracy of estimated breeding values (EBVs) and rates of response to selection. In the context of CT scanning it is of note that it was possible to refine the VIA prediction for the primal weights by calibrating the VIA system against CT measurements in the loin region. The refined predictions increased the accuracy of predictions of primal joints on average by 16% (Rius-Vilarrasa *et al.*, 2009c.)

3. Use of CT scanning in commercial sheep breeding programs

As shown above, CT scanning is a minimally invasive *in vivo* technique that can provide highly accurate estimates of carcass composition and as such is expected to increase rates of gain over those seen using US information (Jopson *et al.*, 1997, 2004). CT scanning is more expensive than ultrasound and so its incorporation into sheep breeding programs has been as part of a two-stage selection strategy in combination with ultrasound scanning. The theory of such a scheme is that all selection candidates are firstly ultrasound scanned and the best 15-20% of males are then CT scanned. Reference CT scanning is used to provide carcass lean, fat and bone weights and leg and loin muscularity for each animal CT scanned. US and CT scan data collected is then used along with live weights and other information collected on-farm in genetic evaluations to derive estimated breeding values for a range of traits and lean tissue growth index scores. These EBVs and index scores are used to help selecting animals for breeding.
Using ultrasound scan data one can expect prediction accuracies (R^2) in the order of 65% and 50% for fat weight and muscle weight, respectively, with heritabilities for US-measured muscle and fat depth of 0.29 and 0.38, respectively. The accuracies of CT- based predictions of the same tissues from just 3 reference scans are 0.99 and 0.97 in meat sheep, and there are high heritabilities (0.46 and 0.40) for CT-measured lean and fat weight (Young *et al.*, 2001,. The selection response can simply be predicted using following equation:

SR = SD x h^2, with SR being the selection response, SD, the selection differential (defined as the average difference between the parent generation and the selected parents) and h^2 the heritability. Considering the accuracy of the selection we would need to multiply SR by the accuracy (r_{ua}, which is strictly speaking the accuracy of using the measure u to predict an individual's breeding value), or the correlation between u and an individual's breeding value. To keep it simple we could use above given accuracies and conclude that SR based only on US would be ca. 50-60% of the SR obtained when measurements are fully based on CT. Considering that measuring all selection candidates with CT would be not practical and a two stage selection scheme is applied the advantage of CT based selection is much smaller. However, using data from industry flocks it has recently been shown that response to selection is 7% (CT -measured muscle weight), 10% (CT-measured fat weight) and 20% (CT measured muscularity) higher when CT scanning is used together with ultrasound scanning compared to ultrasound alone (Moore *et al.*, 2011).

In the UK CT scanning has been in use in terminal sire sheep breeding programs since 2000 (Table 1) especially in Texel, Suffolk, Charollais, Hampshire Down, Meatlinc and Beltex sheep. Each year approximately 400-500 lambs in total are CT scanned either using the fixed CT scanner near Edinburgh or more recently a mobile CT scanner (in 2009 and 2010) that can provide a CT scanning service to breeders located at distances from the fixed scanner that previously discouraged them from using CT scanning.

In addition to above considered CT-derived traits describing carcass composition other traits outlined in section 2.3 could also serve as selection traits in sheep breeding programs using existing variation between animals (Figure 9). A pre-requisite for their use are estimations of their genetic parameters.

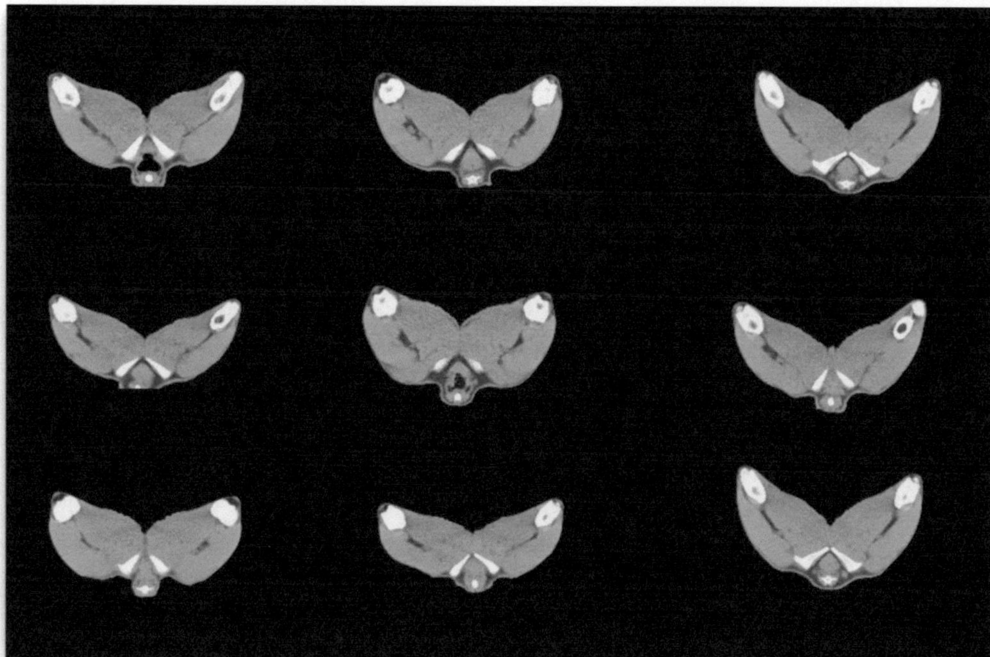

Fig. 9. Examples for Gigot shape variation in sheep

	2000	2001*	2002	2003	2004	2005	2006	2007*	2008*	2009**	2010**	total
Texel	353	0	107	148	204	137	124	83	89	108	198	1551
Suffolk	353	0	59	100	156	168	107	36	27	128	98	1232
Charollais	129	0	0	58	122	92	134	100	20	107	117	879
Hampshire Down	30	0	0	25	25	0	46	21	0	36	27	210
Meatlinc	57	0	20	25	30	26	0	0	28	24	0	210
Beltex									50	34	20	104
total per year	922	0	186	356	537	423	411	240	214	437	460	4186

*The outbreak of diseases in the UK and associated movement restrictions lead to low numbers in some of the years

** In 2009 and 2010 a mobile scanning service was offered. About 50% of the sheep were scanned with the mobile scanner. Since 2009 SAC uses also a 16 slice scanner (GE, LightSpeed, rented from Burgess Diagnostics Limited) as a mobile scanner built into a truck to provide CT scanning service to the sheep breeders. This meant that the transport time and costs could be minimised and consequently enable more animals to be CT scanned.

Table 1. The number of commercial sheep scanned at the SAC/BioSS CT Unit in Edinburgh (including mobile CT scanning)

Summary. Because of the capabilities described, CT is a valuable tool for various fields of animal science (health, nutrition, genetics and breeding) and livestock production (management on-farm, abattoirs, supermarkets), and can replace labour-intensive and expensive *post-mortem* dissection in experimental designs, whilst *in vivo* CT also allows longitudinal studies over time. Much of the focus in animal research has been on using CT to improve carcass composition and muscularity in terminal sire sheep although the estimation of changes in different tissues over the reproductive life cycle in accordance with different physiological states has generated new information on the depletion and repletion of body tissues to fuel lactation for lamb growth. As shown above CT scanning is a minimally invasive *in vivo* technique that can provide highly accurate estimates of body or carcass composition, muscle shape and density and provides data on spine and pelvic characteristics all of potential importance in sheep breeding and production. Further work is required to develop a synergistic approach to use CT-scanning together with US and VIA for the genetic improvement of carcass quality, with a two-fold role of CT, as a benchmarking system and as integrated part of the breeding system.

4. References

Allen, P. (2005). Evaluationg video image analysis systems for beef carcass classification. *Proceedings of the 8th Annual Langford Food Industry Conference, University of Bristol, 18th-19th of May 2005*

Allen, P. & Finnerty, N. (2001). Mechnical grading of Beef Carcasses. *National Food Centre Research Report, Teagasc* 45, 1-26.

Allen, P. & Leymaster, K.A. (1985). Machine Error in X-Ray Computer-Tomography and Its Relevance to Prediction of Invivo Body-Composition. *Livestock Production Science* 13, 383-398.

Amer, P.R., Nieuwhof, G.J., Pollott, G.E., Roughsedge, T., Conington, J. & Simm, G. (2007). Industry benefits from recent genetic progress in sheep and beef populations. *Animal* 1, 1414-1426.

Belk, K.E., Scanga, J.A., Tatum, J.D., Wise, J.W. & Smith, G.C. (1998). Simulated instrument augmentation of USDA yield grade application to beef carcasses. *Journal of Animal Science* 76, 522-527.

Bilbe, E., Conington, J., McLean, K.A., Lambe, N.R. & Bünger, L. (2005). Using CT to assess pelvic dimensions linked to dystocia and maternal behaviour score in Scottish-Blackface ewes. *Proceedings of the Annual BSAS Meeting 2005*

Binns, S.H., Cox, I.J., Rizvi, S. & Green, L.E. (2002). Risk factors for lamb mortality on UK sheep farms. *Preventive Veterinary Medicine* 52, 287-303.

Brady, A.S., Belk, K.E., LeValley, S.B., Dalsted, N.L., Scanga, J.A., Tatum, J.D. & Smith, G.C. (2003). An evaluation of the lamb vision system as a predictor of lamb carcass red meat yield percentage. *Journal of Animal Science* 81, 1488-1498.

Cannell, R.C., Belk, K.E., Tatum, J.D., Wise, J.W., Chapman, P.L., Scanga, J.A. & Smith, G.C. (2002). Online evaluation of a commercial video image analysis system (Computer Vision System) to predict beef carcass red meat yield and for augmenting the assignment of USDA yield grades. *Journal of Animal Science* 80, 1195-1201.

Cross, H.R. & Whittaker, A.D. (1992). The role of instrument grading in a beef value-based marketing system. *Journal of Animal Science* 70, 984-989.

Cunha, B.C.N., Belk, K.E., Scanga, J.A., LeValley, S.B., Tatum, J.D. & Smith, G.C. (2004). Development and validation of equations utilizing lamb vision system output to predict lamb carcass fabrication yields. *Journal of Animal Science* 82, 2069-2076.

Donaldson, C.L., Lambe, N.R., Macfarlane, J.M., McLean, K.A., Maltin, C.A., Knott, S. & Bunger, L. (2011). Breed and sex effects on spine characteristics in sheep. *Proceedings of the British Society of Animal Science* Submitted,

Emmans, G.C., Kyriazakis, I., and Fisher, C. (2000). Consequences of selecting for growth and body composition characteristics in poultry and pigs. *The challenge of genetic change in animal production.* (Hill, W.G., Bishop, S.C., McGuirk, B., Mckay, J.C., Simm, G., and Webb, A.J., eds) pp. 39-53, British society of animal science ,

Fernandez, X., Monin, G., Talmant, A., Mourot, J. & Lebret, B. (1999). Influence of intramuscular fat content on the quality of pig meat - 2. Consumer acceptability of m. longissimus lumborum. *Meat Science* 53, 67-72.

Glasbey, C.A. & Young, M.J. (2002). Maximum a posteriori estimation of image boundaries by dynamic programming. *Journal of the Royal Statistical Society Series C-Applied Statistics* 51, 209-221.

Hill, W.G., Bishop, S.C., McGuirk, B., Mckay, J.C., Simm, G., and Webb, A.J. (2000). The challenge of genetic change in animal production. Foreword to publication. *The challenge of genetic change in animal production.* (Hill, W.G., Bishop, S.C., McGuirk, B., Mckay, J.C., Simm, G., and Webb, A.J., eds) pp. iiiBritish society of animal science ,

Hopkins, D.L. (1996). The relationship between muscularity, muscle:bone ratio and cut dimensions in male and female lamb carcasses and the measurement of muscularity using image analysis. *Meat Science* 44, 307-317.

Hopkins, D.L., Safari, E., Thompson, J.M. & Smith, C.R. (2004). Video image analysis in the Australian meat industry - precision and accuracy of predicting lean meat yield in lamb carcasses. *Meat Science* 67, 269-274.

Jones, H.E., Lewis, R.M., Young, M.J. & Simm, G. (2004). Genetic parameters for carcass composition and muscularity in sheep measured by X-ray computer tomography, ultrasound and dissection. *Livestock Production Science* 90, 167-179.

Jones, H.E., Lewis, R.M., Young, M.J. & Wolf, B.T. (2002). The use of X-ray computer tomography for measuring the muscularity of live sheep. *Animal Science* 75, 387-399.

Jopson, N.B., Amer, P.R. & McEwan.J.C. (2004). Comparison of two-stage selection breeding programmes for terminal sire sheep. *Proc. NZ Society of Animal Production* 64, 212-216.

Jopson, N.B., Mcewan, J.C., Fennessy, P.F., Dodds, K.G., Nicoll, G.B. & Wade, C.M. (1997). Economic benefits of including computed tomography measurements in a large terminal sire breeding programme. *Proc. Assoc. Advmt. Anim. Breed. Genet.* 12, 72-76.

Karamichou, E., Richardson, R.I., Nute, G.R., McLean, K.A. & Bishop, S.C. (2006). Genetic analyses of carcass composition, as assessed by X-ray computer tomography, and meat quality traits in Scottish Blackface sheep. *Animal Science* 82, 151-162.

Krause, W. (1999). Delivery of diagnostic agents in computed tomography. *Advanced Drug Delivery Reviews* 37, 159-173.

Lambe, N.R., Young, M.J., Brotherstone, S., Kvame, T., Conington, J., Kolstad, K. & Simm, G. (2003). Body composition changes in Scottish Blackface ewes during one annual production cycle. *Animal Science* 76, 211-219.

Macfarlane, J.M., Lambe, N.R., Bishop, S.C., Matika, O., Rius-Vilarrasa, E., McLean, K.A., Haresign, W., Wolf, B.T., McLaren, R.J. & Bunger, L. (2009a). Effects of the Texel muscling quantitative trait locus on carcass traits in crossbred lambs. *Animal* 3, 189-199.

Macfarlane, J.M., Lewis, R.M., Emmans, G.C., Young, M.J. & Simm, G. (2009b). Predicting tissue distribution and partitioning in terminal sire sheep using X-ray computed tomography. *Journal of Animal Science* 87, 107-118.

Macfarlane, J.M., Lewis, R.M., Emmans, G.C., Young, M.J. & Simm, G. (2009c). Predicting tissue distribution and partitioning in terminal sire sheep using x-ray computed tomography. *Journal of Animal Science* 87, 107-118.

Macfarlane, J.M. & Simm, G. (2007). Genetic improvement programme for meat type sheep: an experience from the United Kingdom. *Proceedings of the 3rd International Symposium about Goat and Sheep Meat Type - 3rd SINCORTE, in João Pessoa, Paraiba, Brazil, November 2007*

Macfarlane, J.M., Young, M.J., Lewis, R.M., Emmans, G.C. & Simm, G. (2005). Using X-ray computed tomography to predict intramuscular fat content in terminal sire sheep. *Proceedings of the 56th Annual Meeting of the European Association for Animal Production. June, Uppsala, Sweden.* 264

Mann, A.D., Young, M.J., Glasbey, C.A. & McLean, K.A. (2008). STAR: Sheep Tomogram Analysis Routines (V.4.8). *BioSS software documentation, University of Edinburgh*

Masri, A.Y., Lambe, N.R., Macfarlane, J.M., Brotherstone, S., Haresign, W., Rius-Vilarrasa, E. & Bunger, L. (2010). The effects of a loin muscling quantitative trait locus (LoinMAX (TM)) on carcass and VIA-based traits in crossbred lambs. *Animal* 4, 407-416.

Mcsporran, K.D. & Fielden, E.D. (1979). Studies on Dystocia in Sheep .2. Pelvic Measurements of Ewes with Histories of Dystocia and Eutocia. *New Zealand Veterinary Journal* 27, 75-78.

Moore, K., McLean, K.A. & Bunger, L. (2011). The benefits of Computed Tomography (CT) scanning in UK sheep flocks for improving carcase composition. *Proceedings of the Annual BSAS Meeting, Nottingham*

Murray, A., Pommier, S., Gibson, L.L. & Robertson, W. (2004). Influence of intramuscular fat (IMF) on pork quality. *Advances in Pork Production* 15, 16

Navajas, E.A., Glasbey, C.A., McLean, K.A., Fisher, A.V., Charteris, A.J.L., Lambe, N.R., Bünger, L. & Simm, G. (2006a). *In vivo* measurements of muscle volume by automatic image analysis of spiral computed tomography scans. *Animal Science* 82, 545-553.

Navajas, E.A., Lambe, N.R., Bünger, L., Glasbey, C.A., Fisher, A.V., Wood, J.D. & Simm, G. (2006b). Genetics of carcass shape and eating quality in sheep. *Proceedings of the 9th Langford Food Industry Conference: New Developments in Sheepmeat Quality*

Navajas, E.A., Lambe, N.R., McLean, K.A., Glasbey, C.A., Fisher, A.V., Charteris, A.J.L., Bunger, L. & Simm, G. (2007). Accuracy of in vivo muscularity indices measured by computed tomography and their association with carcass quality in lambs. *Meat Science* 75, 533-542.

Navajas, E.A., Lambe, N.R., Sawalha, R.M., Bünger, L. & Simm, G. (2006c). Genetic parameters of *in vivo* muscularity in two divergent sheep breeds: preliminary results. *Proceedings of the 8th World Congress on Genetics applied to Livestock Production , Brazil*

Pollott, G.E. and Stone, D.G.(2006). *The breeding structure of the British sheep industry 2003.*Defra,

Rius-Vilarrasa, E., Bunger, L., Brotherstone, S., Macfarlane, J.M., Lambe, N.R., Matthews, K.R., Haresign, W. & Roehe, R. (2010). Genetic parameters for carcass dimensional measurements from Video Image Analysis and their association with conformation and fat class scores . *Livestock Science* 128, 92-100.

Rius-Vilarrasa, E., Bunger, L., Brotherstone, S., Matthews, K.R., Haresign, W., Macfarlane, J.M., Davies, M. & Roehe, R. (2009a). Genetic parameters for carcass composition and performance data in crossbred lambs measured by Video Image Analysis. *Meat Science* 81, 619-625.

Rius-Vilarrasa, E., Bunger, L., Maltin, C., Matthews, K.R. & Roehe, R. (2009b). Evaluation of Video Image Analysis (VIA) technology to predict meat yield of sheep carcasses on-line under UK abattoir conditions. *Meat Science* 82, 94-100.

Rius-Vilarrasa, E., Roehe, R., Macfarlane, J.M., Lambe, N.R., Matthews, K.R., Haresign, W., Matika, O. & Bunger, L. (2009c). Effects of a quantitative trait locus for increased muscularity on carcass traits measured by subjective conformation and fat class scores and video image analysis in crossbred lambs. *Animal* 3, 1532-1543.

Rivero, M.A., Ramirez, J.A., Vazquez, J.M., Gil, F., Ramirez, G. & Arencibia, A. (2005). Normal anatomical imaging of the thorax in three dogs: computed tomography and macroscopic cross sections with vascular injection. *Anat. Histol. Embryol.* 34, 215-219.

Roberts, N., Cruzorive, L.M., Reid, N.M.K., Brodie, D.A., Bourne, M. & Edwards, R.H.T. (1993). Unbiased Estimation of Human-Body Composition by the Cavalieri Method Using Magnetic-Resonance-Imaging. *Journal of Microscopy-Oxford* 171, 239-253.

Shackelford, S.D., Wheeler, T.L. & Koohmaraie, M. (2003). On-line prediction of yield grade, longissimus muscle area, preliminary yield grade, adjusted preliminary yield grade, and marbling score using the MARC beef carcass image analysis system. *Journal of Animal Science* 81, 150-155.

Simm, G.(1998). *Genetic improvement of cattle and sheep*.Farming Press Books,

Simm, G. & Dingwall, W.S. (1989). Selection Indexes for Lean Meat Production in Sheep. *Livestock Production Science* 21, 223-233.

Simm, G., Lewis, R.M., Grundy, B. & Dingwall, W.S. (2002). Responses to selection for lean growth in sheep. *Animal Science* 74, 39-50.

Speakman, J.R.(2001). *Body composition analysis of animals-A handbook of non-destructive methods*.Cambridge University Press, Cambridge.

Stanford, K., Richmond, R.J., Jones, S.D.M., Robertson, W.M., Price, M.A. & Gordon, A.J. (1998). Video image analysis for on-line classification of lamb carcasses. *Animal Science* 67, 311-316.

Steiner, R., Wyle, A.M., Vote, D.J., Belk, K.E., Scanga, J.A., Wise, J.W., Tatum, J.D. & Smith, G.C. (2003). Real-time augmentation of USDA yield grade application to beef carcasses using video image analysis. *Journal of Animal Science* 81, 2239-2246.

Vote, D.J., Belk, K.E., Tatum, J.D., Scanga, J.A. & Smith, G.C. (2003). Online prediction of beef tenderness using a computer vision system equipped with a BeefCam module. *Journal of Animal Science* 81, 457-465.

Walling, G.A., Visscher, P.M., Wilson, A.D., McTeir, B.L., Simm, G. & Bishop, S.C. (2004). Mapping of quantitative trait loci for growth and carcass traits in commercial sheep populations. *Journal of Animal Science* 82, 2234-2245.

Wegener, O.H.(1993). *Whole body computed tomography*. ed 2, Blackwell Scientific Publications, Boston.

Young, M.J., Simm, G. & Glasbey, C.A. (2001). Computerised tomography for carcass analysis. *Proceedings of the British Society of Animal Science 2001* 250-254.